A Clinical
Manual of
Urology

Appleton Clinical Manuals

A Clinical Manual of Urology

Philip M. Hanno, M.D.
Associate Professor of Urology
University of Pennsylvania School of Medicine
Philadelphia, Pennsylvania

Alan J. Wein, M.D.
Professor and Chairman
Department of Urology
University of Pennsylvania School of Medicine
Philadelphia, Pennsylvania

 APPLETON-CENTURY-CROFTS/Norwalk, Connecticut

0-8385-1261-5

87 88 89 90 91 / 10 9 8 7 6 5 4 3 2 1

Prentice-Hall of Australia, Pty. Ltd., Sydney
Prentice-Hall Canada, Inc.
Prentice-Hall Hispanoamericana, S.A., Mexico
Prentice-Hall of India Private Limited, New Delhi
Prentice-Hall International (UK) Limited, London
Prentice-Hall of Japan, Inc., Tokyo
Prentice-Hall of Southeast Asia (Pte.) Ltd., Singapore
Whitehall Books Ltd., Wellington, New Zealand
Editora Prentice-Hall do Brasil Ltda., Rio de Janeiro

Library of Congress Cataloging-in-Publication Data

A Clinical manual of urology.

  (Appleton clinical manuals)
  Includes bibliographies.
  1. Urology—Handbooks, manuals, etc. 2. Genito-
urinary organs—Diseases—Handbooks, manuals, etc.
I. Hanno, Philip M. II. Wein, Alan J. III. Series.
[DNLM: 1. Urology—handbooks. WJ 39 C641]
RC872.9.C57 1987   616.6   86-20617
ISBN 0-8385-1261-5

PRINTED IN THE UNITED STATES OF AMERICA

Contributors

Marc P. Banner, M.D.
Associate Professor of Radiology
University of Pennsylvania School of Medicine
Philadelphia, Pennsylvania

Victor L. Carpiniello, M.D.
Assistant Clinical Professor of Urology
University of Pennsylvania School of Medicine
Philadelphia, Pennsylvania

Robert S. Charles, M.D.
Instructor in Urology
University of Pennsylvania School of Medicine
Philadelphia, Pennsylvania

John W. Duckett, M.D.
Professor of Urology
University of Pennsylvania School of Medicine
Director of Pediatric Urology
Children's Hospital of Philadelphia
Philadelphia, Pennsylvania

John W. Francfort, M.D.
Instructor in Vascular Surgery
Case Northwestern University School of Medicine
Chicago, Illinois

James M. Galvin, Ph.D.
Assistant Professor of Radiation Therapy
Director of Clinical Medical Physics
University of Pennsylvania School of Medicine
Philadelphia, Pennsylvania

Donna Glover, M.D.
Assistant Professor of Medicine
Section of Hematology-Oncology
University of Pennsylvania School of Medicine
Philadelphia, Pennsylvania

Nathan P. Goldin, M.D.
Department of Urology
Eastern Virginia Medical School
Norfolk, Virginia

Robert A. Grossman, M.D.
Associate Professor of Nephrology
University of Pennsylvania School of Medicine
Philadelphia, Pennsylvania

Philip M. Hanno, M.D.
Associate Professor of Urology
University of Pennsylvania School of Medicine
Philadelphia, Pennsylvania

Ruth Hanno, M.D.
Assistant Professor of Medicine
Division of Dermatology
University of South Florida
Tampa, Florida

Joseph A. Jacobs, M.D.
Clinical Assistant Professor of Urology
Hospital of the University of Pennsylvania
Philadelphia, Pennsylvania

Robert E. Krisch, M.D.
Associate Professor of Therapeutic Radiology
University of Pennsylvania School of Medicine
Philadelphia, Pennsylvania

Philip Littman, M.D.
Professor of Radiation Medicine
Brown University
Providence, Rhode Island

Bruce Malkowicz, M.D.
Instructor in Urology
University of Pennsylvania School of Medicine
Philadelphia, Pennsylvania

Terrence R. Malloy, M.D.
Professor of Urology
University of Pennsylvania School of Medicine
Philadelphia, Pennsylvania

Kathleen Murphy, M.D.
Instructor in Urology
University of Pennsylvania School of Medicine
Philadelphia, Pennsylvania

Ali Naji, M.D., Ph.D.
Assistant Professor of Surgery
University of Pennsylvania School of Medicine
Philadelphia, Pennsylvania

Leonard Perloff, M.D.
Associate Professor of Surgery
University of Pennsylvania School of Medicine
Philadelphia, Pennsylvania

Howard M. Pollack, M.D.
Professor of Radiology and Urology
University of Pennsylvania School of Medicine
Philadelphia, Pennsylvania

John F. Redman, M.D.
Professor and Chairman
Department of Urology
University of Arkansas for Medical Sciences
Little Rock, Arkansas

Roger E. Schultz, M.D.
Staff Urologist
Naval Hospital
Portsmouth, Virginia

Howard M. Snyder, M.D.
Associate Professor of Urology
University of Pennsylvania School of Medicine
Assistant Director of Pediatric Urology
Children's Hospital of Philadelphia
Philadelphia, Pennsylvania

David R. Staskin, M.D.
Assistant Professor of Urology
Boston University School of Medicine
Boston, Massachusetts

William F. Tarry, M.D.
Assistant Professor of Pediatric Urology
West Virginia University Medical Center
Morgantown, West Virginia

Keith N. Van Arsdalen, M.D.
Assistant Professor of Urology
University of Pennsylvania School of Medicine
Philadelphia, Pennsylvania

Alan J. Wein, M.D.
Professor and Chairman
Department of Urology
University of Pennsylvania School of Medicine
Philadelphia, Pennsylvania

Jeffrey P. Weiss, M.D.
Clinical Assistant Professor of Medicine
Temple University School of Medicine
Philadelphia, Pennsylvania

Contents

Preface

This book is intended primarily for the busy student and house officer rotating on the urology service. The purpose of this text is not to provide a heavily referenced compendium of urologic practice complete with controversies and "the answer" to each. Rather, we have tried to concisely summarize agreed upon (for the most part) material in such a way that pathophysiology, presentation, evaluation, and treatment referable to a given problem can be easily understood. While "answers" may vary from institution to institution, we hope they will be consistent with the content presented. Although the practices and philosophy of the University of Pennsylvania staff may be evident, moreso in some sections than in others, we have tried to keep "dogma" to a minimum, allowing others to add their input without the intellectual disruption (to the reader) of major disagreements.

We hope students, nonurologists, and first-year urology residents find this text a readily accessible, quickly read, and portable initial reference and starting point for more in-depth reading. Each author has been encouraged to carefully select and list suggested references at the end of each section rather than to use exhaustive citations throughout.

Our thanks are due to the contributors for trying to inform rather than persuade, and to the editors for their encouragement and forebearance.

Philip Hanno
Alan Wein
July 1986

1

Anatomy of the Urogenital Tract

John F. Redman

I. INTRODUCTION

An understanding of function, either normal or abnormal, must be preceded by an understanding of structure. The study of the anatomy of the genitourinary system involves knowledge of not only the organs and collecting structures of that system but also of the innervation, vasculature, and lymphatic associations as well. Because urology is a subspecialty of surgery, anatomy as it applies to urology encompasses more than just the genitourinary tract itself but also the surrounding structures that must be incised to gain operative access.

II. ABDOMINAL WALL MUSCULATURE

All operative approaches to the urinary tract of necessity require incision through the abdominal wall, using either an anterior or a posterior approach. To understand the operative approaches a knowledge of the abdominal wall musculature is needed. For discussion the abdominal wall may be divided into the anterior wall, anterior lateral wall, and posterior lateral wall.

A. Anterior Abdominal Wall

The primary musculature of the anterior abdominal wall is the rectus abdominus muscles (Fig. 1). These are paired segmented muscles that extend from the pubic crest to insertions on the cartilage of the fifth, sixth, and seventh ribs. The muscles are divided into segments by tendinous

1

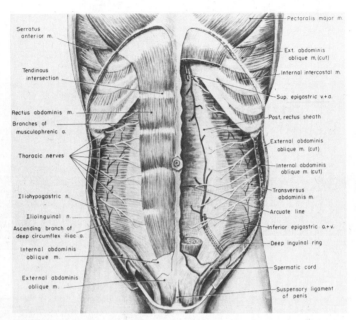

Figure 1. Anatomy of the anterior abdominal wall after reflection of external and internal abdominus oblique musculature. *(Reproduced from Crafts RC: A Textbook of Human Anatomy, ed 2, 1979, p 104.)*

intersections. As regards the surface anatomy, the lateral aspect of the rectus abdominus muscles can be identified in leaner individuals as a vertical depression in the midclavicular line known as the linea semilunaris. The rectus abdominus muscles are encased in a fibrous tissue envelope, the rectus sheath (Fig. 2). The fibrous investments represent continuations of the anterior lateral abdominal musculature, the external abdominus oblique, the internal abdominus oblique, and the transversus abdominus muscles. The most ventral portion of the rectus sheath is formed from the aponeurosis of the external oblique muscle. Dorsal to this investment is the aponeurosis of the internal oblique muscle, which splits at the lateral edge of the rectus muscle, the ventral portion melding with the external oblique aponeurosis and the dorsal portion melding with the aponeurosis of the transversus abdominus muscle. At a variable position halfway between the umbilicus and pubis all of the aponeuroses are found dorsal to the rectus abdominus muscles (Fig. 3). This arched termination of the heavy fascial sheath is known as the arcuate line. In the midline the recti are separated by the dense joining of these fascial layers known as the linea alba, which varies in thickness.

B. Anterior Lateral Abdominal Wall

The anterior lateral abdominal musculature comprises the external abdominus oblique, the internal abdominus oblique, and the transversus abdominus oblique.

1. The external abdominus oblique takes origin from the fifth to the twelfth ribs and interdigitates with the origin of the serratus anterior and latissimus dorsi muscles. The fibers are oriented in a caudal and medial direction. The muscle per se inserts to the outer anterior half of the iliac crest. Its aponeurosis inserts by the anterior rectus sheath to the xyphoid, the linea alba, the symphysis pubis, and the pectineal line. The bridge between the anterior superior iliac spine and the pubic tubercle has been termed the inguinal ligament. At the level of the pubic tubercle the aponeurosis of the external oblique is thinned for the penetration of the spermatic cord known as the superficial inguinal ring. A thin continuation of the aponeurosis continues over the cord as the external spermatic fascia (Fig. 4).

2. The internal abdominus oblique arises from the lumbodorsal or thoracolumbar fascia, the anterior two-thirds of the iliac crest, and the lateral two-thirds of the inguinal ligament. The upper half of the fibers course in an oblique and cranial direction, inserting into the inferior borders of the cartilage of the last three or four ribs. The lower half of the fibers course almost horizontally to terminate in the anterior rectus sheath, ultimately inserting into the linea alba. A continuation of

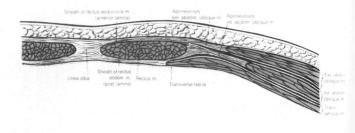

Figure 2. Detail of the rectus sheath cranial to the umbilicus. Note that the aponeurosis of the internal abdominus oblique muscle contributes to both the anterior and posterior rectus sheath. *(Reproduced from Crafts RC: A Textbook of Human Anatomy, ed 2, 1979, p 129.)*

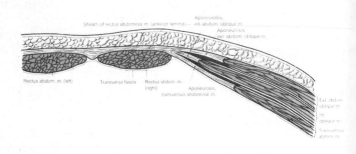

Figure 3. Configuration of the anterior rectus sheath caudal to the arcuate line. *(Reproduced from Ferner H, Staubesand J: Sobotta Atlas of Human Anatomy, 1983, vol 2, p 110.)*

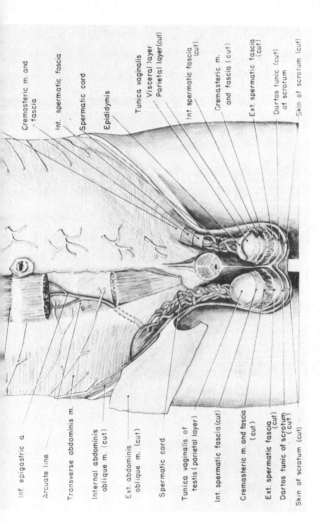

Inf epigastric a.

Arcuate line

Transverse abdominis m.

Internal abdominis
oblique m. (cut)

Ext. abdominis
oblique m. (cut)

Spermatic cord

Tunica vaginalis of
testis (parietal layer)

Int. spermatic fascia (cut)

Cremasteric m. and fascia
(cut)

Ext. spermatic fascia
(cut)

Dartos tunic of scrotum
(cut)

Skin of scrotum (cut)

Cremasteric m. and
fascia

Int. spermatic fascia

Spermatic cord

Epididymis

Tunica vaginalis
Visceral layer
Parietal layer(cut)

Int. spermatic fascia
(cut)

Cremasteric m.
and fascia (cut)

Ext. spermatic fascia
(cut)

Dartos tunic (cut)
of scrotum

Skin of scrotum (cut)

Figure 4. Contributions to the spermatic cord from the anterior abdominal wall musculature and fascia. *(Reproduced from Crafts RC: A Textbook of Human Anatomy, ed 2, 1979, p 139.)*

5

the internal oblique is the cremaster muscle, which extends caudally and invests with its fascia the spermatic cord.

3. The transversus abdominus muscle arises from the costal cartilages of the lower ribs, from the lumbodorsal fascia and the anterior two-thirds of the inner lip of the iliac crest and the lateral one-third of the inguinal ligament. The fibers course transversely and insert on the linea alba and then the pubic crest and the pectineal line.

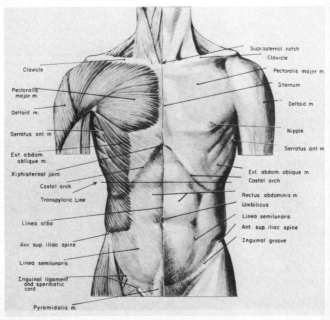

Figure 5. A. Superficial anatomy on left. On right superficial anterior abdominal wall musculature. *(Reproduced from Crafts RC: A Textbook of Human Anatomy, ed 2, 1979, p 61.)*

C. Posterior Lateral Abdominal Wall

The posterior lateral abdominal wall musculature may be divided into three groups, a superficial group, an intermediate group, and a deep group.

1. The superfical group consists of the external oblique and latissimus dorsi (Fig. 5). The intermediate group consists of the serratus posterior inferior, internal oblique, and sacrospinalis (Fig. 6). The deep group consists of the transversus abdominus, quadratus lumborum, and psoas (Fig. 7).

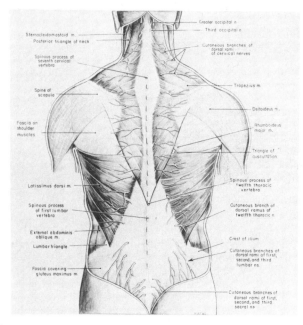

Figure 5. B. Posterior lateral abdominal wall showing position of the latissimus dorsi. *(Reproduced from Crafts RC: A Textbook of Human Anatomy, ed 2, 1979, p 61.)*

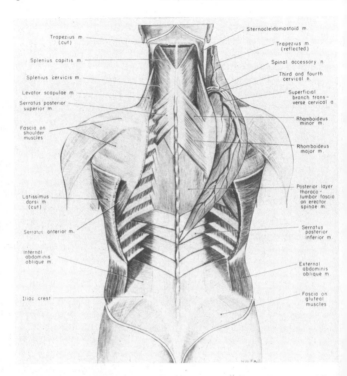

Figure 6. Intermediate group of abdominal wall musculature. *(Reproduced from Crafts RC: A Textbook of Human Anatomy, ed 2, 1979, p 65.)*

2. Consider the musculature that has not been previously described.
   a. The latissimus dorsi is a large triangular-shaped muscle that originates in the posterior layer of the lumbodorsal fascia. Muscular fascicles also arise from the external lip of the crest of the ileum as well as from the caudal three or four ribs.
   b. The serratus posterior inferior arises by an aponeurosis from the spinous processes of the last

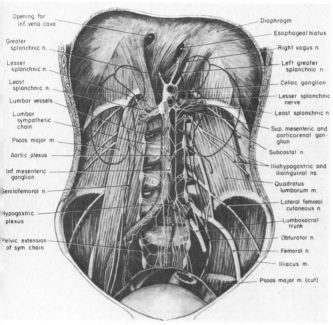

Figure 7. Deep group of anterior abdominal wall musculature. *(Reproduced from Crafts RC: A Textbook of Human Anatomy, ed 2, 1979, p 261.)*

two thoracic vertebra and the first two or three lumbar vertebra. They progress in a cranial lateral direction and insert into the inferior borders of the last four ribs just distal to their angles.

c. The sacrospinalis, also known as the erector spinae, arises from the sacrum and the spinous processes of the lumbar and lower thoracic vertebra near the juncture with the thoracic vertebra and divides into three muscular columns that insert in various ways on the dorsal medial aspects of the ribs.

d. The quadratus lumborum arises from the iliac crest

and inserts into the inferior border of the last rib in its medial aspect and into the transverse processes of the first four lumbar vertebra.

e. The psoas major arises from the transverse processes of all lumbar vertebra as well as from their bodies, lying ventral to the quadratus lumborum as it passes into the pelvis to insert into the lesser trochanter of the femur.

III. ADRENAL GLAND

A. Gross Structure

The adrenal glands are thin, cadmium yellow structures located above the kidneys bilaterally. They are contained within the intermediate stratum of retroperitoneal connective tissue surrounded by its specialization of Gerota's fascia. The right adrenal gland has a triangular appearance whereas the left adrenal gland has a more elongated leaf-life appearance (Fig. 8).

B. Microscopic Anatomy

The adrenal glands are composed of two distinct sections—the outer adrenal cortex, which makes up the bulk of the gland, and the inner adrenal medulla. The gland is surrounded by a thin, fibrous capsule. The adrenal cortex is composed of three distinct layers—an outer zona glomerulosa, a middle zona fasciculata, and an inner zona reticularis. The centrally located medulla consists primarily of chromaffin cells (Fig. 9).

C. Blood Supply

The adrenal gland is supplied generally by three arteries. An adrenal artery from the renal artery supplies the lower portion. The medial aspect is supplied by a branch from the aorta. A superior artery derives from the inferior phrenic artery. The venous drainage on the left side is by the left adrenal vein, which empties into the left renal artery. On the right side an extremely short adrenal vein drains directly into the vena cava.

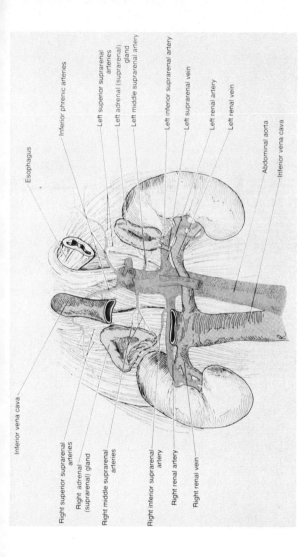

Figure 8. Position and morphology of the adrenal glands. *(Reproduced from Tortora GJ, Anagnostakos NP: Principles of Anatomy and Physiology, ed 3, 1981, p 423.)*

Inferior vena cava

Esophagus

Inferior phrenic arteries

Left superior suprarenal arteries

Left adrenal (suprarenal) gland

Left middle suprarenal artery

Left inferior suprarenal artery

Left suprarenal vein

Left renal artery

Left renal vein

Abdominal aorta

Inferior vena cava

Right superior suprarenal arteries

Right adrenal (suprarenal) gland

Right middle suprarenal arteries

Right inferior suprarenal artery

Right renal artery

Right renal vein

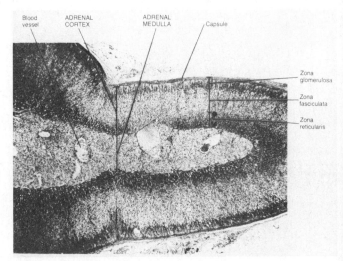

Figure 9. Longitudinal photomicrograph showing layers of the adrenal cortex and the medulla. *(Reproduced from Tortora GJ, Anagnostakos NP: Principles of Anatomy and Physiology, ed 3, 1981, p 423.)*

    D. Innervation

        The innervation of the adrenal gland is by the celiac and renal plexuses.

    E. Lymphatics

        The lymphatics follow the venous drainage and drain into the periaortic lymph nodes.

IV. KIDNEY

    A. Anatomy

      1. The kidneys are paired, bean-shaped organs located retroperitoneally lateral to the psoas muscle (Fig. 10). This position is somewhat oblique, with the lower pole of the kidney displaced lateral to the muscle. The kidney is a relatively large organ in the adult, measuring approximately 11.5 cm in length, 6 cm in width,

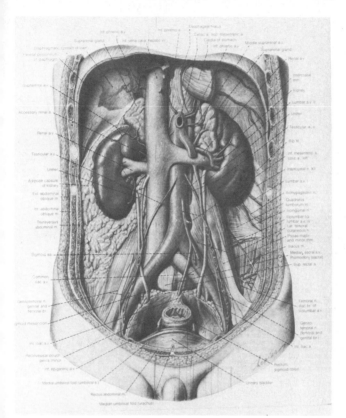

Figure 10. Position of the kidneys and retroperitoneum in relation to the great vessels. *(Reproduced from Ferner H, Staubesand J: Sobotta Atlas of Human Anatomy, 1983, vol 2, p 180.)*

and 2.5 to 3 cm in thickness. Near the center of the medial convex border of the kidney is a shallow depression, the hilum, through which pass the renal vasculature, nerves, lymphatics, and the renal pelvis. The interior of the kidney is a space called the renal sinus

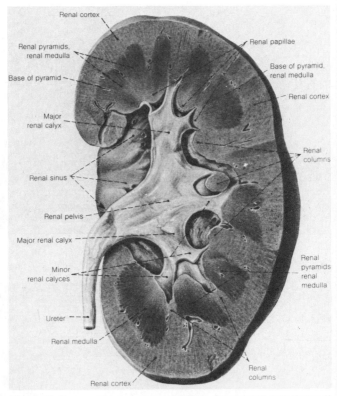

Figure 11. Cross sectional anatomy of kidney. *(Reproduced from Ferner H, Staubesand J: Sobotta Atlas of Human Anatomy, 1983, vol 2, p 179.)*

and is occupied by the major renal collecting structures, minor calyces, major calyces, pelvis and the larger renal vasculature, and fat (Fig. 11).

2. The kidneys, along with the adrenal gland, are encased in retroperitoneal connective tissue. This intermediate stratum of retroperitoneal connective tissue, as opposed to outer stratum (transversalis fascia) and inner

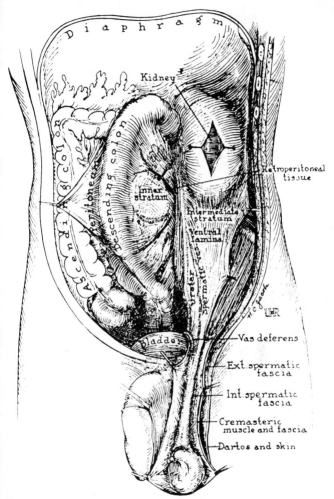

Figure 12. Anatomy of retroperitoneal connective tissue. Note the continuity of the intermediate stratum through the internal ring as a component of the cord. *(Reproduced from Tobin CE, Benjamin JA, Wells JC: Surg Gynecol Obstet 83: 586, 1946.)*

stratum (supporting connective tissue of the peritoneum) (Fig. 12), is further thickened around the
kidney and is known as Gerota's fascia. The fatty
tissue that is external to Gerota's fascia is known as
paranephric fat. Fatty tissue within Gerota's fascia is
known as perinephric fat. Posterior to the kidney the
fatty layer is thick. Anterior to the kidney it is relatively thin. Because of these coverings other organs do
not directly encroach on the kidneys, but knowledge of
the organ relationships to the kidneys is of clinical
significance. The right lobe of the liver, the descending duodenum, and the hepatic flexure of the colon are
in proximity to the right side of the kidneys. The stomach, the spleen, the splenic flexure of the colon, the
pancreas, and the jejunum are close to the left side of
the kidneys (Fig. 13).

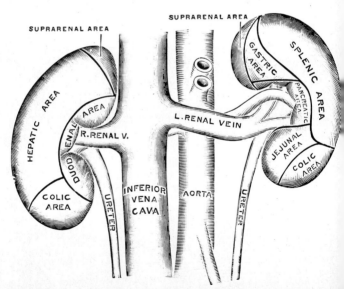

Figure 13. Position of visceral relationships of kidney. *(Reproduced from Gray H: Anatomy of the Human Body, ed 29, 1973, p 1279.)*

3. If the kidney is sectioned sagitally, it will be noted that it is covered by a thick renal capsule that is penetrated by capsular vessels. The substance of the kidney as usually seen is divided into cortex and medulla (columns of Bertine). The medulla is composed of pyramids that end in papilla that terminate in minor calyces or drain into the pelvis of the kidney itself.

B. Renal Blood Supply

1. Since the major function of the kidney is to regulate the composition and volume of the blood, the vasculature of the kidney is most important. Both renal arteries transport approximately one-fourth of the total cardiac output. Although there may be great variation in renal vasculature, a general pattern is noted. It should be stated that renal arteries are end arteries and the more proximal a renal artery is occluded the greater amount of tissue will be devascularized. Basically, the renal artery is a singular large artery, although there may be two or more arising from the lateral aspect of the aorta just caudal to the superior mesenteric artery. Prior to entering the renal hilum the artery branches into an anterior and posterior division. The arteries are found posterior to the renal vein and anterior to the renal pelvis. The posterior division of the renal artery generally does not branch until it enters the renal substance and supplies the posterior segment of the kidney. The anterior division divides into three or four branches and provides superior, anterior, and inferior segmental arteries and usually an apical artery. The kidney is thus considered to be divided into superior, anterior, inferior, and apical segments. Within the substance of the kidney the arteries branch into interlobar, arcuate, and interlobular arteries.

2. The veins generally accompany the arteries. They differ from the arteries in that they intercommunicate. If an intrarenal vein is ligated, the segment drained by the vein will drain through another venous channel. On the posterior lateral surface of the kidney a whitish depression known as Brodel's white line will be noted. This line does not represent a vascular plane but in-

stead is the line of division between the anterior and posterior row of pyramids. The left renal vein is unique in that two major branches enter it; cranially the venous drainage of the left adrenal, and caudally the left ovarian or spermatic veins.

C. Microscopic Anatomy

1. In general the cortex of the kidney is composed of nephrons, whereas the medulla is composed primarily of collecting ducts. The primary functioning unit of the kidney is the nephron, which consists of the renal

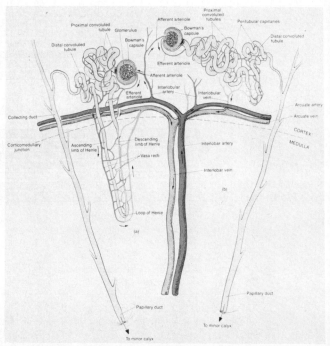

Figure 14. Anatomy of the nephron and its vascular relationships. *(Reproduced from Tortora GJ, Anagnostakos NP: Principles of Anatomy and Physiology, ed 3, 1981, p 672.)*

corpuscle and the collecting tubules (Fig. 14). The renal corpuscle consists of Bowman's capsule and the glomerulus, the proximal tubule, which has a convoluted and straight portion, a thin limb of Henle, a distal tubule, which has a straight portion, called the macula densa, and a convoluted portion, and a collecting duct.

2. The glomerulus or capillary tuft, which fits within Bowman's capsule, is fed by an afferent arteriole that arises from the interlobular artery. Blood is drained from the capillary tuft by an efferent arteriole that then supplies blood to the remainder of the nephron through peritubular capillaries. Long loops of vessels called the vasa recta also proceed alongside the loop of Henle. Peritubular capillaries eventually form interlobar veins, draining through arcuate veins to the interlobar veins and then to the segmental veins. Bowman's capsule itself consists of two layers, as if the balloon-shaped end of the nephron had been invaginated by the glomerular tuft (Fig. 15). The outer layer is called the parietal layer and is composed of simple squamous epithelium. The visceral layer consists of epithelial cells that are called podocytes. These foot processes give off smaller processes; termed pedicels, they cover the endothelium of the glomerulus, which is perforated by endothelial pores. The space between the visceral and parietal layers of epithelium is known as Bowman's space and is contiguous with the lumen of the proximal convoluted tubule.

3. The proximal convoluted tubule is the longest part of the nephron. The wall of the proximal convoluted tubule consists of cuboidal epithelium that is covered by microvilli.

4. The descending limb of Henle descends into the medulla, proceeding in hairpin fashion; the turn is the loop of Henle. The descending limb of Henle is thicker in diameter and consists of cuboidal and columnar epithelium.

5. It becomes convoluted as it reaches the cortex and is known as the distal convoluted tubule. The cells of the

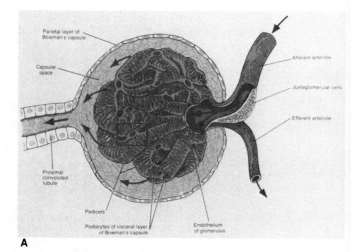

A

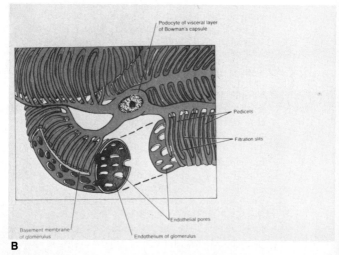

B

Figure 15. A. Anatomy of the glomerulus. **B.** Detail of Bowman's capsule. *(Reproduced from Tortora GJ, Anagnostakos NP: Principles of Anatomy and Physiology, ed 3, 1981, p 673.)*

distal tubule are also cuboidal epithelium. The distal tubule terminates in a straight collecting duct that passes through the renal pyramids and opens into the papilla in terminal ducts of Bellini.

6. Although the distal convoluted tubule is so termed because of its distance from Bowman's space, it also lies adjacent to the afferent arteriole. This particular closeness modifies cells of both the afferent arteriole and the distal convoluted tubule. The modified smooth muscle cells of the tunica media of the afferent arteriole are known as juxtaglomerular cells. A modification of the cells of the distal convoluted tubule is known as the macula densa. Together these modified cells are collectively known as the juxtaglomerular apparatus. There are two types of nephrons—cortical nephrons, in which the glomerulus and the remainder of the nephron are contained wholly within the cortex, and juxtamedullary nephrons, in which the glomerulus is close to the cortical medullary junction but the other parts of the nephron are found within the substance of the medulla.

D. Innervation

The renal nerve supply is derived from the renal plexus of the autonomic nervous system, which overlies the aorta just cranial to the renal arteries. The nerves accompany the renal arteries and enter the kidney at the hilum and continue along the course of the vessels. The nerve supply consists of the sympathetic nerve supply which originates as preganglionic fibers in the 12th thoracic and upper lumbar segments. The synapses occur in the renal ganglion. Parasympathetic innervation is from the vagal portion of the parasympathetic. The ganglia are located within the walls of the kidney themselves. Sensory fibers from the kidney are primarily from the renal pelvis and accompany the sympathetic nerves.

E. Lymphatics

The lymphatic vessels of the kidney form three plexuses. One of the plexuses is located within the substance of the kidney, one beneath the fibrous capsule, and the third in the perinephric fat. The latter two communicate freely. The lymphatics from the intrarenal plexus join to form larger lymphatic trunks that exit at the hilum. The lymphatics follow the course of the renal vein and drain into the lumbar nodes.

V. CALYCES, RENAL PELVIS, AND URETER

A. Gross Structure

1. The major collecting structures of the urinary tract begin at the renal papilla. The collecting part itself is termed a minor calyx. The number varies from 7 to 13. Each calyx may enclose more than one papilla. Under the mucosa of the papilla is a circular layer of smooth muscle. The calyces are connected by necks termed infundibula to form two to three major calyces that coalesce to form the funnel-shaped renal pelvis.

2. The ureters are approximately 25 to 30 cm in length and extend from the renal pelvis to the bladder. For discussion the ureter may be divided into an abdominal portion and a pelvic portion. The ureters from the renal pelvis to the bladder are contained in the intermediate stratum of retroperitoneal connective tissue. The gonadal vessels, which are also contained within this connective tissue in a ventral location, cross the ureters. The pelvic portion of the ureter is located dorsal to the obliterated umbilical artery (lateral umbilical ligament) and the vascular leash proceeding to the bladder. In females the uterine artery also crosses ventral to the ureter. In the male the vas deferens crosses ventral to the ureter. The three areas of relative narrowing of the ureter are the ureteropelvic junction, the site of crossing of the iliac vessels, and the ureterovesical junction.

B. Microscopic Anatomy

On cross section, the ureter appears to be composed of three layers. The body of the ureter is surrounded by fibroadiposal tissue, which represents the intermediate stratum of retroperitoneal connective tissue and its specialized thickening, the periureteric fascia. The innermost portion of the ureter is mucosa that is composed of transitional epithelium. The bulk of the wall of the ureter is composed of muscularis that is generally said to be composed of an inner longitudinal and an outer circular layer. The differentiation between the two layers is not so pronounced since they tend to run obliquely and mesh together. In the terminal portion of the ureter the muscularis is primarily longitudinal. At the ureterovesical juncture itself the bladder musculature reflects onto the ureter and is separated from the ureteric musculature by loose connective tissue that has been termed Waldeyer's sheath.

C. Blood Supply

The ureteric blood supply is predominantly longitudinal but derives from several adjacent structures. The renal calyces, pelvis, and upper ureter derive their blood supply from the renal arteries. The central portion of the ureter may receive blood from the gonadal vessels. The more distal portions of the ureter are supplied from the aorta near its bifurcation, the common iliacs, the internal iliacs, and ureteric branches of the superior and inferior vesical arteries. In the female, blood supply may be derived also from the uterine artery. The venous drainage accompanies the arterial supply.

D. Innervation

Innervation is autonomic and derives from the inferior mesenteric, testicular, and pelvic plexuses. The afferent supply of the ureter is contained in the 11th and 12th thoracic and 1st lumbar nerves. Nerves basically follow the course of the blood vessels to the ureter.

E. Lymphatics

The lymphatic drainage of the ureter generally accompanies the arteries and thus drain to lymph nodes adjacent to the renal artery in the upper portion. In the central portion drainage is to the lateral aortic nodes and in the terminal portion, the internal iliac nodes.

VI. BLADDER

A. General

The urinary bladder is a hollow muscular organ that when filled with urine is spherical; its shape has great variability, however, depending on its degree of filling. In the adult it is basically a pelvic organ. In the child it occupies a more abdominal position. The bladder is traditionally described as having four surfaces, a superior surface, two inferior lateral surfaces, and a posterior or basal surface. The superior surface of the bladder is covered by peritoneum. The posterior surface of the bladder or base of the bladder lies on the ventral aspect of the rectum in the male and on the vagina of the female. The remainder of the bladder is surrounded by an intermediate stratum of retroperitoneal connective tissue. The potential space between the inferior lateral surface of the bladder has been termed the prepubic space or space of Retzius. The apex of the bladder is connected to the umbilicus by a fibrous cord termed the urachus or medial umbilical ligament. On either side of the medial umbilical ligament are two other fibrous ligaments, called the lateral umbilical ligaments, which are obliterated umbilical arteries. In the male the base of the bladder is supported by the prostate and a thickening of endopelvic fascia that bridges the pubis and the bladder, termed the puboprostatic ligaments. A similar condensation of fascia termed the pubovesical or pubourethral ligament is located in the female. In the male between the base of the bladder and the rectum lie the seminal vesicles and more medially the ampulla of the vas deferens.

B. Gross Anatomy

In most general descriptions of gross anatomy of the bladder wall three muscular layers—an outer longitudinal, a middle circular, and an inner longitudinal layer are listed. It is probable that the arrangement most closely approaches a meshwork of musculature (Fig. 16). Although an internal sphincter is frequently spoken of, a ring of musculature as such does not exist (Fig. 17). Instead is noted a prominent detrusor band that thickens towards the

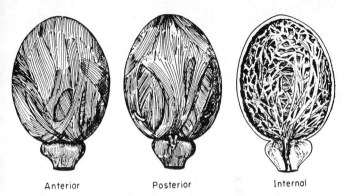

Anterior   Posterior   Internal

Figure 16. Detail of bladder musculature. *(Reproduced from Woodburne RT: J Urol 100:479, 1968.)*

prostate as it progresses caudally where it divides and spreads around the neck of the bladder and the base of the prostate. A further bundle of musculature that progresses from the anterior vesical neck posteriorly has been termed the bundle of Heiss. Over the inner musculature of the

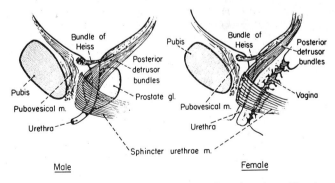

Figure 17. Detail of vesical neck and urethral musculature in males and females. *(Reproduced from Woodburne RT: J Urol 100:479, 1968.)*

bladder is a well-developed submucosal layer that is composed primarily of transitional epithelium. The trigone is the triangular-shaped internal base of the bladder. It is formed by the ureteric musculature as it both crosses the midline to blend with ureteric muscle of the opposite side and spreads towards the vesical neck. The muscular band that forms the base of the trigone is termed the interureteric ridge. The ureteral orifices themselves appear slit-like, the appearance varying with the site of entrance of the ureter into the bladder.

C. Blood Supply

The arterial supply of the bladder is derived primarily from the internal iliac artery; it further branches to supply a superior vesical artery and an inferior vesical artery. The upper portion of the bladder is supplied by the superior vesical artery whereas the lower portion of the bladder is supplied by the inferior vesical artery. Variably a middle vesical artery will be found. In addition, vessels may be supplied from the obturator or inferior gluteal arteries. In the female, uterine and vaginal arteries may also provide some supply to the bladder. The venous drainage does not follow the arteries but forms a complicated plexus primarily on the inferior surface and the base of the bladder. The venous drainage terminates in the internal iliac veins.

D. Innervation

The sympathetic nerve supply of the bladder arises from the 11th and 12th thoracic and 1st and 2nd lumbar segments of the cord. The nerves pass to the lateral sympathetic chain, where they form the superior vesical plexus, which is known as the presacral nerve and is located over the bifurcation of the aorta. The hypogastric nerves derive from the presacral nerve and enter the pelvis to form the hypogastric ganglia on the lateral wall of the rectum. Postganglionic fibers from these ganglia innervate the bladder. The parasympathetic nerve supply arises from the 2nd, 3rd, and 4th segments at the level of the 12th thoracic vertebra. They pass through the pelvic plexus to synapse in the bladder wall. The external sphincter receives somatic supply by the pudendal nerve, which is derived from S2 and S4.

E. **Lymphatics**

The bladder wall is rich in lymphatics. The lymphatics intercommunicate and drain into the vesical, internal iliac, external iliac, and common iliac lymph nodes.

VII. PROSTATE

A. **General**

The prostate is a chestnut-shaped glandular structure that lies between the neck of the bladder and the external sphincter. It is traversed throughout its length by the posterior urethra. The prostate is fixed to the pelvic floor by investments of the parietal fascia and the endopelvic fascia. Two dense condensations of the endopelvic fascia that affix the prostate to the pubis are the puboprostatic ligaments. The prostate is encased in an intermediate stratum of retroperitoneal connective tissue that contains a rich plexus of veins that are received from the dorsal vein of the penis beneath the pubic symphysis. Posteriorly the prostate is separated from the rectum by Denonvillier's fascia, which represents the connective tissue remaining from the obliterated peritoneal cul-de-sac between the rectum and the prostate.

B. **Gross Anatomy**

The prostate is covered by a firm fibrous capsule. The prostate is traditionally divided into five lobes—an anterior, posterior, median, and two lateral lobes. The posterior aspect of the prostate is traversed by the terminal portions of the vas deferens, which exit in the ejaculatory ducts in the posterior urethra. The posterior urethra, which traverses the prostate, houses a small mound on its dorsal aspect termed the verumontanum. In the middle portion of the verumontanum is a small pit, the utricle. The ejaculatory ducts exit on the verumontanum.

C. **Microscopic Anatomy**

On cross section the prostate is encased in a fibrous capsule. Its glandular structure resembles a sponge, with the major ducts of the gland exiting into the floor of the urethra. The glands are surrounded by fibromuscular stroma. The glands are distributed into external glands and periurethral glands. The external glands are the predominant glandular structures of the prostate.

D. Blood Supply

Primary vascularization of the prostate is from the prostatic artery, which derives from the inferior vesical artery. Two main groups of arteries occur, a capsular group and a urethral group. Some accessory vessels to the prostate are supplied from the middle hemorrhoidal and internal pudendal arteries. The venous drainage of the prostate is through a prostatic plexus that joins the venous drainage of the penis in Santorini's plexus and then drains into the hypogastric veins. It is of note that the prostatic plexus connects with the prevertebral veins (Batson's plexus).

E. Innervation

Innervation of the prostate is through sympathetic fibers from L1 and L2 and from the third and fourth sacral nerves through the sacral plexus.

F. Lymphatics

Prostatic lymphatics egress via the vesical, hypogastric, external iliac, and sacral lymph nodes.

VIII. URETHRA

A. Male Urethra

1. In the male the urethra runs from the vesical neck to the tip of the penis (Fig. 18). It is generally divided into two portions—a posterior urethra and the anterior urethra. The posterior urethra is that portion that traverses the prostate. The anterior urethra may be divided into three parts—the bulbous urethra, the pendulous or penile urethra, and the glandular urethra. The urethra itself is contained within an erectile body termed the corpora spongiosa, which is held to the corpora cavernosa of the penis by Buck's fascia. Numerous mucous glands, the urethral glands, open into the lumen.

2. The posterior urethra is lined by transitional epithelium. The major portion of the anterior urethra is

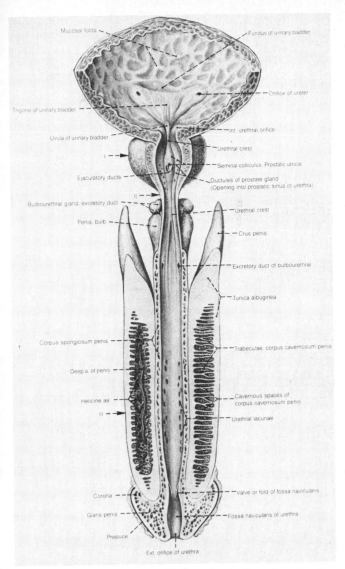

Figure 18. Relationships of urethra to bladder and penis. *(Reproduced from Ferner H, Staubesand J: Sobotta Atlas of Human Anatomy, 1983, vol 2, p 193.)*

lined by stratified columnar epithelium. As it passes through the glans the urethra is dilated to form the fossa navicularis, which is lined by squamous epithelium.

3. The blood supply to the anterior urethra is from a branch to the pudendal artery, the bulbourethral artery.
4. The lymphatic drainage of the deep urethra is to the hypogastric lymph nodes. Drainage to the anterior urethra is to the inguinal lymph nodes, the deep inguinal nodes, and the external iliac nodes.

B. Female Urethra
The female urethra is related on its dorsal aspect closely to the ventral aspect of the vagina. Its position in relation to the bladder is somewhat analogous to the posterior urethra in the male. It is also lined by transitional epithelium.

IX. ENDOSCOPIC ANATOMY

A. **Although endoscopy of body passages and cavities** has burgeoned over the past several years, urology was one of the first fields to incorporate this examination modality. Although much of the urinary collecting structures can be negotiated and visualized, the most frequently visualized is the lower tract, which may be examined with a variety of rigid and flexible endoscopes.

B. **On negotiation of the urethra from the meatus to the bladder neck,** three fusiform dilatations of the urethra are noted. The most distal is the fossa navicularis as the scope passes through the glans penis. Within the fossa navicularis there are several small pits known as lacunae. The large one in the midline is known as lacuna magna. On the floor of the urethra are noted numerous small orifices. These represent the orifices of the urethral glands or Littre's glands. The second dilatation of the urethra is the bulbous urethra. After negotiating the bulbous urethra, the bellows-like membranous portion of the urethra is noted. This represents the passage of the urethra through the urogenital diaphragm and marks the beginning of the posterior urethra. On the floor of the urethra and almost in its central portion is the verumontanum. In the central portion of the veru is noted the pit-like utricle. On either side the ejaculatory ducts may varyingly be noted. The vesical neck is noted just ahead. With enlargement of the prostate the lateral lobes encroach laterally and a median lobe may be noticed that requires deflection of the endoscope upward to go over the lobe into the bladder. On the floor of the bladder is noted the trigone, with the orifices forming apices of the base of the triangle and the base itself being the inner ureteric ridge. The underlying detrusor under the mucosa gives a gridlike appearance to the wall of the bladder. With hypertrophy of the detrusor frank trabeculations may be seen. With protrusion of the mucosa through these trabeculations cellules or even diverticula may be formed.

X. TESTIS AND EPIDIDYMIS

A. General

The testes are paired ovoid structures that measure 4.5 cm in length, 3 cm in width, and 2 cm in depth. Adjacent to the testicle on its posterior aspect is an elongated structure termed the epididymis (Fig. 19). The testes reside dependently in the scrotum, with their long axis being vertical. The scrotum is divided into two compartments. The contents of the scrotum comprise the investments of the testis and epididymis. Immediately adjacent to the testis is the remnant of the patent processes vaginalis termed the visceral and parietal layers of tunica vaginalis. They encompass approximately three-fourths of the anterior lateral aspects of the testis and epididymis. Surrounding these structures is the internal spermatic fascia, which is contiguous with the transversalis fascia of the abdominal wall. This is covered by the cremasteric muscle and fascia contiguous with the internal oblique musculature. This in turn is covered by the external spermatic fascia which is contiguous with the investing fascia of the external oblique aponeurosis. The testicular and spermatic cord investments are covered by the dartos tunic of the scrotum which is contiguous with the superficial fascia (Scarpa's

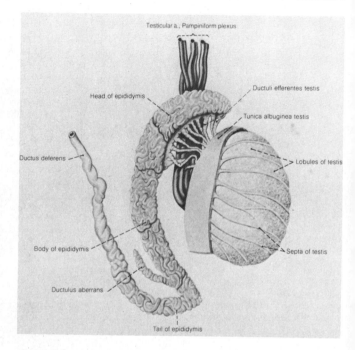

Figure 19. Gross anatomy of the testicle following the removal of the tunica albuginea and relationships to the ductuli efferentes and the epididymis. *(Reproduced from Ferner H, Staubesand J: Sobotta Atlas of Human Anatomy, 1983, vol 2, p 191.)*

fascia of the anterior abdominal wall, Colle's fascia of the perineum, and the dartos tunic of the penis).

B. Gross Anatomy

The testis is surrounded by a dense fibrous covering, the tunica albuginea. On longitudinal section the testis is seen to be divided by fibrous septa into approximately 250 lobules. Each lobule contains one to three convoluted seminiferous tubules that coalesce to form straight seminiferous tubules that then join at the hilum of the testis to a network of tubules called the rete testis. The rete testis in turn drain into the efferent ductules in the epididymis and thus form a single convoluted ductus of the epididymis that in turn forms the lumen of the ductus deferens. The cranial portion of the epididymis is known as the globus major or head of the epididymis. The caudal portion of the epididymis before it turns to become the vas deferens is known as the tail of the epididymis or globus minor. Vestigial appendages are noted on the cranial aspect of the testis and head of the epididymis. These are known, respectively, as the appendix testis and the appendix epididymis.

C. **Microscopic Anatomy**

The bulk of the testis is composed of the seminiferous tubules. The tubules consist of a basement membrane lined with a relatively thick layer of germinal cells that progress from primary spermatocytes to mature spermatozoa. Between the developing germ cells on the base of the tubule are Sertoli (supporting) cells. Between the seminiferous tubules are clusters of triangular (Leydig) cells. The ductus epididymis is lined with a pseudostratified columnar epithelium. Its wall contains smooth muscle.

D. **Blood Supply**

Blood supply to the testicle is by the internal spermatic artery, which arises from the aorta near the ventral midline just caudal to the take-off of the renal arteries. The arteries pass through the retroperitoneal connective tissue, the internal ring, and down the inguinal canal to the testicle. Additional arterial supply to the testicle is by the vasal artery and the external spermatic artery. The vasal artery is derived from the superior vesical artery. Its return is by a plexus of veins, the pampiniform plexus, which coalesce to form a single gonadal vein. The gonadal vein on the right enters the vena cava obliquely usually with a valve. On the left side the gonadal vein enters the left renal vein, usually without a valve.

E. **Lymphatics**

The lymphatic drainage of the testes accompanies the blood supply and drains to paraaortic lymph nodes that are located primarily between the renal vessels and the bifurcation of the aorta.

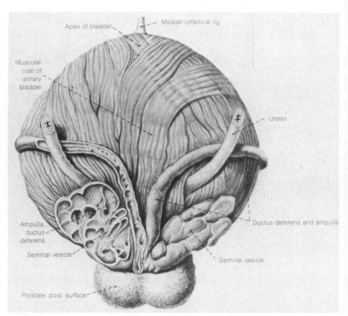

Figure 20. Bladder and prostate viewed posteriorly showing relationships of seminal vesicles and ampulla of vas. *(Reproduced from Ferner H, Staubesand J: Sobotta Atlas of Human Anatomy, 1983, vol 2, p 189.)*

XI. VAS DEFERENS AND SEMINAL VESICLES

From the internal ring the vas proceeds extraperitoneally, posteriorly and medially. It passes between the ureter and behind the base of the bladder, where it becomes dilated and tortuous for several centimeters. This is termed the ampulla of the ductus deferens. The vas terminates in the ejaculatory ducts, which open into the prostatic urethra on either side of the utricle on the verumontanum. A large diverticulum, the seminal vesicle of the vas deferens, has its juncture adjacent with the ampulla of the vas near the ejaculatory ducts just above the base of the prostate (Fig. 20). Seminal vesicles are approx-

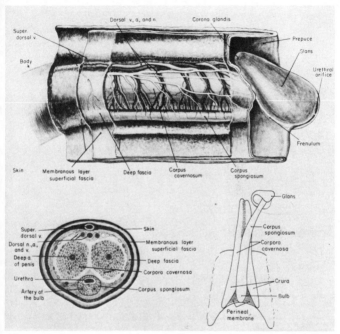

Figure. 21. Gross anatomy of the penis. *(Reproduced from Crafts RC: A Text-book of Human Anatomy, ed 2, 1979, p 324.)*

imately 6 cm long. They are lobulated in appearance. Histologically they are lined by pseudostratified epithelium. The wall of the seminal vesicle is composed of thin circular longitudinal smooth muscle.

XII. PENIS

A. Gross Structure

The penis is comprised of three erectile bodies—a paired corpora cavernosum and the corpora spongiosum, which contains the urethra (Fig. 21). The cylindrical corpora cavernosa invaginate the glans distally. Proximally they diverge at the level of the pubic symphysis to end as the crura of the penis where they are attached to the inferior pubic rami. The corpora spongiosa is in direct contact with the glans penis, and indeed the structures appear similar in composition. At the divergence of the corpora cavernosa the corpora spongiosa becomes more dilated and is known as the bulbous portion of the corpora spongiosa. On cross section it will be noted that the corpora cavernosa and spongiosa are held together as a single bundle by a dense fascia known as Buck's fascia. Covering Buck's fascia is the Dartos tunic, which is in turn covered by the skin. The penile shaft is supported at the level of the pubic symphysis by the suspensory ligament that is contiguous with Buck's fascia.

B. Arterial Supply

The penis derives its blood supply from the internal pudendal artery, which branches at the bulb to form an artery to the bulb. The remainder of the penis is supplied by the deep artery of the penis, which runs the length of the corpora cavernosa through the center of the erectile body. The dorsal artery of the penis lies distally on the dorsum of the penis deep to Buck's fascia. Superficial blood supply to the penis is also supplied from the external pudendal artery.

C. Innervation

The nerve supply generally accompanies the vessels. The innervation to the skin and fascia is by the dorsal nerve of the penis, which is a branch of the pudendal nerve. Branches of the perineal nerve, ilioinguinal nerve, and perineal branches of the posterior femoral cutaneous nerve of the thigh supply additional innervation. Sympathetic nerve supply via the hypogastric plexus supplies the corpora cavernosum. Venous drainage is through the superficial and deep dorsal veins into the prostatic plexus.

D. Lymphatics

Superficial and deep groups of lymphatics drain to the superficial and deep inguinal lymph nodes and from there to the external iliac lymph nodes.

BIBLIOGRAPHY

Crafts RC: Textbook of Human Anatomy, ed 2. New York: Wiley, 1979.

Ferner H, Staubes and J (eds): Sobotta Atlas of Human Anatomy. Baltimore: Urban and Schwartzenberg, 1983, vol 2.

Goss CM (ed): Anatomy of the Human Body, ed 29. Philadelphia: Lea & Febiger, 1973.

Tobin CE, Benjamin JA, Wells JC: Continuity of the fasciae lining the abdomen, pelvis, and spermatic cord. Surg Gynecol Obstet 83:586, 1946.

2

Signs and Symptoms: The Initial Examination

Keith N. Van Arsdalen

I. INTRODUCTION

A. Definition
Urology is a surgical specialty devoted to the study and treatment of disorders of the genitourinary tract of the male and the urinary tract of the female. In addition to the surgical correction of acquired and congenital abnormalities, the urologist is often involved with the diagnosis and treatment of many "medical" disorders of the genitourinary tract.

B. Importance to Other Branches of Medicine
1. Approximately 15% of patients initially presenting to a physician will have a urologic complaint or abnormality.
2. There is a wide overlap with other specialties and frequent interaction with other physicians, including family practitioners, internists, pediatricians, geriatricians, endocrinologists, nephrologists, neurologists, obstetricians and gynecologists, and general, vascular, and trauma surgeons.
3. It is important that all physicians be aware of the specific diagnostic and therapeutic measures that are available within this specialty.

II. UROLOGIC MANIFESTATIONS OF DISEASE

A. Direct

The most obvious manifestations of urologic disease are those signs and symptoms that are directly related to the urinary tract of the male and female or to the genitalia of the male. Hematuria and scrotal swelling are examples in this category.

B. Manifestations Referred to or from Other Organ Systems

1. Symptoms from the genitourinary tract may be referred to other areas within the genitourinary tract or to contiguous organ systems.
   a. A stone in the kidney or upper ureter may produce ipsilateral testicular pain.
   b. This same stone may be associated with symptoms of nausea and vomiting.
   c. The gastrointestinal tract is probably the most common site to manifest symptoms from primary urologic problems. This is most probably due to the common innervation of these systems as well as the close direct relationship between the various component organs.
2. Primary urologic disorders may also be manifest in different organ systems and by seemingly unrelated signs and symptoms. Bone pain and pathologic fractures secondary to metastatic carcinoma arising in the genitourinary tract are examples in this regard.
3. Similarly, primary disease in other organ systems may result in secondary urologic signs and symptoms that initially lead the patient to the urologist. Most commonly these are related to inflammatory or neoplastic processes arising in:
   a. the lower lobes of the lungs
   b. the gastrointestinal tract
   c. the female internal genitalia

C. Systemic

Fever, weight loss, and malaise may be nonspecific systemic manifestations of acute and chronic inflammatory disorders, renal failure, and genitourinary carcinoma with or without metastases.

D. Asymptomatic

Lastly, it should be remembered that extensive disease may exist within the genitourinary tract without any signs or symptoms being manifest. Large renal calculi or neoplasms may only be found incidentally during other examinations. Far advanced renal deterioration may occur prior to the detection of silent reflux or obstruction.

III. HISTORY

A. Symptoms

1. A symptom is any departure from normal appearance, function, or sensation as experienced by the patient. Symptoms are reported to the physician or uncovered by careful history taking, with varying degrees of importance and/or significance attached to each symptom by both parties.

   a. The chief complaint, history of the present illness, and past medical history are delineated in a standard fashion.

   b. The character, onset, duration, and progression of the symptom is carefully defined. It is important to note what factors exacerbate or ameliorate the problem.

2. Urologic symptoms are generally related to:

   a. Pain and discomfort

   b. Alterations of micturition

   c. Changes in the gross appearance of the urine

   d. Abnormal appearance and/or function of the external genitalia

B. Pain

1. Pain within the genitourinary tract generally arises from distention or inflammation of a part or parts of the genitourinary system. Pain may be experienced directly in the involved organ or referred as noted above. Referred pain is a relatively common symptom of genitourinary disease.

2. Renal Pain

   a. The kidney and its capsule are innervated by sensory fibers traveling to the T10–L1 aspect of the spinal cord.

    b. The etiology of renal pain may be due either to capsular distention or inflammation or due to distention of the renal collecting system.

    c. Renal pain may be a dull aching sensation felt primary in the area of the costovertebral angle or it may be of a sharp, colicky nature felt in the area of the flank, with radiation around the abdomen into the groin and ipsilateral testicle. The latter is due to the common innervation of the testicle and the kidney.

    d. The nature of the primary disease process within the kidney often determines the type of sensation that is experienced and may depend upon the degree and rapidity of capsular and/or collecting system distention.

3. Ureteral Pain

    a. The upper ureter is innervated in a similar fashion to that described above for the kidney. Therefore, upper ureteral pain has a similar distribution to that of renal pain.

    b. The lower ureter, however, sends sensory fibers to the cord through ganglia subserving the major pelvic organs. Therefore, pain derived from the lower ureter is generally felt in the suprapubic area, bladder, penis, or urethra.

    c. The most common etiologic mechanism for ureteral pain is sudden obstruction and ureteral distention.

    d. Acute renal and ureteral colic are among the most severe types of pain known to humankind.

4. Bladder Pain

    a. Pain within the bladder may be derived from retention of urine and overdistention or from inflammatory processes.

    b. The pain of overdistention is generally felt within the suprapubic area, resulting in severe local discomfort.

    c. The pain due to bladder inflammation is generally felt as a sharp burning pain that is often referred to the tip of the penile urethra in males and the entire urethra in females.

5. Prostate Pain
   a. Sensory fibers from the prostate mostly enter the sacral aspect of the spinal cord.
   b. Prostate pain is most commonly due to acute inflammation and is generally perceived as discomfort in the lower back, rectum, and perineum.
   c. Irritative symptoms arising from the bladder may overshadow the purely prostate symptoms.
6. Penile Pain
   a. Penile and urethral pain is generally directly related to a site of inflammation.
7. Scrotal Pain
   a. Pain within the scrotum generally arises from disorders of the testis and/or epididymis.
   b. The most common etiologic factors include trauma, torsion of the spermatic cord, torsion of the appendix testis or appendix epididymis, and acute inflammation, particularly epididymitis. The pain in these cases is generally of rapid onset, if not sudden, and severe in nature.
   c. Hydroceles, varicoceles, and testicular tumors may also be associated with scrotal discomfort but generally of a more insidious nature and of less severity in most cases.

C. **Alterations of Micturition**
   1. Definitions and Problems
      a. A variety of specific terms have been developed to describe alterations related to the act of micturition. This section will attempt to define a variety of these terms.
      b. It must be emphasized at this point that a variety of disease processes may result in similar symptoms at the level of the lower urinary tract and although these terms are used to describe specific symptoms in this area, they do not necessarily pertain to specific etiologies.
   2. Changes in Urine Volume
      a. *Anuria* and *oliguria* are terms that refer to the varying degrees of decreased urinary output that may be secondary to prerenal, renal, or postrenal fac-

tors. In all cases it is essential to rule out urethral and/or ureteral obstruction as postrenal causes for these problems.

b. *Polyuria* refers to an increase in the volume of urine excreted on a daily basis. The etiologic mechanisms include increased fluid intake, exogenous or endogenous diuretics, or abnormal states of central or peripheral osmoregulation.

3. Irritative Symptoms

a. *Dysuria* is a term that refers simply to painful or difficult urination. The burning sensation that occurs during micturition associated with either bladder, urethral, or prostatic inflammation is generally used synonomously. This discomfort is generally felt in the entire urethra in females and in the distal urethra in males.

b. *Strangury* is a subtype of dysuria in which intense discomfort accompanies frequent voiding of small amounts of urine.

c. *Frequency* refers to the increased number of times one feels the need to urinate. This may be secondary to a true decrease in bladder capacity resulting from a loss of elasticity and edema due to inflammation or secondary to a decrease in the effective bladder capacity due to a failure of the bladder to empty completely with persistence of a large residual urine.

d. *Nocturia* is essentially the nighttime equivalent of urinary frequency, that is, there is a decreased real or effective bladder capacity that forces the patient to arise at night to urinate.

e. *Nycturia* refers to the excretion of larger volumes of urine at night than during the day and is secondary to mobilization of dependent fluid that accumulated when the patient was in the upright position. Nycturia may result in nocturia even in the presence of a normal bladder capacity if large quantities of fluid are mobilized.

f. *Urgency* refers to the sudden severe urge to void that may or may not be controllable.

    g. The irritative symptoms noted above are most commonly associated with inflammation of the lower urinary tract, i.e., the bladder and prostate. Acute bacterial infections probably represent the most common etiologic mechanism. It should be noted, however, that the irritative symptoms may be secondary to the presence of a foreign body, nonspecific inflammation, radiation therapy or chemotherapy, neoplasms, and neurogenic bladder dysfunction.

4. Bladder Outlet Obstructive Symptoms

    a. *Hesitancy* refers to the prolonged interval necessary to voluntarily initiate the urinary stream.

    b. *Straining* refers to the need to increase intraabdominal pressure in order to initiate voiding.

    c. *Decreased force* and *caliber* of the urinary stream refer to the physical changes of the urinary stream that may be noted due to increased urethral resistance.

    d. *Terminal dribbling* refers to the prolonged dribbling of urine from the meatus after the completion of micturition.

    e. *Sense of residual urine* is the complaint of a sensation of incomplete emptying of the bladder that the patient recognizes after micturition.

    f. *Prostatism:* All of the above symptoms may be noted with any type of bladder outlet obstruction, i.e., secondary to benign prostatic hypertrophy, prostatic carcinoma, or urethral stricture disease. The most common cause of these symptoms, however, is benign prostatic enlargement and hence this complex of symptoms has often been referred to as "prostatism."

    g. *Urinary retention:* The retention of urine within the bladder may occur on a chronic, gradual basis due to progressive obstruction and bladder decompensation, and large amounts of urine may be retained with minor changes in symptomatology. Acute urinary retention may occur as a complication of chronic urinary retention or de novo. Sudden acute urinary retention may be associated with severe suprapubic discomfort.

h. *Interruption* of the urinary stream: Sudden painful interruption of the urinary stream may be secondary to the presence of a bladder calculus that ball valves into the bladder neck causing abrupt blockage of the urinary flow.

i. *Bifurcation* of the urinary stream: The symptom of a double stream or spraying of the urinary stream may be secondary to urethral stricture disease.

5. Incontinence

a. *True or total incontinence* occurs when there is constant dribbling of urine from the bladder. It may be due to the configuration of the bladder, such as with extrophy or epispadias, or due to ectopia of the ureteral orifices distal to the bladder neck in females. The most common cause, however, is secondary to injury to the sphincter mechanisms of the bladder neck and urethra due to trauma, surgery, or childbirth. Neurogenic disorders affecting the bladder outlet may also have similar effects.

b. *False or overflow incontinence* is seen with total bladder decompensation where the bladder acts as a fixed reservoir and the only outflow of urine is an overflow phenomenon with constant dribbling through the bladder outlet.

c. *Urgency incontinence* results when the sensation of urgency becomes so severe that involuntary bladder emptying occurs. This is commonly secondary to severe inflammation of the urinary bladder. This type of incontinence may also be due to uninhibited bladder contractions.

d. *Stress incontinence* is secondary to distortion of the normal anatomic relationship between the bladder and the urethra such that sudden increases in intraabdominal pressure (laughing, straining, etc.) are transmitted unequally to the bladder and the urethra, resulting in elevated bladder pressure without a concomitant rise in urethral pressure. Most commonly, this is related to laxity of the pelvic floor, particularly following childbirth, but it may also be noted in women who have not had children.

e. It is important to differentiate the various types of incontinence as each is treated differently. Historical factors are very important in separating these different entities.

6. *Enuresis* refers to involuntary urination and bedwetting that occurs during sleep (see Chapter 24).

D. Changes in the Gross Appearance of the Urine

1. Cloudy Urine

a. Cloudy urine (*phosphaturia*) is most commonly due to the benign process of precipitation of phosphates in an alkaline urine. This may be noted after meals or after consumption of large quantities of milk and is generally intermittent in nature. Patients are otherwise asymptomatic. Acidification of the urine with acetic acid at the time of urinalysis causes prompt clearing of the specimen.

b. *Pyuria* is a urinary tract infection in which large quantities of white blood cells may cause urine to have a cloudy appearance. Microscopic examination of the urine sample will demonstrate the inflammatory nature.

c. *Chyluria* refers to the presence of lymph fluid mixed with the urine. It is an unusual cause of cloudy urine.

2. *Pneumaturia* refers to the passage of gas along with urine while voiding. There may be associated pyuria or frank fecal contamination of the urine, as this phenomenon is almost exclusively due to the presence of a fistula between the gastrointestinal and urinary tracts. On occasion, the presence of a gas-forming infection within the urinary tract may produce similar symptoms, although this is very unusual.

3. Hematuria

a. The passage of bloody urine is always alarming and generally the patient makes a prompt visit to the physician. Prompt investigation is always warranted, including a properly performed urinalysis to be certain that the red discoloration of the urine is indeed secondary to the presence of blood. For a differential diagnosis of the causes of red urine, see the following section.

b. Although hematuria is always a danger signal, a clue to its significance may lie in whether there is associated pain or whether the bleeding is essentially painless. Pain such as occurs in association with cystitis or passage of a urinary tract calculus may indicate that the bleeding is in fact benign in nature. Painless hematuria, however, is always felt to be secondary to a urinary tract neoplasm until proven otherwise. This differentiation is not infallible and therefore all urinary tract bleeding warrants investigation to be certain that there is not an associated neoplasm in addition to the more obvious cause for painful bleeding.

c. The probable site of bleeding within the urinary tract may be ascertained by determining whether the bleeding is initial, i.e., at the beginning of the stream only, terminal, i.e., at the end of the stream only, or total, i.e., throughout the entire stream. Initial hematuria generally indicates some type of anterior urethral bleeding that is flushed out by the initial passage of the bladder urine through the urethra. Terminal hematuria is often secondary to posterior urethral, bladder neck, or trigone bleeding and is noted when the bladder finally compresses these areas at the end of micturition. Total hematuria indicates that the bleeding occurs at the level of the bladder or above such that all of the urine is mixed with blood and is therefore bloody throughout the time of the stream.

4. *Colored urine* may result from a variety of foods, medications, and medical disorders. The colors may range from almost clear to black, with all other colors of the spectrum noted in between. (See Table 3 for common causes of colorful urine.)

E. **Abnormal Appearance and/or Function of the Male External Genitalia**
   1. Impotence (see Chapter 17)
   2. Infertility (see Chapter 18)
   3. Penile Problems
       a. Cutaneous lesions. A variety of exophytic and ulcerative lesions may be noted by the patient. The relationship of the onset of these lesions to recent sexual activity should be explored. The physical characteristics of these lesions should be noted at the time of physical examination. The combination of historical and physical factors as well as associated physical findings such as adenopathy will provide a working diagnosis for the treatment of these lesions. (See Chapter 19.)
       b. Penile curvature. Bending of the penis, particularly during erection, is noted in association with scarring and fibrosis of the tunica albuginea. These plaque-like structures may be noted on physical examination. The process is essentially idiopathic and has been referred to as Peyronie's disease.
       c. Urethral discharge. The character of the urethral discharge should be described as well as its onset in relationship to sexual activity as noted above. The presence of the discharge should be confirmed on physical examination and a microscopic examination performed and a culture obtained.
       d. Bloody ejaculate. Like hematuria, this is also a frightening experience that usually causes the patient to seek prompt attention. This problem, however, is generally secondary to benign congestion and/or inflammation of the seminal vesicles. The process is usually self-limited or treatable with antibiotics and does not initially require an extensive evaluation.
   4. Scrotal Problems
       a. Cutaneous lesions. The hair-bearing skin of the scrotum is susceptible to the variety of skin diseases that may occur anywhere else on the body.

TABLE 1. CAUSES OF SCROTAL SWELLING

Structure Involved	Pathology
Scrotal Wall	Hematuria
	Urinary extravasation
	Edema from cardiac, hepatic, or renal failure
Testis	Carcinoma
	Torsion of testes or appendix testis
Epididymis	Epididymitis
	Tumor
	Torsion of appendix epididymis
Spermatic Cord	Hydrocele surrounding testis or involving cord only
	Hematocele
	Hernia
	Varicocele
	Lipoma

Fungal infections and venereal warts may also be noted commonly.

b. Scrotal swelling and masses. The presence of scrotal swelling or a scrotal mass may be noted incidentally by the patient while bathing, while

TABLE 2. DIFFERENTIAL DIAGNOSIS OF SCROTAL DISCOMFORT AND SOLID MASS LESIONS

	Torsion	Epididymitis	Tumor
Age	Birth to 20 years	Puberty to old age	15 to 35 years
Pain			
Onset	Sudden	Rapid	Gradual
Degree	Severe	Increasing severity	Mild or absent
Nausea/Vomiting	Yes	No	No
Examination			
Testis	Swollen together	Normal early	Mass
Epididymis	and both tender	Swollen, tender	Normal
Spermatic cord	Shortened	Thickened, often tender as high as inguinal canal	Normal
Urinalysis	Normal	Often infection	Normal

performing a self-examination, or due to the presence of associated discomfort. A variety of lesions may produce unilateral or bilateral scrotal enlargement. These range from normal structures that are misinterpreted by the patient to testicular neoplasms. The differential diagnosis is as noted in Table 1.

A combination of historical information, particularly with regard to onset of the mass, progression, and associated pain and the physical examination is helpful in differentiating some of the more confusing lesions. (See section on physical examination and Table 2.)

IV. THE PHYSICAL EXAMINATION

A. General Information

1. The problems delineated in the history will determine how extensive a physical examination is necessary. A complete physical examination is obviously necessary for someone who will undergo some type of urologic surgery; in most instances, however, a limited examination of the genitourinary tract is usually sufficient at the time of the initial examination.

2. The commonly taught techniques of physical examination, including inspection, palpation, percussion, and auscultation, are also used during the urologic examination. Each has varying degrees of usefulness depending upon the organ being evaluated. The process of transillumination with a high-intensity, small-diameter light source is useful in evaluating pediatric abdominal masses as well as scrotal masses in the child and the adult. Particular aspects of the physical examination will be noted below.

B. Kidneys and Flanks

1. *Inspection.* Inspection of the flanks is best carried out with the patient in the sitting or standing position facing straight ahead and the examiner located behind the patient facing the area in question. Scoliosis may be

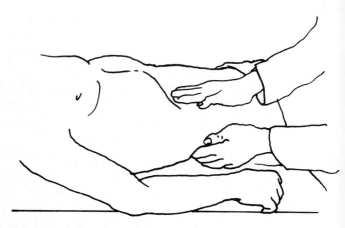

Figure 1. With the patient in the supine position, one hand is used to raise the flank while the abdominal hand palpates deeply beneath the costal margin.

evident in the patient with an inflammatory process directly or indirectly involving the psoas muscle with resultant spasm. Bulging of the flank may be noted if there is an underlying mass, although this is only evident in most cases if the mass is extremely large or if the patient is very thin. Edema of the flank may be noted if there is an underlying inflammatory process.

2. *Palpation and Percussion.* A method of bimanual renal palpation has been described with the patient in the supine position (Fig. 1). The examiner lifts the flank by placing one hand beneath this area and subsequently palpates deeply beneath the ipsilateral costal margin anteriorly. This technique is successful in children and thin adults but generally yields little information under most other circumstances. A large mass may be palpable. *Percussion* is a useful technique, particularly in the area of the costovertebral angle to elicit tenderness due to underlying capsular inflammation or distention (Fig. 2).

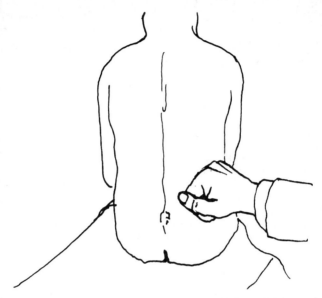

Figure 2. Gentle percussion with the heel of the hand in the angle between the lumbar vertebrae and the 12th rib is useful in eliciting underlying tenderness due to obstruction or inflammation.

3. *Auscultation*. This technique is particularly useful in evaluating patients with possible renovascular hypertension. An underlying bruit may be noted in the area of the costovertebral angle due to renal artery stenosis, aneurysm formation, or arteriovenous malformation.
4. *Transillumination*. This technique, which may differentiate a solid from a cystic mass in neonates or infants, has largely been replaced by ultrasonography, which much more clearly defines these lesions.

C. Abdomen and Bladder
1. *Inspection*. The abdominal examination and bladder examination are best carried out with the patient in the

supine position. The full or overdistended bladder may be visible on general inspection of the abdomen with the patient in this position.

2. *Palpation and Percussion.* It is generally possible to palpate or percuss the bladder above the level of the symphysis pubis if it contains 150 ml or more of urine (Fig. 3). It should be remembered that in the child, the bladder may be percussible or palpable with much smaller volumes of urine relative to its size, due to the fact that it is more of an intraabdominal organ in the child than the true pelvic organ it is in the adult.

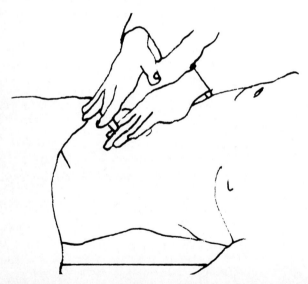

Figure 3. Percussion over the bladder may be particularly useful when palpation is difficult due either to obesity or failure of the patient to relax during the examination. The bladder may be percussed if it contains greater than 150 ml of urine in the adult.

D. Penis

1. *Inspection.* Inspection of the penis will reveal obvious lesions of the skin and will define whether the patient has been circumcised. If the patient has been circumcised, the glans penis and meatus may be inspected directly. In the uncircumcised patient, the foreskin should be retracted and the glanular surface of the foreskin as well as the glans and meatus should then be inspected. The number and position of ulcerative and/or exophytic lesions should be noted if they are present. The position and size of the urinary meatus should be defined.

   a. Foreskin. Phimosis is present when the orifice of the foreskin is constricted, preventing retraction of the foreskin over the glans. Paraphimosis is present when the foreskin, once retracted over the glans, cannot be replaced to its normal position covering the glans.

   b. Penile meatus. The normal meatus should be located at the tip of the glans. Hypospadias is present when the meatus opens anywhere along the ventral aspect of the penis or in the perineum. Epispadias is present when the meatus is located on the dorsal aspect of the penis.

2. *Palpation.* Palpation of the penile shaft is important to identify and define the limits of areas of fibrous induration that may be found in patients with Peyronie's disease who complain of penile curvature during erection. The urethra should also be palpated for areas of induration that may be associated with periurethritis and urethral stricture disease. The urethra can also be "stripped" from the penile–scrotal junction towards the meatus looking for a urethral discharge which can then be collected for microscopic examination and culture.

E. Scrotum and Scrotal Contents

1. *Inspection.* The inspection of the scrotum and the remainder of this portion of the physical examination is

best carried out with the patient initially in the standing position. Lesions of the scrotal skin are readily evident in this position. One also generally notes that if two testicles are present, one usually hangs lower than the other. In most cases, the left testicle is lower than the right. In cases of congenital absence or failure of descent of one or both testicles, the involved side may demonstrate hypoplastic scrotal development. It is always important to note the presence or absence of the testes. Scrotal masses and the "bag of worms" appearance of an underlying large varicocele may be identified on initial inspection.

2. *Palpation.* The contents of each hemiscrotum should be palpated in an orderly fashion. First the testes should be examined, then the epididymides, then the cord structures, and finally the area of the external inguinal ring to inspect for the presence of an inguinal hernia (Fig. 4).

   a. Each testis should be in the dependent portion of the scrotum when the patient is relaxed and in a warm environment. The long axis of the testicle should be in a vertical direction and the size of the testis should be noted. The long axis of the testicle should normally be greater than or equal to 4 cm in adult males.

   b. Each epididymis is adherent to the posterolateral aspect of the testicle. The head of the epididymis is noted to be near the superior pole of the testicle, the body of the epididymis near the middle portion of the testicle, and the tail of the epididymis represents the most inferior aspect of this structure. The examiner should palpate each portion of the epididymis, looking primarily for areas of tenderness or induration.

   c. The spermatic cord varies somewhat in thickness and often this depends upon the presence or absence of what has been termed a "lipoma of the cord." One should be particularly attentive for the presence or absence of enlarged venous structures,

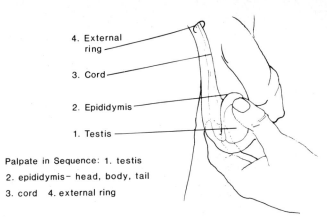

4. External ring

3. Cord

2. Epididymis

1. Testis

Palpate in Sequence: 1. testis
2. epididymis— head, body, tail
3. cord   4. external ring

Figure 4. Palpation of the scrotal contents should be carried out in an orderly, routine fashion. One should begin palpating the testes, followed by the epididymides, the cord structures, and finally the external rings. Palpating each structure from side to side is useful for detecting differences in testicular size and for identifying varicoceles. All of the scrotal structures may be examined between the thumb and the index and middle fingers.

i.e., a varicocele, descending with the cord. If a varicocele is detected, the patient should also be examined in the supine position to be certain that the varicocele decompresses. If it does not, one must suspect inferior vena cava or renal vein obstruction. Changes in the size of the cord between the standing to the supine position or when using the Valsalva maneuver with the patient in the upright position indicate the presence of a small varicocele. The vas deferens should be palpated. This structure normally has the thickness of a pencil lead and has a distinct, smooth firmness.

d. Lastly, with the patient in the standing position, palpation of the inguinal canal may be carried out. Increasing intraabdominal pressure by asking the patient to cough or by using the Valsalva maneuver

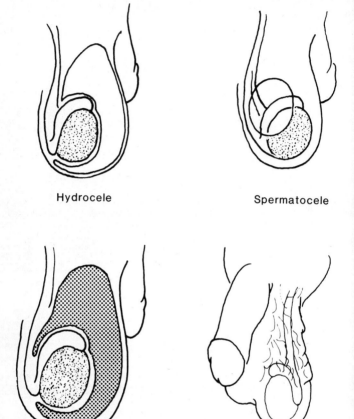

Hydrocele

Spermatocele

Hematocele

Varicocele

Figure 5. A variety of fluid-filled masses may develop within the scrotum. Hydroceles and spermatoceles (and occasionally bowel in a hernia sac) will transilluminate. Hydrocele fluid is contained within the tunica vaginalis and essentially surrounds the testicle. A spermatocele generally occurs above or adjacent to the upper pole of the testis and represents a cyst of the rete testis or epididymis. A hematocele is a collection of blood within the tunica vaginalis due usually to trauma or surgery. Occasionally bleeding will occur spontaneously associated with bleeding disorders. A varicocele represents dilated veins of the pampiniform plexus as discussed in the text. Hematoceles and varicoceles will not transilluminate.

will help to define the presence of an inguinal hernia.

3. Abnormal Scrotal Masses and Transillumination (Figs. 5 and 6)

   a. The presence of an abnormal mass within the scrotum is best defined by careful palpation. It should be noted whether the mass arises from the testicle, is contained within the testicle, arises from the epididymis, is located in the cord, or tends to surround most of the scrotal structures. It is important to note the character of the mass, i.e., whether it is hard, firm, or cystic in nature.

   b. All scrotal masses should be transilluminated and this may be accomplished with a small penlight. Any mass that radiates a reddish glow of light through the lesion, represents a cystic, fluid-filled structure. Caution is advised in defining the benignity of these lesions, however, in that benign and malignant lesions may coexist. A hydrocele surrounding a testicular tumor is a not uncommon example.

   c. See Table 2 for a differential diagnosis of scrotal masses.

F. The Rectum and Prostate

1. *Position.* A variety of positions have been described for performing a rectal examination. I have found that having the patient lie on the examining table in the lateral decubitus position with the legs flexed at the hips and knees and the uppermost leg pulled higher towards the chest than the lowermost leg affords the most comfortable position for the patient and the examiner (Fig. 7). Alternatively, one may have the patient bend over the examining table while in the standing position such that he then rests the weight of his upper body on his elbows. Probably more important than the position, however, is the necessity that the gloved examining finger be adequately lubricated and that slow, gentle pressure be applied as the finger traverses the anal sphincter. A rectal examination can be

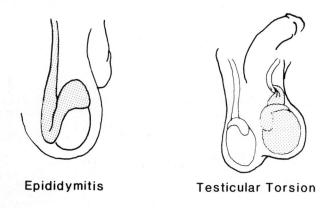

Epididymitis   **Testicular Torsion**

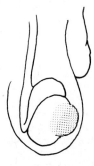

Testicular Tumor

Figure 6. Solid scrotal masses may be painful or painless and may involve the testis, the epididymis, or both. Table 2 further differentiates the three lesions depicted in this figure.

an extremely painful or a painless experience depending upon the skill and patience of the examiner. It is important at the time of the examination not only to palpate the prostate gland but to palpate the entire inside of the rectum in search of other abnormalities.

Lying Position

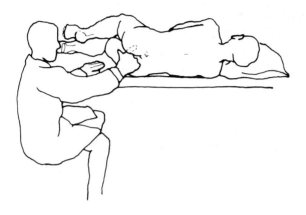

Standing Position

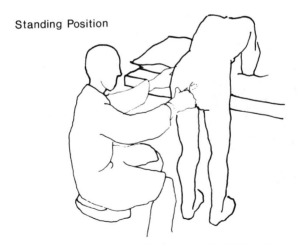

Figure 7. Two positions are illustrated for performing the digital rectal examination. I have generally found that the patient appears to be more comfortable lying on his side than in the standing position.

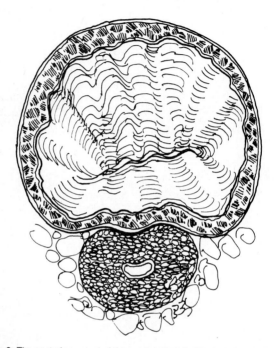

Figure 8. The posterior aspect of the prostate is palpable on rectal examination. The surface is normally smooth, rubbery, and approximately 4 × 4 cm in size. The median furrow may be lost with diffuse enlargement of the gland and the lateral sulci may be either accentuated or obscured. Deviations from normal contour, consistency, or size should be carefully described. Stating that an area is "hard" implies that one is suggesting the presence of carcinoma. The seminal vesicles are not normally palpable. *Remember:* check the entire rectum. Do not miss an occult rectal carcinoma. *(Redrawn, with modifications, from Smith DR: General Urology, ed 11. Los Altos: Lange, 1984, p 40.)*

   2. *Prostate.* During the rectal examination, the posterior aspect of the prostate is palpated (Fig. 8). The significance of this part of the general physical examination cannot be overemphasized. Most types of

prostate carcinoma begin in the posterior lobe of the prostate, which is very accessible to the examining finger.

a. The prostate gland is normally a small, walnut-sized structure with a flattened, heart-shaped configuration. There is a median furrow that runs down the longitudinal axis of the prostate and there are two lateral sulci where the rectal mucosa folds back upon itself after reflecting off the prostate. The consistency of the normal prostate is generally described as "rubbery" in nature and has been likened to the consistency of the thenar eminence when one opposes the thumb and fifth finger.

b. Abnormal consistency of the prostate may be noted on rectal examination and includes nodular abnormalities that may be raised or within the substance of the prostate, areas of induration that may suggest malignancy, or areas of bogginess or fluctuance that may be associated with abscess formation.

c. Prostatic massage may be carried out in order to express prostatic secretions into the urethral lumen. These secretions may then be collected directly if they happen to drain through the penile meatus or they may be collected by having the patient void a small amount of urine directly into a container immediately following the massage. Prostatic massage is generally carried out in a methodical fashion to strip the entire gland from a lateral to a medial aspect bilaterally.

3. *Seminal Vesicles.* Under normal conditions the seminal vesicles are not palpable. They may become evident on a rectal examination, however, if they are enlarged due to obstruction or inflammation.

G. The Vaginal Examination

1. *Inspection.* The vaginal examination is best performed with the patient in the relaxed lithotomy position. Inspection of the vulva may reveal a variety of vene-

real and nonvenereal lesions. The urinary meatus should be identified and its position and size noted. An erythematous, tender lesion arising from the meatus may represent a benign urethral caruncle or possibly a urethral carcinoma. The character of the vaginal mucosa at the introitus should be noted. One may also note the presence of a cystocele or a rectocele while examining the patient in this position. These structures may be accentuated with increases in intraabdominal pressure such as occur with coughing or straining. In fact, this maneuver may elicit some leakage of urine in patients with stress urinary incontinence.

2. *Palpation*. Palpation of the urethra to the level of the bladder neck and trigone may be accomplished during examination of the anterior vaginal wall. Bimanual palpation is useful to define the internal genitalia and to define further the size and consistency of the urinary bladder.

V. THE URINALYSIS AND CULTURE

A. Collection

Proper collection and prompt examination of the urine is essential to gain the most information from the routinely collected specimen.

1. Males

   a. A midstream urine collection is most commonly obtained in men for routine examination. With this technique, the male patient is instructed to retract the foreskin if he is uncircumcised and to gently cleanse the glans. He begins to urinate into the toilet, subsequently inserting a sterile glass container into the urinary stream to collect a urine sample. The container is then removed and the act of voiding is completed.

   b. A variety of other collection techniques afford more information with regard to localization of infection within the urinary tract. Four such specimens may be obtained and analyzed separately by routine microscopic evaluation as well as culture techniques. These have been designated the VB-1, VB-2, EPS, and VB-3 specimens, according to Stamey. The VB-1 is the initial 5 to 10 ml of the stream, which contains bladder urine mixed with urethral contents that are initially washed from the urethra. The VB-2 specimen is essentially the midstream portion of the collection. The EPS specimen represents the expressed prostatic secretions following prostatic massage. Lastly, the VB-3 specimen represents a small voided specimen that mixes bladder urine with the contents contained in the urethra immediately following the expression of prostatic secretions. This collection is particularly useful if inadequate amounts of secretion from the prostate are actually expressed during the prostatic massage. The value of these cultures for localization of urinary tract infection is that the VB-1 represents urethral flora, the VB-2 represents bladder flora, and the EPS and VB-3 represent prostatic flora.

2. Females
   a. The midstream urine collection in females is somewhat more difficult to accomplish and is often considered to be inadequate for even the most routine examination. With this technique, the vulva is cleansed and the stream is initiated into the toilet with subsequent insertion of a collecting container as described above for the male. If this specimen is grossly contaminated or appears infected, then one of the collection methods noted below may be necessary to differentiate these two possibilities. However, if the collection has been done with reasonable care and the specimen is essentially negative on microscopic examination, then I generally consider this technique adequate.
   b. A more proper method of midstream urine collection has been described where the patient is placed

in the lithotomy position and then asked to void. The nurse holds the labia apart to prevent contamination and collects a midstream specimen. This is often awkward if not difficult for both the patient and the nurse, however, and I do not recommend this method of collection.

   c. If there is any question with regard to the problem of contamination versus infection of the midstream specimen as noted above, then catheterization to obtain a true bladder specimen is the preferred technique. One should not hesitate to use this method to properly categorize a patient's problem.

3. Children

   a. Percutaneous suprapubic aspiration of urine from neonates and infants is a particularly useful method of obtaining a truly uncontaminated specimen of urine from the bladder. With this technique, the suprapubic area is cleansed with an antiseptic solution and percutaneous aspiration is performed with a fine-gauge needle. The specimen may then be examined for urinalysis and sent for culture.

   b. A variety of sterile plastic bags with adhesive collars are available that surround the male and female infant's genitalia. They are particularly useful for routine screening urinalyses, but as with the collection of midstream specimens from women, it may be difficult at times to differentiate a truly infected urine from a contaminated specimen due to this collection technique.

   c. Older boys and girls may have urine collected in a fashion similar to that described above for their adult counterparts. One is generally quite hesitant, however, to catheterize young boys due to the possibility of urethral trauma. It is easier and safer to perform this in girls and may be used if necessary.

B. Physical Aspects of the Urine

1. *Color.* The color of the urine is generally a clear light yellow but a wide range of colors have been described

TABLE 3. COMMON CAUSES OF COLORFUL URINE

Colorless	Very dilute urine
	Overhydration
Cloudy/Milky	Phosphaturia
	Pyuria
	Chyluria
Red	Hematuria
	Hemoglobinuria/myoglobinuria
	Anthrocyanin in beets and blackberries
	Chronic lead and mercury poisoning
	Phenolphthalein (in bowel evacuants)
	Phenothiazines (Compazine, etc.)
	Rifampin
Orange	Dehydration
	Phenazopyridine (Pyridium)
	Sulfasalazine (Azulfadine)
Yellow	Normal
	Phenacetin
	Riboflavin
Green–Blue	Biliverdin
	Indicanuria (tryptophan indole metabolites)
	Amitriptyline (Elavil)
	Indigo carmine
	Methylene blue
	Phenols (IV cimetidine (Tagamet), IV promethazine (Phenergan), etc.)
	Resorcinol
	Triampterene (Dyrenium)
Brown	Urobilinogen
	Porphyria
	Aloe, fava beans, and rhubarb
	Chloroquine and primaquine
	Furazolidone (Furoxone)
	Metronidazole (Flagyl)
	Nitrofurantoin (Furadantin)
Brown–Black	Alcaptonuria (homogentisic acid)
	Hemorrhage
	Melanin
	Tyrosinosis (hydroxyphenylpyruvic acid)
	Cascara, senna (laxatives)
	Methocarbamol (Robaxin)
	Methyldopa (Aldomet)
	Sorbitol

as noted earlier. The changes in color may be secondary to foods, medications, as well as intrinsic disease
processes. Table 3 describes the etiologic factors in
relationship to abnormal urine color.

2. *pH*. The normal pH of urine ranges from 4.5 to 8.0.
   Urine is described as having an acid pH if it ranges
   between 4.5 and 5.5. It is referred to as having an
   alkaline pH if it ranges between 6.5 and 8.0.

3. *Specific Gravity*. The specific gravity may be determined in the office by relatively simple techniques and
   gives some idea of the concentrating ability of the
   kidneys and their ability to excrete waste products. A
   variety of substances within the urine, such as intravenous contrast material may detract from the value of
   this test. The osmolality of the urine is a better indicator of renal function but requires standard laboratory
   methods.

C. Dipstick Tests

1. A variety of dipsticks are available to evaluate the
   urine sample. These consist of short plastic strips with
   small marker pads that are impregnated with a variety
   of reagents that react with abnormal substances within
   the urine.

2. In addition to determination of urinary pH, the most
   sophisticated dipsticks now contain reagents for the
   determination of the following:
   a. Protein
   b. Glucose
   c. Ketones
   d. Urobilinogen
   e. Bilirubin
   f. Blood
   g. Hemoglobin
   h. Leukocytes
   i. Nitrites

D. Microscopic Examination

1. A small portion of the collected urine sample is placed
   in a test tube and centrifuged at approximately 5000

rpm for 5 minutes. The supernate is then poured from the tube and the remaining sediment is resuspended in the small quantity of urine that drains back down the side of the tube to the sediment. A drop of the resuspended sediment is placed on a glass slide followed by a cover slip.

2. The wet specimen described above is then examined under low and high power for the presence and number of epithelial cells, red blood cells, white blood cells, bacteria, and casts.

E. Urine Culture

1. If a urine culture is desired, it should be promptly plated in the office or sent immediately to the laboratory to prevent overgrowth of bacteria and falsely elevated bacterial counts.

2. The value of localization cultures has been noted above.

VI. DIAGNOSTIC INSTRUMENTATION

A. General Information

The instrumentation and procedures to be described below may be commonly performed in the office setting under local anesthesia. Some of these techniques, such as cystourethroscopy, placement of retrograde catheters and biopsy of the prostate, may also be performed with regional or general anesthesia.

B. Urethral Catheters (Fig. 9)

1. *Straight Catheters*. The standard straight, red, or Robinson catheter is useful for office catheterization when an indwelling catheter is not warranted. It is useful to collect relatively uncontaminated specimens directly from the bladder as noted above.

2. *Standard Balloon or Foley Catheter*. This type of catheter has a double lumen that permits drainage of urine through the larger lumen and inflation of a balloon located at the tip of the catheter. This allows it to

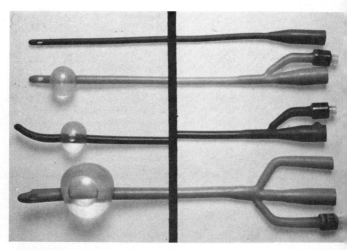

Figure 9. Four types of catheters. From top to bottom: Straight 14F Robinson catheter, 18F Foley catheter with 5-ml balloon, 18F Coudé tip catheter with 5-ml balloon, and 24F three-way irrigating catheter with 30-ml balloon. (*Note:* Catheters have been shortened for photography.)

be retained within the urinary bladder. This type of catheter is useful following certain operative procedures on the urinary tract and to establish temporary, constant urinary drainage for monitoring urine output or for relief of bladder outlet obstruction. These catheters generally have 5- and 30-ml balloons, but the amount of water placed in these balloons is not precisely critical, as each will hold significantly more than its stated volume.

3. *Coudé Catheters.* Red Robinson catheters or balloon retention catheters may each be specially constructed to have a "Coudé-tip configuration." This is essentially a curved tip that allows passage of the catheter beyond certain urethral, prostatic, or bladder neck impediments that may preclude passage of a straight

catheter due to impingement of the catheter tip on these lesions.

4. *Three-way Irrigation Catheters.* This type of catheter has a triple lumen that has an irrigation port, a drainage port, and a port for inflating the balloon used for retention of the catheter within the bladder. Three-way irrigation catheters are particularly useful following transurethral resection of the prostate and in cases of gross hematuria to irrigate the bladder and prevent formation and retention of clots within the bladder.

5. *Technique of Catheter Insertion.* Insertion of a urethral catheter by the physician for either diagnostic or therapeutic reasons always involves sterile technique. Gloves should be applied and the glans and the meatus of the male and the vulva and meatus of the female are then prepared with an antiseptic skin preparation solution. The catheter is then well lubricated with sterile jelly and inserted gently into the meatus. Prior to inflation of the balloon, if a retention catheter is used, one must be certain that the tip of the catheter is within the urinary bladder and that urine is obtained. In cases where urine does not flow freely from the end of the catheter, it is important to irrigate the catheter gently prior to inflation of the balloon to prevent inflation within the urethra. Hematuria and/or sepsis may be noted if this occurs. The catheter is then pulled gently to seat the balloon at the level of the bladder neck. It is then attached to a drainage bag with sterile technique.

C. Urethral Sounds and Filiforms and Followers

1. *General Information.* These two types of instruments are often used to evaluate the urethra in cases of urethral stricture disease or other reasons that preclude passage of a urethral catheter. They may be used in both a diagnostic and therapeutic fashion by the skilled urologist who is familiar with their use.

2. *Urethral Sounds.* These metal objects come in a variety of sizes and shapes (Fig. 10). They must be passed carefully to prevent disruption of the lower urinary tract. They are never inserted with force and must pass

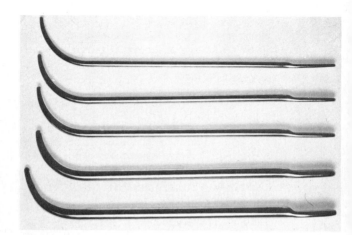

Figure 10. Van Buren urethral sounds. Five sounds are pictured, ranging from 18F to 30F in size.

smoothly into the urinary bladder, where rotation of the tip of the sound is confirmed with each passage.

3. *Filiforms and Followers.* These instruments are also useful for establishing access to the urinary bladder and for dilating urethral strictures (Fig. 11). The tiny filiform aspect of this set is used to gain access initially to the urinary bladder. These filiforms have a variety of different shapes at their tip that allow them to be manipulated through or around a variety of abnormal urethral configurations. It may be necessary to pass several filiforms simultaneously before access can be gained to the bladder. Once it is established that one of these filiforms has passed easily into the bladder, the follower may be then attached to the protruding threaded end and passed as a unit with the filiform into the bladder. Using serially larger followers, it is possible to dilate the urethra. Each follower has an eye in the end and a hollow center so that urine can be obtained as the follower is passed. In cases of severe

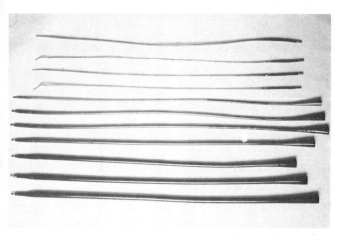

Figure 11. Filiforms and followers. Four small filiforms are at the top of the photograph. Followers from 10F to 20F are also shown.

urethral stricture disease, it may be best to leave the follower in place prior to insertion of a Foley catheter. If the urethra dilates easily, the followers can be removed and a Foley catheter inserted immediately.

D. Cystourethroscopy and Associated Techniques

1. *Equipment.* The standard cystourethroscope consists of a sheath, a bridge, and a lighted telescope for visualization (Fig. 12). An irrigation port is attached to the sheath that allows gravity directed inflow of fluid to distend the urethra and bladder and to aid in visualization. The bridge essentially attaches the telescope to the sheath and may contain a variety of working ports through which urethral catheters, biopsy forceps, and alligator forceps may be passed. The lighted telescopes generally have 30- and 70-degree viewing angles that allow complete inspection within the bladder.
2. Technique of Insertion
   a. Males. Insertion of the cystourethroscope into the

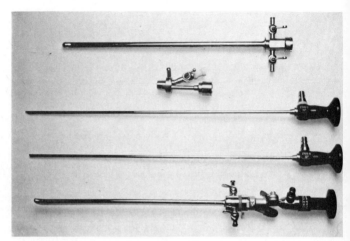

Figure 12. Cystoscope and components. The cystoscope consists of a sheath (*top*), a bridge (below sheath), and two interchangeable lenses with 30- and 70-degree viewing angles. The components of the Storz cystoscope are shown as is the assembled ACMI cystoscope (*bottom*).

male is best performed under direct vision following antiseptic preparation and draping. The cystourethroscope is assembled and a flow of fluid is obtained. The instrument is then introduced into the meatus and passed under direct vision through the anterior urethra. Some narrowing and voluntary constriction of the external sphincter may be noted, but this is passed with slow gentle pressure. With the patient in the lithotomy position, it is necessary to lower the eyepiece and redirect the tip of the instrument beneath the symphysis pubis, through the prostate, and into the bladder. The bladder can then be emptied and inspected with both lenses.

b. Females. The female patient is also placed in the lithotomy position. After proper cleansing and draping, the cystourethroscope may be inserted into the bladder either under direct vision or with the obturator in the cystoscope sheath. Once again, the bladder is inspected with both lenses and the urethra is inspected with the 30-degree lens.

3. Procedures

a. Inspection. In most cases, the urethra and bladder are merely inspected under local anesthesia with these endoscopic techniques in the office setting. This allows the urologist to ascertain the presence or absence of urethral pathology, the degree of anatomic obstruction, and the state of the bladder mucosa and underlying musculature. It is also possible to note the presence or absence of efflux from the ureteral orifices as well as judge their location and configuration. At the time of inspection of the bladder, bladder urine may be obtained for culture or cytology. The bladder may also be washed by barbotage techniques and the saline washings sent for cytology.

b. Bladder biopsies. These may be taken under local anesthesia using cold cup biopsy forceps. Generally, however, there is some degree of associated discomfort and if biopsies are necessary, they are usually best performed under spinal or general anesthesia to ensure an adequate specimen.

c. Retrograde ureteral catheterization. The placement of small (sizes 4F to 7F) ureteral catheters may be performed without difficulty under local anesthesia. These catheters may be passed just within the ureteral orifice for retrograde injection of contrast or they may be passed to the level of the kidney for relief of obstruction within the ureter, to obtain renal washings, or for the injection of contrast material for radiographic studies. They may be removed immediately or left temporarily in place.

d. A variety of resectoscopes and specialized endoscopes are available to perform more sophisticated procedures on the urethra, bladder, and prostate as well as the ureter and kidney. These are therapeutic rather than diagnostic procedures and require regional or general anesthesia. Their use is not considered further herein.

E. Needle Biopsy of the Prostate

1. *General Information.* Needle biopsy of the prostate may be performed under local anesthesia in the office or in the outpatient setting. Generally two techniques exist—the transperineal and the transrectal routes. There are a variety of needles available for performing the biopsy, including skinny needles that may be used for aspiration and cytologic examination. The Vim–Silverman and Tru-Cut needles obtain cores of tissues for standard pathologic sectioning and examination.

2. *Accuracy of Needle Biopsy Techniques.* Needle biopsy techniques are the most accurate means of determining if a prostate nodule represents a benign or a malignant lesion. The advantage of the transrectal method is that it is possible to place the tip of the needle directly on the nodule, thus ensuring greater accuracy. There is, however, an increased risk of sepsis due to the potential contamination of the biopsy tract with feces. The transperineal technique is slightly less accurate than the transrectal technique but has the distinct advantage of a decreased chance of urosepsis. Skinny-needle aspiration techniques may eventually become the most accurate and the safest methods of obtaining specimens from the prostate.

VII. SUMMARY

The surgical subspecialty of urology deals with a well-defined organ system within the body. The urologist diagnoses and treats a wide variety of medical and surgical disorders that may have local or systemic ramifications for the patient. The history, physical examination, and urinalysis serve as the cornerstones of the initial evaluation of these patients. In addition, a variety of unique diagnostic and therapeutic instruments are available for use in the office or outpatient setting to aid in caring for those with urologic diseases. The frequency with which these problems are seen by generalists and other specialists necessitates that all practitioners have some familiarity with this field.

BIBLIOGRAPHY

Carlton CE: Initial evaluation including history, physical examination, and urinalysis. In Harrison JH, Gittes RF, et al (eds): Campbell's Urology, ed 4. Philadelphia: W.B. Saunders, 1978, pp 203–221.

DeGowin EL, DeGowin RL: Bedside Diagnostic Examination. New York: Macmillan, 1969, pp 552–583.

Leadbetter GW: Diagnostic urologic instrumentation. In Harrison JH, Gittes RF, et al (eds): Campbell's Urology, ed 4. Philadelphia: W. B. Saunders, 1978, pp 358–374.

Smith DR: General Urology, ed 11. Los Altos: Lange, chapters 2 & 3, 1984.

Stamey TA: Pathogenesis and Treatment of Urinary Tract Infections. Baltimore: Williams & Wilkins, 1980, pp 1–51.

3

Diagnostic Uroradiology

Howard M. Pollack
Marc P. Banner

I. OVERVIEW OF DIAGNOSTIC IMAGING

Radiology and endoscopy are the two diagnostic pillars upon
which the speciality of urology is built. Uroradiology con-
stitutes that branch of radiology concerned with urinary tract
imaging. All parts of the urinary tract may be visualized by
one or more of the many available uroradiologic studies. Each
study has a particular role and each will provide some knowledge not revealed by the others. Since there is a great deal of
potential overlap in the information obtained, it is well to be
familiar with the particular virtues and limitations of each
method. As physicians are, more and more, being held
accountable, at least in part, for the costs of procedures ordered or performed, a comparison of procedural charges is
included in this section. Since absolute costs vary, a unit
system is employed with the charge for the intravenous
urogram arbitrarily designated as one cost unit. All other
charges are compared to the urogram.

II. EXCRETORY UROGRAPHY (INTRAVENOUS
UROGRAM: IVU: IVP) (Cost Units—1)

A. Purpose
The IVU provides a noninstrumental method of visualizing the kidneys, ureters, and bladder and is the basic
diagnostic radiologic study of the urinary tract. No other
radiologic or urologic examination surpasses urography as
a screening procedure for the entire urinary tract.

B. Basic Considerations

1. *Contrast Agents.* Present urographic contrast media are substituted benzoic acid derivatives. Those in most common usage are the sodium or methylglucamine salts of diatrizoate (Renografin; Hypaque) and iothalamate (Conray). Newer nonionic contrast media, such as Metrizamide and Iopamidol, are currently under investigation but as yet are not available for routine use in urography.

2. *Physiology.* The contrast molecules exist for the most part unbound in the plasma and are therefore excreted almost entirely by glomerular filtration. Only a small amount is bound to serum albumin. This fraction is excreted by the liver.

C. Technique

1. *Preparation.* A thorough bowel prep is necessary to eliminate overlying soft tissue densities that may interfere with optimal visualization of the urinary tract. Vigorous dehydration is not necessary, but withholding of fluids overnight is advantageous for optimal urinary concentration of the opaque medium. An empty stomach is also helpful in the event of vomiting after contrast administration.

2. *Plain Film of the Abdomen* (Scout film; Preliminary film; KUB; "Flat plate"). This is an essential component of every radiographic examination of the genitourinary tract. Important findings such as soft tissue masses, calcifications, and bony changes will be disclosed on this study. In fact, many urinary tract calculi are obscured by excreted contrast material and are therefore seen only on the KUB. In addition, retained barium in the colon or even the presence of a fetal skeleton if seen on the preliminary film may contraindicate the injection of contrast material and justify terminating or postponing the urogram.

3. *Contrast Administration.* The contrast is administered intravenously, either as a rapid bolus injection, a slow steady injection or a drip infusion. This is more often a question of individual preference rather than a matter

of scientific selection. In the average sized adult, 100 ml of contrast are usually administered.

4. *Filming*. A variable number of films constitute an intravenous urogram. Immediately after the contrast has been injected, tomograms are made to visualize the renal parenchyma (nephrographic phase). Within 3 minutes, contrast is usually visible in the collecting systems and several films are taken to visualize the calyces, pelves, and ureters (pyelographic phase) (Fig. 1). Films of the bladder (often including a postvoiding film) conclude the examination.

5. Modifications of the Urogram
    a. Emergency urography. This is usually performed for suspected renal colic or renal trauma. It is usually impossible to prepare the bowel adequately, so the urogram is often not of the highest quality. Nonetheless, with careful attention to technique and appropriate filming, it is usually possible to identify acute ureteral obstruction or major renal injury if present. In patients suffering trauma, often the only information desired is the status of the contralateral (noninjured) kidney. In patients with renal colic, films taken in the middle of the night rarely alter patient management; it is usually possible to delay the examination for a few hours (i.e., until 8:00 A.M.) until the full resources of the radiology department are available to provide for the patients' complete diagnostic needs.
    b. Hydration (diuretic) urography. This study is reserved for those patients suspected of having intermittent hydronephrosis in whom an initial (dehydrated) urogram revealed no obstruction. With forced diuresis a borderline ureteropelvic junction or ureteral narrowing may become inadequate to carry the increased urine load and result in hydronephrosis.
    c. Urography in hypertension. Films taken at 1-minute intervals following the bolus administration of contrast may reveal differential excretion as well as other findings suggestive of unilateral renal vascular insufficiency.

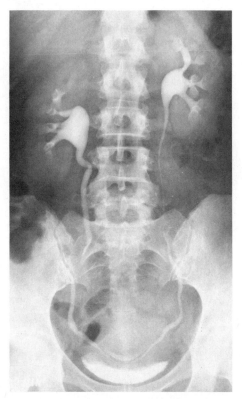

Figure 1. Normal intravenous urogram. A 10-minute postinjection abdominal film from an intravenous urogram demonstrates visualization of both renal collecting systems, ureters, and a normal partially filled urinary bladder.

D. Complications of Urography

1. *Immediate Complications.* There are three types of immediate complications.
   a. Minor side effects. These consist of nausea, vomiting, arm pain, and lightheadedness. Such reactions

   are fairly frequent but never serious, except for the
   possibility of aspiration following vomiting.
   b. Allergic reactions. About 5% of patients demonstrate an allergic or histamine type reaction to contrast media. This generally consists of erythema,
   urticaria, or, in severe cases, facial or glottic
   edema. In patients with a seafood or iodine sensitivity, the reaction rate is approximately 15%. It
   is slightly higher yet in those who have a proved
   history of an allergic reaction to previous contrast
   administration. Treatment is reserved for the more
   severe of these reactions and consists primarily of
   antihistamines. Steroids and/or epinephrine may
   be employed as needed. Pretreatment with antihistamines or steroids is thought by some to be useful
   in patients with a documented previous allergic
   reaction, but its efficacy has yet not been proved.
   c. Chemotoxic or idiosyncratic reactions. These are
   the most serious reactions but also the rarest. Manifestations include convulsions, pulmonary edema,
   cardiovascular collapse, intravascular clotting, or
   thrombolysis and cardiac arrest. They occur in perhaps 1 of every 7500 patients, of whom the majority are successfully managed with prompt effective
   treatment. The mortality rate for contrast administration is approximately 1 per 50,000 patients.
   An allergic history is usually not obtained in patients experiencing this type of reaction and there is
   little that can be done to anticipate which patients
   will experience this complication.
2. *Delayed Complications.* Although contrast agents are
   among the safest pharmaceuticals employed in clinical
   medicine, they may aggravate preexisting renal disease in a small percentage of patients with underlying
   azotemia by a process not yet understood. Nephrotoxicity is almost unknown when kidney function is normal. Patients with diabetic nephropathy—especially if
   it has begun in childhood—and those whose creatinines are 3 mg/dl or greater seem to be the most vul-
   nerable. This nephrotoxicity is usually reversible.

E. Indications

Unless there is a specific reason to avoid doing so, the vast majority of patients requiring urologic imaging will be best served by having intravenous urography performed, because of that study's unsurpassed ability to screen the entire urinary tract. Some exceptions might be patients with scrotal pathology, infertility, or renal insufficiency in whom other imaging studies might be more appropriate.

F. Contraindications

1. Absolute Contraindications—None
2. Relative Contraindications
   a. Previous reactions to the contrast medium employed or to oral cholecystography. By this is meant a documented allergic or idiosyncratic reaction and not merely nausea, vomiting or syncope. Such patients *can* receive contrast again but the indication should be firm and it may be worthwhile to premedicate them.
   b. Multiple myeloma. Patients with multiple myeloma may have transient oliguria, possibly secondary to the precipitation of protein-contrast aggregates in the renal tubules. This can be prevented, however, by rigorous hydration before and immediately following the study.
   c. Renal insufficiency. The more advanced the renal disease, the less likely is the intravenous urogram to be satisfactory. Therefore, rather than perform a relatively useless study, it is often advisable to seek alternative methods of imaging such patients. In this category are patients with creatinine values greater than 4 mg/dl or a blood urea nitrogen (BUN) greater than 50 mg/dl. The possibility of contrast nephrotoxicity must also be kept in mind, but it is a relatively small risk unless the nephropathy is attributable to diabetes mellitus.
   d. Fluid and electrolyte imbalance. Patients who are severely dehydrated or have marked electrolyte imbalance may also be at risk for posturographic oliguria. Therefore it is well to attempt to correct

all such underlying disturbances before contrast is administered. This is especially true if the patient also has associated congestive heart failure.

e. Multiple consecutive contrast studies. Patients who receive intravenous contrast on two or more consecutive days expose themselves to a risk of renal insult which is greater than the combined risk of two random contrast examinations. If studies such as computed tomography (CT), angiography, coronary arteriography, and urography are all indicated, it is well to separate any two of these studies by at least 24 and preferably 48 hours, during which time the patient should be thoroughly hydrated. Once the body burden of contrast has been eliminated, it is safe to continue with the next contrast study. To order such studies consecutively without regard to the cumulative effect on the kidney is inviting trouble.

Neither allergy, pregnancy, nor diabetes mellitus is an absolute contraindication to urography.

II. RETROGRADE UROGRAPHY (RETROGRADE PYELOGRAPHY) (Cost Units—4 [Radiologic = 1; Urologic = 1.5; Cystoscopy O.R. Room Charge = 1.5])

A. Purpose

To investigate lesions of the ureter and renal collecting system that cannot be adequately defined by excretory urography.

B. Technique

1. Preliminary cystoscopy is required.
2. Using a small ureteral catheter, a ureteral orifice is identified and catheterized. The catheter is advanced to the level of the renal pelvis and contrast is instilled. The same contrast agents employed for intravenous urography are used for retrograde pyelography.

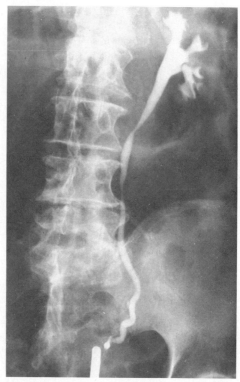

Figure 2. Normal left retrograde pyeloureterogram. Through a cystoscope a ureteral catheter is positioned in the left ureteral orifice and the left ureter and renal collecting system is gravitationally filled with contrast.

3. A preliminary abdominal plain film is essential. Following the injection of contrast material, several films are obtained (Fig. 2), at the conclusion of which the upper urinary tract is allowed to drain for several minutes and a postdrainage film is exposed. The use of fluoroscopy is an important adjunct to retrograde pyelography. In most hospital settings, however, this

requires the insertion of a ureteral catheter in one part of the hospital and the subsequent transport of the patient to the radiology department.

C. Complications

1. If anesthesia is used for cystoscopy, the patient is at risk for any of the complications of general anesthesia.
2. Instrumental perforation of the ureter is uncommon and when it does occur usually leads to no serious sequelae, nor does contrast extravasation outside of the collecting system result in any harm.
3. Since infected bladder urine may be carried to the upper urinary tract, pyelonephritis may, on rare occasion, complicate retrograde pyelography. An overly vigorous injection of contrast material in an infected urinary tract may disseminate bacteria throughout the blood stream as well as the kidney. Fortunately, the normal antegrade flow of urine is usually enough to wash out any bacteria that may have been introduced. However, in the presence of a urinary tract obstruction, the risk increases.
4. Ureteral edema has been reported when relatively large ureteral catheters are employed and allowed to stay in the ureter for long periods of time. This can result in temporary obstruction.
5. Absorption of contrast agents from the upper urinary tract occurs regularly. As much as 10 or 15% of the agent injected can be reabsorbed. In patients truly sensitive to the contrast agent, therefore, the use of the retrograde approach does not confer immunity against a systemic reaction. Other drugs administered by this route will also undergo the same degree of reabsorption.

D. Indications

1. When the urogram is inadequate to define ureteral, renal, pelvic, or calyceal anatomy (e.g., suspected small calyceal filling defects, origin or termination of upper urinary tract fistulae, etc.).
2. When urography is contraindicated.
3. As an adjunct to upper urinary tract manipulation from

below (e.g., ureteral brushing for cytology, stent insertion, etc.).

E. Contraindications

1. Untreated urinary tract infection.
2. Patients who cannot or should not be cystoscoped (e.g., patients recovering from recent bladder or urethral surgery, etc.).
3. Retrograde pyelography may be impossible in some patients, such as those with very large prostates in whom the gland overlies the ureteral orifices and prevents proper catheter placement. At times, even though the orifice is identifiable, it may not be possible to catheterize it, such as may occur with tortuous ureters or following ureteral reimplantation.

IV. ANTEGRADE PYELOGRAPHY (Cost Units—1.5)

A. Purpose

To visualize the upper urinary tract when excretory urography is unsatisfactory and retrograde pyelography cannot be done.

B. Technique

The renal pelvis is punctured with a 22-gauge Chiba ("skinny") needle by means of a direct posterior approach. Localization is provided by means of contrast excreted after an intravenous injection or, in the event of a nonvisualizing kidney, with ultrasound. The procedure is carried out and films exposed under fluoroscopic control (Fig. 3).

C. Complications

1. Inadvertent puncture of neighboring structures. Although puncture of the renal vein, kidney parenchyma, or liver and spleen may occur, few if any complications result because of the extremely fine size of the needle.
2. Some extravasation usually occurs with every antegrade pyelogram. However, the puncture site is very small and rapidly seals after the needle has been removed.

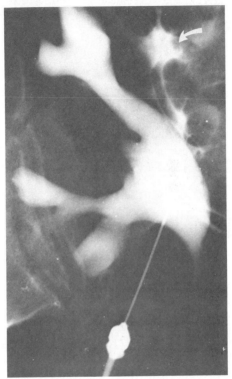

Figure 3. Antegrade pyeloureterogram. A thin needle has been percutaneously inserted into the renal pelvis of a transplanted kidney. After the installation of contrast material, extravasation is seen to occur through a leak in the renal pelvis (*arrow*).

    3. Localization of the renal pelvis is occasionally difficult and time consuming and on rare occasions may fail completely.

D. Indications
    1. For the further delineation of the site or nature of upper urinary tract obstruction if retrograde pyelography has failed.

2. For the further delineation of the site or nature of upper urinary tract obstruction if retrograde pyelography is impossible (e.g., ureteral diversion).
3. For the performance of upper urinary tract urodynamics (Whitaker test).

E. Contraindications.
1. Bleeding diathesis.
2. Diffuse skin infection over the lumbar area.
3. Nondilated collecting system. This is not an absolute contraindication, but because it may be very difficult to puncture a nondilated collecting system, antegrade pyelography is not usually done under these circumstances.
4. Patients who cannot lie prone comfortably.

V. CYSTOGRAPHY (STATIC CYSTOGRAM) (Cost Units—1)

A. Purpose
To visualize the urinary bladder by the retrograde instillation of contrast medium.

B. Technique
After a preliminary KUB, a urethral catheter is passed and contrast is instilled into the bladder. Films of the filled bladder are made in multiple projections (Fig. 4). The bladder is then allowed to empty through the catheter, after which a drainage film is obtained.

C. Complications
Complications of cystography are rare. Excessively forceful injection may result in bladder rupture. The results of traumatic urethral catheterization must also be considered as potential complications.

D. Indications
1. Trauma. One of the major indications for cystography is suspected bladder trauma. Since the intravenous urogram is unreliable in such an evaluation, a properly performed cystogram is indispensible in excluding a bladder rupture.

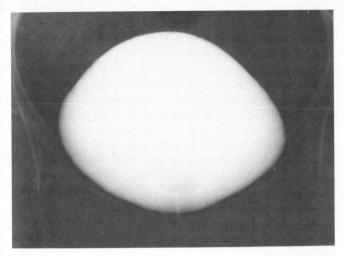

Figure 4. Normal cystogram. A retrograde cystogram has been performed by means of a Foley catheter in the urinary bladder. The contrast-filled urinary bladder has a normal size and shape. It is smooth without evidence of filling defect or extravasation.

2. The evaluation of bladder diverticula. The ability of bladder diverticula to drain properly is best evaluated by cystography.
3. Evaluation of fistulae beginning or terminating in the urinary bladder.
4. Evaluation of postoperative healing following open bladder surgery.
5. Cystography adds very little to the diagnosis of bladder tumors and is not commonly performed for this purpose.

E. Contraindications

Contraindications to passage of a urethral catheter may make attempts at cystography unadvisable, but there are no contraindications to cystography itself.

VI. VOIDING CYSTOURETHROGRAPHY (VCU, ANTEGRADE URETHROGRAPHY) (Cost Units—1.2)

A. Purpose
1. To demonstrate the anatomy of the lower urinary tract during the physiologic act of micturition.
2. To establish the presence or absence of vesicoureteral reflux.

B. Technique
Voiding cystourethrography may be performed in males or females. In either sex it is best performed under fluoroscopy. The bladder is catheterized and filled with water-soluble contrast medium. When the patient has a strong desire to void the catheter is withdrawn and the patient voids. Filming is carried out by means of either serial fluoroscopic spot films or videotape recording (Fig. 5).

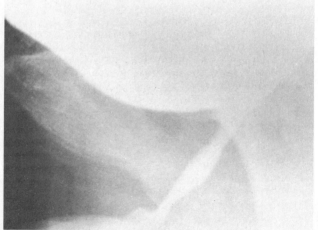

Figure 5. Normal voiding cystourethrogram. A lateral view of the bladder and urethra during voiding demonstrates a normal funnel-shaped bladder neck and tubular urethra in this 34-year-old woman.

C. **Complications**

These are essentially the same as those listed under cystography.

D. **Indications**

1. Recurrent urinary tract infections, especially in children, in whom reflux is not uncommon.
2. Evaluation of the posterior urethra in the male and the entire urethra in the female. By means of VCU, posterior urethral pathology may be demonstrated. VCU is especially valuable in evaluating urethral stricture disease, posterior urethral valves in the infant male, and the postoperative urethra. In the female it is the primary method of visualizing urethral diverticula.
3. For the evaluation of certain voiding dysfunctions (e.g., detrusor–external sphincter dyssynergia, neuropathic bladder, etc.). Sometimes VCU is combined with simultaneous pressure-flow recordings (videourodynamics).
4. For the evaluation of an ectopic ureter thought to insert into the urethra. Reflux into such ectopic ureters is fairly common.

E. **Contraindications**

There are no contraindications to VCU except in the unusual instance of the patient who cannot be catheterized. On occasion, however, the examination cannot be satisfactorily performed because of the patient's voluntary or involuntary inability to void at the time.

VII. RETROGRADE URETHROGRAPHY (Cost Units—1)

A. **Purpose**

To provide detailed visualization of the anterior urethra in the male. The procedure has little or no application in the female. Unlike VCU, retrograde urethrography incompletely visualizes the posterior urethra because of the resistance to retrograde flow provided by the external sphincter.

B. Technique

1. The most distal 1 to 2 cm of the urethra is occluded by means of a partially inflated Foley catheter balloon placed in the fossa navicularis and the remainder of the anterior urethra is filled with water-soluble contrast medium.

2. Spot films of the urethra fully distended with contrast are taken.

C. Complications

1. Infection. Reflux of contrast from the urethra to the surrounding cavernous bodies (i.e., corpus spongiosum) may occur during retrograde urethrography. Such reflex is usually minimal and without clinical consequence except in the presence of urethritis, when bacteria may be forced into the bloodstream.

2. Pulmonary embolism is a very real consideration unless water-soluble contrast media are used. For this reason, oily contrast agents are contraindicated for retrograde urethrography.

D. Indications

1. The most common indication is for the detailed delineation of suspected or known urethral stricture (Figs. 6A,B).

2. The procedure is indispensible in suspected urethral trauma. When urethral injury is suspected, retrograde urethrography should be routinely performed before attempting passage of a urethral catheter.

3. Retrograde urethrography may also be helpful in demonstrating urethral diverticula, fistulae, and neoplasms.

E. Contraindications

1. Acute urethritis, as discussed above.

2. Patients who are contrast sensitive may manifest sensitivity if contrast is absorbed during the procedure.

VIII. LOOPOGRAPHY (Cost Units—1)

Anastomosis of the ureters to an isolated segment (''loop'') of ileum or, less commonly, transverse colon, is the most common method of establishing permanent urinary diversion. Ra-

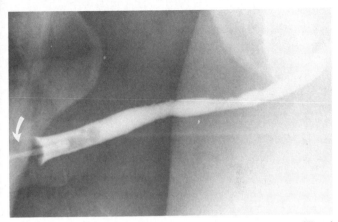

Figure 6. A. A retrograde urethrogram in a 42-year-old man demonstrates filling of the anterior urethra. The bulbous urethra appears suspiciously irregular but is not visualized in great detail in this view. Note the occlusive Foley balloon in the distal urethra (*arrow*).

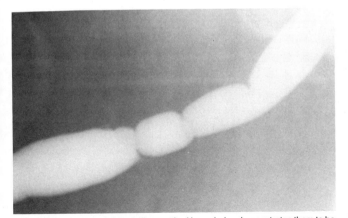

Figure 6. B. A close-up of the bulbar urethral irregularies demonstrates them to be attributable to a series of short diaphgram-like strictures, in all probability postinflammatory.

diologic examination of such bowel segments or conduits is referred to as "loopography."

A. Purpose
1. To visualize the conduit and evaluate it for intrinsic disease (e.g., filling defects, capacity, peristalsis, etc.).
2. To visualize the upper urinary tracts by reflux. Reflux is normal with ileal conduits because the thin small bowel wall precludes an antireflux ureteroileal anastomosis. Large bowel conduits, however, may be of an antirefluxing nature.

B. Technique
1. Following a plain abdominal film the study of the urinary conduit is carried out under fluoroscopy. By placing gentle traction on the catheter with its inflated balloon just underneath the anterior abdominal wall, contrast material is prevented from exiting the stoma. The conduit is then filled with water-soluble contrast medium by gravity or hand injection until the bowel is well distended. Spot films are made, with particular attention given to the presence or absence of reflux. The catheter is then removed and the conduit and upper urinary tracts evaluated for emptying.

C. Complications
There are few complications. Pyelonephritis may accompany forceful reflux of infected conduit urine, however.

D. Indications
1. Patients with loop diversion whose upper urinary tracts show deterioration by serial IVU (i.e., worsening hydronephrosis, renal calculi, etc.). In such patients the absence of reflux may indicate ureteroileal or ureterocolonic obstruction.
2. Patients with untoward urinary symptoms or laboratory findings (i.e., recurrent pyelonephritis, diminishing urinary output, increasing creatinine level, etc.).
3. Patients with suspected conduit disorders (e.g., anastomotic leaks, periloopal abscesses, etc.).

E. Contraindications

There are no contraindications to a retrograde study of a urinary conduit.

IX. ANGIOGRAPHY (Cost Units—6–8)

A. Basic Considerations

Angiography refers to the radiologic study of both the arterial and venous systems. There are various anatomic subdivisions. Those pertinent to the study of the urinary tract include:

1. Arterial
   a. Aortography
   b. Renal arteriography
   c. Adrenal arteriography
2. Venous
   a. Inferior vena cavography
   b. Renal phlebography
   c. Adrenal phlebography
   d. Gonadal phlebography

B. Purpose

1. To visualize the arterial and/or venous systems with contrast medium.
2. To catheterize veins for biochemical sampling.
3. For therapeutic vascular dilatation.
4. For therapeutic embolization.

C. Technique

There are several methods of performing angiography.

1. *Direct Puncture*. Here a needle is placed percutaneously through the flank into the aorta. This is known as translumbar aortography (TLA). TLA is for the most part reserved for those instances in which the retrograde catheterization of the femoral and iliac vessels is felt to be inadvisable.
2. Percutaneous Arterial Catheterization (Seldinger Technique)
   a. Arterial
   b. Venous. By means of a percutaneous puncture— usually into the femoral artery or femoral vein—a

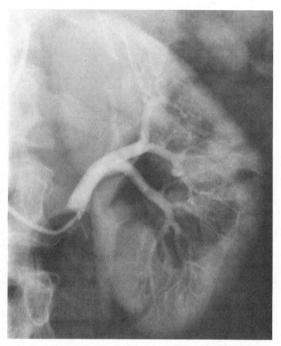

Figure 7. A. Left selective renal arteriogram—arterial phase. The main renal artery, its anterior and posterior divisions as well as the segmental and interlobar branches are clearly visualized. Note the catheter in the left renal artery.

needle is inserted into the desired blood vessel and a guidewire is passed through it. The needle is removed and a catheter is passed over the guidewire until its tip is satisfactorily placed within the vascular system. Contrast is then injected.

3. Selective Angiography
   a. Selective renal arteriography. This is the most common method of performing renal arteriography. A catheter is inserted retrograde into the aorta

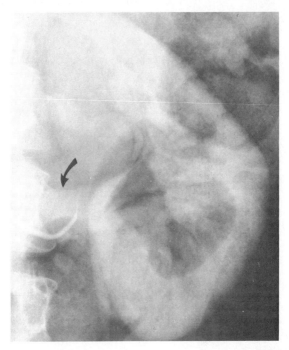

Figure 7. B. Left selective renal arteriogram—venous phase. Eight seconds after the contrast has been injected the renal parenchyma is well visualized, as is the left main renal vein (*arrow*).

as described and then manipulated until its tip comes to lie in the renal artery. Ten or twelve milliliters of contrast media are injected and serial x-ray filming follows. Because of the rapid transit of the contrast through the vascular system, films must be exposed quite rapidly, often at the rate of several per second. Three phases of renal arteriography can be recognized: arterial (Fig. 7A), nephrographic, and venous (Fig. 7B).

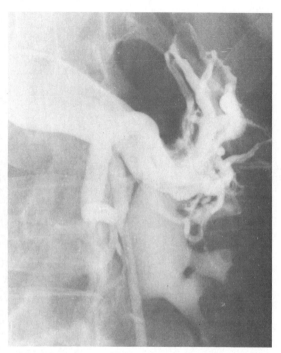

Figure 7. C. Selective left renal phlebogram. Contrast has been retrogradely injected into the main left renal vein, opacifying the main intrarenal branches.

      b. Selective renal phlebography. The renal vein is
         selectively catheterized percutaneously and con-
         trast injected. Usually the renal artery needs to be
         temporarily occluded or constricted with epi-
         nephrine to slow blood flow and preclude the over-
         ly rapid washout of contrast from the renal vein
         (Fig. 7C).
   4. *Digital Subtraction Angiography (DSA)*. This is a
      relatively new modality in which electronic subtrac-
      tion and computerized image manipulation are carried

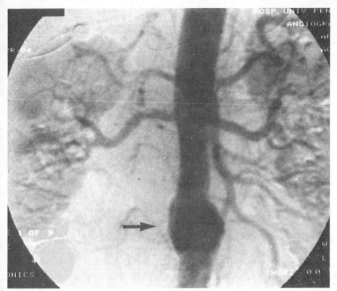

Figure 7. D. Digital subtraction angiogram. A selective intraaortic injection of 5 ml of contrast material provides clear visualization of the aorta and both main renal arteries, including the major tributories. Note the presence of an aortic aneurysm (*arrow*).

out to provide visualization of the arterial tree after intravenous injection (or after relatively small intraarterial injections) (Fig. 7D).

D. Complications

Angiography is relatively safe when performed by trained personnel. There are certain well-recognized complications, however.

1. Vascular Complications Related to the Puncture
   a. Minor—transient spasm, small hematomas, pain, etc.
   b. Major—bleeding, thrombosis, dissection, arteriovenous fistula, and aneurysm formation.

2. Physiologic complications secondary to the effect of contrast injected directly into the kidney. These are transient and rarely lasting. Properly performed by currently recommended techniques, there is no permanent or lasting deleterious effect on renal function following the injection of contrast material into the renal artery.
3. Systemic Effects of Contrast (see II.D).

E. Indications
1. Renal
   a. Hypertension. Angiography may be employed diagnostically both to image the arterial supply to the kidney and also to sample renal vein blood for renin.
   b. Neoplasms. Angiography is employed in the diagnosis of renal masses suspected of being neoplastic, and for the embolization of renal neoplasms if found. In these cases, the inferior vena cava should also be assessed for the presence of tumor thrombus.
   c. Renal trauma. Angiography is necessary to exclude traumatic occlusion of the renal artery when contrast is not excreted by the injured kidney on the emergency urogram. In addition, if post-traumatic arterial bleeding is a problem, embolization may be carried out.
   d. For the evaluation of vascular abnormalities such as aneurysms and arteriovenous malformations.
   e. In suspected embolism of the renal arterial tree or thrombosis of the renal artery or renal vein.
   f. To provide a preoperative arterial "road map" when extensive intrarenal surgical dissection is contemplated. This is especially valuable when there is a high risk of anomalous vascular supply such as in a horseshoe kidney.
   g. In the preoperative evaluation of potential renal donors.
2. Adrenal
   a. Angiography may be helpful in determining the nature of adrenal masses.

      b. Ablation of adrenal function by embolization or overinjection of the adrenal veins.

      c. For adrenal vein sampling of functioning adrenal tumors.

  3. Other

      a. Gonadal phlebography is sometimes employed in the search for a nonpalpable undescended testis.

      b. Gonadal phlebography is also valuable in evaluating varicoceles and in treating them by means of venous occlusion with balloons or sclerosing agents.

F. Contraindications

  1. Bleeding diathesis.

  2. Hypercoagulation states such as polycythemia vera constitute relative contraindications. Extremely small instruments should be used in these patients because of the risk of thrombosis.

X. ULTRASONOGRAPHY (Cost Units—1.7)

A. Purpose

Ultrasound can be used to image most parts of the genitourinary system.

  1. Advantages

      a. It is not invasive.

      b. It is not function dependent.

      c. Contrast media are not required.

      d. Structures not amenable to imaging by other techniques may be imaged by ultrasound (e.g., prostate).

  2. Disadvantages

      a. Inferior resolution compared to, for example, IVU.

      b. Certain structures cannot be visualized, for example, the nondilated ureter.

B. Technique

Two types of sonographic imaging may be employed in the urinary tract: real-time imaging and static imaging. Static imaging has greater resolution and a wider field of view. Real-time allows consistent modification of transducer position to obtain optimal projections (Fig. 8).

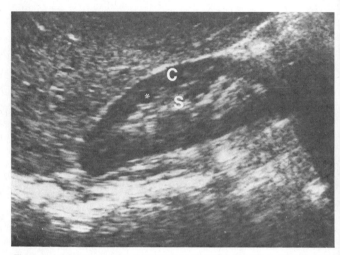

Figure 8. Longitudinal supine ultrasonogram of normal right kidney. Note the renal cortex (C), the relatively sonolucent renal medulla (*asterisk*), and the echogenic renal sinus (S).

C. Complications
There are no known complications.

D. Indications
1. Kidney
   a. Renal masses. Ultrasound can detect the presence of a fluid-filled renal mass with greater than 98% accuracy. Because most renal masses are either tumors or cysts, ultrasound is extremely valuable in their evaluation.
   b. Impaired renal function. The number, size, shape and location of the kidneys as well as the status of the renal pelvis can be determined accurately. Dilated renal pelves and calyces usually indicate obstructive uropathy.
   c. Unilateral nonvisualization at urography. The cause for a nonvisualizing kidney may frequently

be revealed by ultrasonography. In many cases, however, the study must be supplemented by other imaging modalities such as retrograde pyelography.

d. To screen patients at risk for the presence of hydronephrosis. Ultrasonography is extremely accurate in detecting volume changes in the upper urinary tract. False positives are not uncommon, but false negatives are rare.

e. Aspiration biopsy procedures. Ultrasound can outline the kidney and ascertain its depth below the skin, thus facilitating percutaneous renal biopsy with an aspiration biopsy needle guide. Ultrasound is also very helpful in guiding needles into renal cysts or dilated renal collecting systems.

f. Renal pelvic filling defects. These are most commonly caused by nonopaque calculi, urothelial neoplasms, and blood clots. Renal calculi are markedly echogenic, produce acoustic shadowing, and are readily detectable by ultrasound. Clots and tumors may also be demonstrated.

g. Evaluation of perinephric collections. Fluid collections around the kidney consist of abscesses, urinomas, hematomas, or, in the case of a transplanted kidney, lymphoceles. Although these can all be recognized as echo-free masses in the perinephric space or around the kidney, differentiating one from the other is usually not possible by ultrasound alone.

h. Renal surveillance. Kidneys at risk for the development of specific diseases can be periodically monitored by ultrasound, e.g., the contralateral kidney following nephrectomy for Wilms' tumor, evaluation of family members of patients with hereditary disorders such as polycystic disease, tuberous sclerosis, etc. The status of existing diseases such as hydronephrosis may also be monitored to determine if the process is static, improving, or worsening.

2. *Ureter*. Ultrasound has limited usefulness in ureteral disorders. However, dilated ureters may be seen, ureteroceles demonstrated within the bladder, and small calculi imaged, especially in the pelvic ureter.

3. *Bladder*. Uses of ultrasonography include the measurement of residual urine, guidance for suprapubic aspiration, staging of bladder tumors, and evaluation of intravesical masses and diverticula.

4. *Prostate and Seminal Vesicles*. Ultrasonography of the prostate can sometimes estimate prostatic size and distinguish benign from malignant enlargement. Intrarectal transducers may be used to scan the prostate through the rectal wall.

5. *Scrotum and External Genitalia*. Ultrasound can differentiate solid from cystic scrotal masses. This is helpful when inflammation or neoplasm of the testis or epididymis is associated with a secondary hydrocele that prevents adequate palpation of the underlying lesion.

XI. COMPUTED TOMOGRAPHY (Cost Units—2.5)

A. Basic Principles

An x-ray beam is rotated about the patient and the amount of transmitted radiation is measured. Adjacent areas are compared. A computer processes the data and formats them as a digitized matrix of dots corresponding to an anatomic cross section of the body. The darkness of each dot is a function of the amount of radiation detected. A number of cross sections, each about 1 cm thick, is made through the anatomic areas of interest. Although many visceral structures can be recognized by their suggestive CT appearance, others have similar densities. To enhance structural differences, contrast material is frequently given. This is the same type as is used for urography and other urologic studies. Following administration of contrast material multiple images are repeated. Many pathologic lesions can be recognized on the basis of their appearance before and after contrast. The advantage of CT over ordinary radiography is not so much a difference in the type of information obtained but rather CT's greater contrast resolution, which is approximately ten times that possible with film radiography. CT's useful display of tomographic cross-sectional anatomy, relatively un-affected by surrounding high x-ray absorbing tissues such as bone, is another distinct advantage.

B. Purpose
To visualize the urinary tract, primarily in thin cross-sectional slices.

C. Technique
Preparation is the same as for any procedures in which contrast is to be administered. Obscuration from bowel content is not a problem with CT but retained barium should be evacuated prior to the study because it can produce artefacts. After a series of preselected non–contrast enhanced CT scans through an area of interest, certain sections are repeated following contrast administration (Fig. 9). The contrast may be given as a rapid bolus or

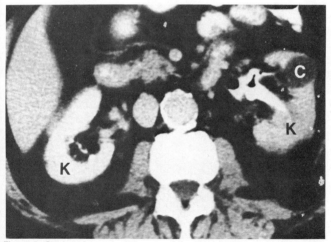

Figure 9. Computed tomographic scan of the kidneys (K) reveals them to be normal in size, shape, and density. Note the low-density cyst (C) in the anterior portion of the left kidney.

as a slow intravenous drip. The bolus has the advantage of producing higher blood levels, differentiating renal cortex from medulla, and in a rough manner comparing the blood flow to each kidney.

D. Complications

There are no complications specific to CT. The complications are limited to those described under contrast media.

E. Indications

CT has had a major impact on uroradiologic diagnosis. It has a number of important uses.

1. Renal Masses
   a. Diagnosis. CT is very accurate in differentiating cystic from solid lesions of the kidney. In the detection of renal cysts it is almost as accurate as ultrasonography. It has the advantages of being able to detect the presence of fresh blood so that certain hemorrhagic lesions and hematomas are immediately recognizable. Renal neoplasms also have a suggestive appearance on CT. In certain respects CT is competitive with ultrasonography in evaluating renal masses but in other respects the two procedures are complementary.
   b. Staging of Renal Neoplasms. CT provides evidence of renal vein or IVC tumor thrombus, lymphadenopathy, and liver metastases. It is therefore very helpful in the preoperative evaluation of neoplasms.
2. *Perinephric Effusions.* Perinephric abscess, urinoma, and hematoma can be readily recognized by CT.
3. *Trauma.* CT is very informative in assessing the extent of renal trauma and its possible complications. It is not necessary, however, in most cases because ordinary intravenous urography is generally adequate to evaluate the patient with suspected renal trauma. CT is best reserved for more complicated cases.
4. *Retroperitoneal Masses.* CT is the best method of evaluating most retroperitoneal masses, including neoplasms.

5. *Retroperitoneal Lymph Nodes.* CT is the most reliable method presently available to evaluate enlarged retroperitoneal lymph nodes. This is an important part of the staging of many urologic tumors, including those arising in the testis, bladder, and prostate.

6. *Retroperitoneal Fibrosis.* In suspected cases of retroperitoneal fibrosis, CT is the single most imporant diagnostic study.

7. *Renal Pelvic Filling Defects.* Many renal pelvic defects are attributable to nonopaque calculi. CT is exquisitely sensitive in detecting such calculi even though they are nonopaque on film radiography. In addition, some of the other causes for filling defects, including blood clots and neoplasms, may also be detected by CT.

8. *Adrenal Gland.* CT is the study of choice for the evaluation of any patient with suspected adrenal pathology.

XII. RADIONUCLIDE IMAGING (Cost Units—1.0)

A. Basic Principles

The flow of radioisotopes through the kidney and other genitourinary (GU) structures may be monitored so that, in turn, vascular perfusion, parenchymal integrity, and, in the case of the kidney, outflow tract anatomy, may be imaged. By means of radiopharmaceuticals designed for specific physiologic functions, tissue isotopic distribution is imaged by means of a gamma camera that measures emitted gamma radiation as a function of time and spatial distribution. In this way, organ function may also be ascertained. Examples of some of the radiopharmaceuticals employed are iodine-131-Hippuran, technetium-99m-Pertechnetate, Tc-99m-DTPA, Tc-99m-Glucoheptonate, Tc-99m-DMSA, and gallium-67-Citrate.

B. Purpose

1. To estimate renal function.
2. To image the urinary tract.
   a. Blood flow.
   b. Structural anatomy. Radionuclide estimation of re-

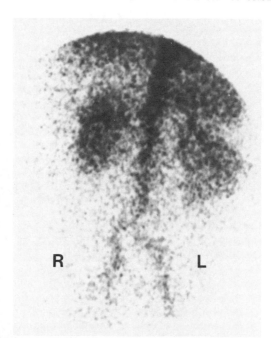

Figure 10. A. Radionuclide renal scintiscan—vascular phase. This image taken with Tc-99m-DTPA was made 10 seconds after the injection of the radionuclide. Note the aorta and both common iliac arteries. Both the right and left kidneys are normally perfused.

nal function is often the method of choice, whereas radionuclide anatomic imaging is often employed only when radiographic methods are not suitable.

C. Technique

Techniques vary depending upon the information desired. In general, a tracer dose of radioactive isotope bound to a specific pharmaceutical agent is administered and the patient is placed beneath a gamma camera, where images are generated at intervals dependent upon the information sought. For flow studies images are taken as frequently as

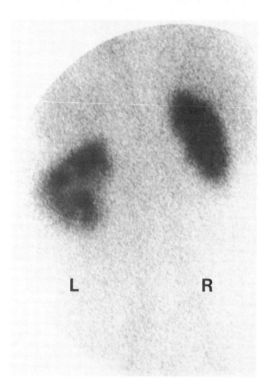

Figure 10. B. Radionuclide renal scintiscan—nephrographic phase. This was imaged 5 minutes after radionuclide administration. Here the parenchyma of both kidneys is homogeneously depicted. Radioactivity is no longer visualized in the vascular tree but the renal collecting systems and ureters have not yet filled. (Note that this image is reversed since it was made in a posterior projection.)

every few seconds (Fig. 10A). For anatomic information images are obtained by accumulating counts for several minutes (Figs. 10B,C). These images may be taken sequentially for as long as several hours, and under certain circumstances may even be delayed up to 24 or 48 hours. When evaluating renal function, small radiation detectors

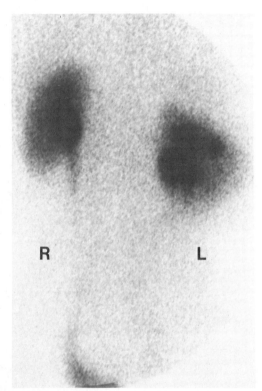

Figure 10. C. Radionuclide renal scintiscan—excretory phase. This demonstrates radioactivity in a dilated right and left renal collecting system. The right ureter is seen in part and it appears somewhat dilated.

placed directly over the kidneys may be used to generate time–radioactivity curves. This is known as a renogram.

D. Complications

There are no known complications of nuclear medicine diagnostic procedures. The radiation doses involved are minimal and, in many cases, are less than those for comparable radiographic studies.

E. Indications

1. Measurement of Renal Function

    a. Total renal function. Using radionuclides, approximation of glomerular filtration rate (GFR) and renal plasma flow can be obtained. Appropriate radionuclides are given by bolus injection and one or more blood samples are taken at predetermined intervals. The determination of residual radioactivity in each sample permits the construction of a radioactivity disappearance curve that can be used to accurately measure clearance of the nuclide.

    b. Separate renal function. With computer-enhanced scanning techniques the contribution of each kidney to total renal plasma flow and total GFR can be estimated fairly accurately. The ability to ascertain the function of one kidney has special significance when decisions regarding nephrectomy versus salvage operations must be made. In cases of severe hydronephosis, split renal functions before and after a period of nephrostomy drainage may show a surprising degree of renal functional improvement in the hitherto obstructed kidney.

2. *Hypertension.* Differential renal blood flow studies detect approximately 85% of cases of renal artery stenosis but the study is complicated by an approximately 10% false-positive rate, primarily in patients with essential hypertension. Another difficulty with isotope screening in hypertension is the fact that there may be difficulty distinguishing unilateral renal vascular lesions from unilateral renal parenchymal disease.

3. *Renal Functional Impairment.* Radionuclide imaging is more sensitive than urography in providing images of the kidney when renal function is diminished and is sometimes used in lieu of radiographic methods in evaluating patients with renal failure of unknown cause. Anatomic detail is much less satisfactory than that provided by urography, however. In cases of suspected obstructive uropathy, radionuclide studies are often not specific enough to compete with the

other imaging modalities, specifically ultrasonography.

4. *Contraindications to Contrast Media.* Although radionuclide methods are not as specific as radiographic
studies, they represent an acceptable alternative in an
attempt to gain some gross information about renal
anatomy and differential function. Patients with renal
failure and those with demonstrated contrast sensitivity fall into this group.

5. *Evaluation of Renal Transplant Failure.* Isotopic
methods of imaging the kidney are very helpful in
evaluating renal transplant complications, including
obstruction, extravasation, and stenosis of the arterial
anastomosis.

6. *Questionable or Intermittent Obstruction.* The presence of intermittent obstruction, especially at the
ureteropelvic junction, is often difficult to document.
Using radionuclide methods the rate of emptying of
the collecting system after a diuretic challenge can be
evaluated and compared to standard emptying
profiles.

7. *Renal Masses* (Fig. 11). Occasionally it is difficult or
impossible to differentiate between a renal mass or
pseudomass (pseudotumor) by intravenous urography. In these cases the use of radionuclides to provide
a functional image of the renal parenchyma can be
extremely important in showing whether there is a
pathologic mass in the renal parenchyma. In the presence of an abnormality there is a photon-deficient
area in the kidney (''cold spot''). With pseudotumors
no such defect is noticed.

8. *Extravasation of Urine.* Small urinary leaks may
sometimes be undetectable with contrast studies. Because small amounts of radionuclide can be detected
readily with modern gamma cameras scanning techniques, however, small or early extravasations can be
imaged much more readily with radionuclide studies
than with film radiography.

9. *Vesicoureteral Reflux.* Vesicoureteral reflux is usually demonstrated initially by voiding cystourethro-

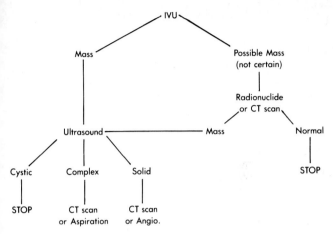

Figure 11. Workup for renal mass.

graphy. Once demonstrated, however, it may be followed periodically by radionuclide cystourethrography, which is more sensitive than VCU and imposes less of a radiation burden on the patient.

10. *Testicular Torsion.* When testicular torsion is suspected, a radionuclide flow study of the scrotum will demonstrate the viability of the testis and compare its perfusion to the opposite side.

11. *Inflammatory Lesions.* Inflammatory lesions of any organ result in an abnormal uptake of Ga-67. Gallium scanning is therefore useful in uncovering occult inflammatory foci or confirming the presence of a clinically atypical infection such as subacute pyelonephritis. Other agents, such as indium-111, which can be fixed to leukocytes, may also be used.

F. Contraindications

No contraindications exist to the use of radionuclides for diagnostic purposes.

XIII. LYMPHOGRAPHY (Cost Units—7)

A. Purpose

To opacify lymph nodes and lymphatic channels draining the testis, prostate, and urinary bladder. In urology, lymphography is used almost exclusively for the stating of malignancies. Although gross lymphadenopathy can be recognized by CT, lymphography is the most sensitive and perhaps the only method of demonstrating smaller metastatic deposits.

B. Technique

A few drops of a water-soluble dye, such as indigo carmine or patent blue, are injected intradermally into the webbing between the first and second toes. After sufficient dye has been absorbed, the subcutaneous lymphatics draining the area are identified as fine blue streaks on the dorsum of the foot. Under local anesthesia, these dye-stained lymphatics are surgically isolated and cannulated with a No. 30 gauge needle. Using a mechanical injector approximately 6 ml of an oily contrast medium (Ethiodol) is injected into the cannulated lymphatic over the period of 30 to 60 minutes. Water-soluble contrast cannot be used because it diffuses out of the lymph channels before reaching regional lymph nodes. Radiographs of the pelvis taken at 30 to 60 minutes (lymphangiogram) will usually demonstrate the lymphatic channels leading into the hypogastric, external, and common iliac chains. Delayed films of the same area taken at 24 hours will better reveal the nodes themselves (lymphadenogram).

Testicular lymphography may be performed during orchiectomy for testis tumor. After the spermatic cord has been cut, lymph vessels within the cord are cannulated and injected with Ethiodol in much the same fashion as lower extremity lymphography is carried out. Testicular lymphography has the advantage of selectively opacifying the testicular lymphatic chain which is often not seen during ordinary pedal lymphography.

C. Complications

Although as with any iodinated contrast agent there is the slight risk of a sensitivity reaction to Ethiodol, the main complication of lymphography is pulmonary oil embolism. Because of lymphaticovenous communications, some of the oily contrast invariably gains access to the lungs. The tiny oil droplets are found in the pulmonary alveoli and remain there until phagocytized. It is not uncommon for pulmonary perfusion to be adversely affected for some days following lymphography. In patients with normal pulmonary function this presents no significant risk. However, in patients with impaired pulmonary ventilatory capacity the pulmonary oil deposits constitute a potentially serious hazard.

D. Indications

Patients with malignant disease of the prostate, bladder, and testis. Although CT has to a large extent replaced lymphography in the staging of genitourinary neoplasms, there is still an occasional need for lymphography when it is necessary to ascertain the presence or absence of small metastatic lymphatic foci. Failure of certain lymphatic channels to fill represents a potential diagnostic pitfall of lymphography. Such nonvisualized portions of the lymphatic chain can occur under normal circumstances and do not always represent unequivocal evidence of obstruction by tumor.

E. Contraindications

Lymphography should be undertaken with caution in patients with pulmonary disease and is contraindicated in those with significant functional impairment.

XIV. MAGNETIC RESONANCE IMAGING (MRI)

A. Background

Magnetic resonance imaging was introduced in 1973 and is the newest diagnostic imaging modality. In addition to topographic anatomic display, this new nonionizing modality is capable of providing information about the chemical composition and blood flow of a given organ.

B. Technique

MRI is based on the magnetic properties of nuclei with an odd number of protons and neutrons. Hydrogen is the most abundant such nucleus in biologic tissue. The magnetic moments of individual hydrogen nuclei either align with or against the direction of an externally imposed magnetic field. When energy in the form of a radio frequency signal interacts with such a magnetized sample, the parallel orientation of the magnetic vector of the protons is displaced by an amount determined by the strength and duration of the radio frequency pulse. The pulse also induces a rapid repetitive "flipping" or "resonance" of the protons in a coherent fashion between their two energy states. When the pulse is terminated, the resonance decays very rapidly and the net magnetization vector returns to its original orientation at a less rapid rate. MRI derives information by utilizing four parameters: proton density, bulk motion or flow, and T-1 or T-2 relaxation values. It permits direct imaging in coronal, sagittal, as well as transaxial planes with multiple sections scanned simultaneously.

C. Future Considerations

MRI adds an additional dimension to radiologic diagnostic technique. Its precise role in the specialty of urology remains to be determined.

BIBLIOGRAPHY

Elkin E: Radiology of the Urinary System. Boston: Little, Brown, 1980.

Friedland GW, Filly R, et al (eds): Uroradiology: An Integrated Approach. New York: Churchill Livingstone, 1983.

Lalli AF. Tailored Urologic Imaging. Chicago: Year Book, 1980.

Ney C, Friedenberg RM (eds): Radiographic Atlas of the Genitourinary System, ed 2. Philadelphia: J.B. Lippincott, 1981.

Pollack HM: Radiologic Examination of the Urinary Tract. Hagerstown, Md: Harper & Row, 1971.

Sherwood T, Davidson AJ, Talner LB: Uroradiology. Oxford, England: Blackwell, 1980.

Witten DM, Myers GH, Jr, Utz DC: Emmett's Clinical Urography, ed 4. Philadelphia: W.B. Saunders, 1977.

4

Lower Urinary Tract Infections in Women

David R. Staskin

I. INCIDENCE

A. Epidemiology

1. Dysuria accounts for over five million office visits per year—up to 50% of urologic practice and 2 to 10% of general practice. Forty-eight percent of women have one episode; 40% of these see a physician.

2. Thirty to sixty percent of women with frequency and dysuria will have a lower urinary tract infection—approximately one-third with sterile urine, one-third with low colony count (<10,000 cfu/ml) infection, and one-third with more than 100,000 cfu/ml.

3. After their initial infection, 16% within 3 months, 25% within 18 months, and 40% of women within 3 years will be reinfected. Eighty percent of patients with histories of multiple UTIs will be reinfected within 18 months.

4. Sexual activity, pregnancy, and the postpartum period are associated with an increased incidence of initial and complicated infections.

5. Combining the asymptomatic/bacteriuric group and infected group, this represents a prevalance of greater than 2%. Five percent of school girls will have at least one episode of bacteriuria between the 1st and 12th grades, and these females will be more susceptible to UTIs as adults. Ten to twenty-five percent of women will have a urinary tract infection at some point in their lifetime.

PREVALANCE OF URINARY TRACT INFECTION:

Less than 2 years	0.8%
Schoolgirls	1.2%
Pregnancy	3.7%
20 to 40 years	4–6%
(increases by 2% per decade)	
55 to 64 years	10%

6. Five to thirteen percent of female children with recurrent symptomatic UTI and no obstruction will develop renal scarring. Thirteen to twenty-six percent of female children with asymptomatic bacteriuria will develop renal scarring. One-third of children with bacteriuria and 95% of children with renal scarring will have had vesicoureteral reflux. The scarring will have occurred by the age of 6 years in most of the patients. Virtually all pyelonephritic scarring noted in adults is initiated by reflux in childhood.

7. Less than 1% of patients with a UTI will develop chronic pyelonephritis and only a very small percentage of these will require dialysis: yet due to the high prevalance of infection, 10% of dialysis patients have renal failure secondary to infection or its complications.

B. Etiology

1. Fecal flora colonize the introitus.
   a. Usually *Escherichia coli.*
      (1) A few O serotypes (e.g., 01, 02, 06, 018, 075) account for 50 to 70% of infections. These serotypes may become the quantitatively dominating serotype in the fecal flora before infection (prevalance theory).
      (2) Certain *E. coli* O and K antigen types may have increased resistance to the bactericidal effect of serum antibodies and higher hemolytic activity (special pathogenicity theory).
      (3) Specialized bacterial pili are responsible for bacterial adherence.

b. Vaginal defense mechanisms (extrinsic bladder defense mechanisms in women)
  (1) Vaginal cell receptivity may be genetically determined.
  (2) Cervicovaginal antibody
    (a) Complement-mediated lysis
    (b) Enhanced phagocytosis
    (c) Prevention of bacterial adherence
  (3) Vaginal pH less than 4.5 has been proposed as a defense mechanism but this is controversial. Alkaline pH is most often associated with bacterial colonization but has not shown to be statistically significant when comparing infected patients and controls.
  (4) Colonization by nonpathogenic vaginal flora (i.e., *Lactobacillus*) has been proposed by some investigators—the binding of vaginal epithelial sties, preventing colonization by pathogenic strains is the proposed mechanism of defense. Use of *Lactobacillus* (live or extract) has been proposed to colonize or bind ''receptors'' in infection-prone females. Other investigators have disagreed with these data on the basis of vaginal flora studies in infection-prone females and healthy controls.

INTROITAL MULTIPLICATION IS INFLUENCED BY IRRITATION FROM VAGINAL INFECTION, TRAUMA (CHEMICAL IRRITATION), ATROPHY, POOR HYGIENE OR VENTILATION, URINARY OR FECAL INCONTINENCE, OR IMMUNOSUPPRESSIVE STATES.

c. Bladder defense mechanisms (intrinsic bladder defense)
  (1) Voiding: In experimental studies, bacteria were placed in the bladders of normal volunteers and equal sized glass flasks. Mechanical rinsing of the flasks and voiding by the volun-

teers were compared. The flasks had 99% of bacteria removed by mechanical rinsing alone but were not sterilized. The volunteers were able to sterilize their urine with several voids without the need for antibiotic therapy. Emptying alone is an effective but incomplete defense mechanism.

- (2) Mucosal resistance
    - (a) Patients with P blood group antigen (75% of total population appear to have receptors which allow fimbirial attachment by *E. coli* strains).
    - (b) Glycosaminoglycans (polysaccharide) that are secreted by the mucosal cells may be an antiadherence factor.
    - (c) Immunoglobulin A (IgA) and complement C8 and C9 are probably not major factors.
    - (d) Urinary pH, osmolality, urea concentration, and ammonia concentration are probably not significant factors due to accommodation by bacteria, or the presence of a dilute urine.
- (3) Urethral ascent of bacteria—Mechanical factors
    - (a) Cytoscopy 3 to 5%
    - (b) Single catheterization 3% (5 to 6% hospitalized; 0.5 to 1% nonhospitalized)
    - (c) Indwelling catheters
        - i. Data vary as to the time course of bladder bacteriuria with an indwelling catheter. Old data indicated contamination within 3 days. Closed drainage systems with meticulous care have resulted in up to 7 to 10 days without contamination (4 to 7.5% incidence per day).
        - ii. Meatal care with iodine or antibiotics and addition of antiseptic agents to the urinary drainage bag do not ap-

pear to decrease the incidence of infection and predispose to the selection of resistant organisms.

   iii. Antibiotics should be given before the catheterization of infected patients. Antibiotic coverage for a short-term catheterization is controversial and may be used most efficaciously after discontinuation of the catheter. Antibiotic prophylaxis does not decrease the incidence of infection in long-term catheterization and tends to select for resistant organisms. Systemic antibiotic coverage appears to be useful for no more than 4 days in preventing bladder colonization.

  (d) Catheter care

    i. Use a closed drainage catheter system.

    ii. Do not treat asymptomatic bacteriuria unless it is associated with a stone-forming organism.

    iii. Administer an appropriate antibiotic (culture) when changing a catheter or before the removal of catheter.

    iv. Separate infected from noninfected patients.

    v. Use sterile technique when obtaining specimens from the catheter port, or when irrigating the catheter.

(4) Other mechanisms of lower tract infection

  (a) Renal infection

  (b) Hematogenous—usually affects upper tracts first

  (c) Lymphatics—periurethral glands seed the bladder

  (d) Fistula—from a gynecologic or intestinal structure caused by surgery, radiation, infection, inflammatory disease, or tumor

(e) Residual urine or stasis—functional or anatomic obstruction may predispose to infection. Although there is some controversy as to whether residual urine in and of itself predisposes to infection, it certainly makes infection difficult to eradicate as bacteria cannot be effectively "washed out" with urine flow.

(f) Foreign body—nidus for infection
   i. Indwelling catheter
   ii. Stone
   iii. Foreign body

II. SIGNS AND SYMPTOMS

A. Dysuria
1. Painful and difficult micturition

B. Frequency

C. Strangury
1. Dysuria with pelvic musculature contraction

D. Tenesmus
1. Ineffectual painful straining to void

E. Nocturia

F. Nocturnal enuresis

G. Incontinence

H. Urethral Pain

I. Suprapubic pain

J. Fever/Flank Pain/CVA Tenderness
1. Factors other than the site of infection probably determine the location or origin.
2. Fever and flank pain in unselected females with bacteriuria are not specific for pyelonephritis (50% are cystitis only).

III. LABORATORY FINDINGS/ RADIOGRAPHS/CYSTOSCOPY

A. **Urinalysis**

All urinalysis results will be influenced by the degree of inflammatory response, the frequency of voiding, the rate of urine flow, the growth characteristics of the organism, the previous therapy (antibiotic), and the method of collection.

1. Hematuria
   a. Originates from an inflamed epithelium and may be gross or microscopic.
2. Pyuria
   a. Two to ten WBCs per milliliter may be regarded as normal.
   b. Usually greater than 5 WBCs per high power field if infection.
   c. Pyuria without bacteria
      (1) L-forms *Chlamydia,* tuberculosis, viral, stone, foreign body, nephritis, nephrosis, *Candida,* anerobes, interstitial cystitis, ureaplasma, analgesic abuse, carcinoma in situ.
      (2) Rule out urethral or vaginal contamination.
      (3) Dipstick tests relying on the conversion of indoxyl carbonic acid ester, by leukocytes, to indigo blue are 94% sensitive but have false positives, especially with *Trichomonas* or high vitamin C ingestion.
      (4) Streptococcal infections may not have high number of WBCs.
3. Bacteriuria
   a. Approximately 50% of women with asymptomatic bacteriuria have no pyuria.
   b. Gram stain—One organism per high powered field on oil immersion correlates well with 100,000 cfu/ml. Bacteria are rarely seen if not greater than 30,000/ml.
   c. Clean catch midstream specimen
      (1) When screening large populations for inci-

dence of UTI, 100,000 cfu/ml has been determined to be "epidemiologically" useful.
(2) Most patients with UTI have greater than 1
million cfu/ml.
(3) Of women with dysuria, 33 to 45% will have
UTI with positive culture on suprapubic aspiration (SPA) and less than 10,000 organisms
on midstream urine culture.
(4) Twenty percent of true UTIs have less than
100,000 cfu/ml (counts as low as 100 cful/ml
may be significant).
(5) There is an 80% chance of significance if
count is greater than 100,000 cfu/ml on one
specimen.
(6) Ninety-one percent chance if greater than 100
million cfu/ml on two specimens
(7) Ninety-five percent of patients with clinical
pyelonephritis have greater than 100,000
cfu/ml.
    d. Straight catch specimen
       (1) Ninety-five percent chance of significance if
           greater than 100,000 cfu/ml on single
           specimen.
    e. Suprapubic aspirate
       (1) Ninety-five percent chance of significance if
           count is greater than 5000 cfu/ml on single
           specimen.

**B. Use of Intravenous Urogram (IVU), Voiding Cystoure-
throgram (VCUG), and Cystoscopy**
   1. In a study of adult females with lower urinary tract
      symptoms and recurrent UTIs, 5% of patients demon-
      strated an anatomic abnormality on IVU, but in no
      case was surgery required and the therapeutic regimen
      was unaltered. Indication for IVU would be pyelone-
      phritis, unresponsive infections, previous stone dis-
      ease, or hematuria.
   2. VCUG or double-balloon urethrogram are good meth-
      ods for determining the presence of urethral diver-
      ticula. VCUG should also be advocated to rule out

vesicoureteral reflux in children or in adults with resistant infection, pyelonephritis, or neurologic disease.
3. Cystoscopy should be advocated to rule out foreign body, stone, or anatomic abnormality of the urethra or bladder in cases of UTI unresponsive to therapy. Persistent hematuria or urgency and frequency may be signs of bladder carcinoma.

IV. CLINICAL CLASSIFICATIONS

A. Stamey Classification
1. First infection
2. Unresolved bacteriuria during therapy: implies an inability to clear the initial infection due to improper antibiotic selection or the selection or development of a resistant strain.
3. Persistent bacteriuria: brief interval of response to antibacterial treatment followed by reinfection with the same organism, with persistence due to a reservoir of bacteria (stone, urinary tract diverticulum, etc.).
4. Recurrent infection: infection with a new organism; 99% of infections that recur are of this type—they may still be *E. coli* but will be a different serotype.

B. Other Descriptive Terms
1. Asymptomatic bacteriuria
   a. Significant (greater than 1000 to 10,000 bacteria per milliliter)—bacteriuria without symptoms
   b. May or may not have tissue invasion
   c. Fifty percent in a screened population will resolve without therapy but will have a seven times greater chance of infection in the future
   d. Should probably treat all cases but should definitely treat in pregnant females—suspect anatomic abnormality if recurrent
2. Simple infection—first infection or symptoms of cystitis only
3. Complex infection—second UTI in 1 year or upper tract symptoms

4. Urethral syndrome—symptoms of UTI with negative or low count culture by routine methods
   a. Thirty to forty percent of females who have dysuria have a negative culture, but 30% of these patients at 3 months, and 60% at 6 months, will be culture positive.
   b. It is important to rule out:
      (1) Low colony count infections (especially)
      (2) *Chlamydia* (especially)
      (3) *Trichomonas* or other vaginitis (especially)
      (4) *Staphylococcus saprophyticus*
      (5) Yeast
      (6) Interstitial cystitis
      (7) External irritants
      (8) Herpes
      (9) Carcinoma in situ
   c. Treatment is often empiric and based on the differential diagnosis:
      (1) Antibiotics (culture specific for low colony count organisms or tetracycline for *Chlamydia*)
      (2) DMSO
      (3) Chlorpactin   } bladder
      (4) Steroids   } instillations
      (5) Silver nitrate
      (6) Urinary anesthetics
      (7) Estrogens
      (8) Pharmacologic bladder manipulation based on urodynamic findings (e.g., anticholinergics)
5. Interstitial cystitis
   a. A symptom complex of urgency, frequency, and, rarely, urge incontinence with suprapubic or periurethral pain on bladder filling that is somewhat improved by voiding
   b. Possibly autoimmune in nature, but allergic and infectious etiologies have been proposed
   c. Cystoscopy
      (1) Classical Hunner's ulcers (rare)
      (2) Submucosal hemorrhages, cracking of mucosa, and bleeding seen with bladder distension

    d. Decreased functional bladder capacity
    e. Decreased compliance with increased fibrosis
    f. Pathologic changes of normal, thinned, or ulcerated mucosa with nonspecific edema, inflammatory cells, and fibrosis in the submucosa and muscularis
    g. Differential diagnosis
      (1) Carcinoma in situ
      (2) Tuberculosis
      (3) Schistosomiasis
      (4) Perivesical diverticulitis or Crohn's
      (5) Chemical or pharmacologic cystitis
    h. Therapy
      (1) Pharmacologic: intravesical
        (a) Silver nitrate
        (b) DMSO
        (c) Oxychlorosene sodium (Chlorpactin)
        (d) Bladder distension under anesthesia
      (2) Surgical
        (a) Bladder denervation or transection
        (b) Bladder augmentation
        (c) Urinary diversion (with or without cystectomy)

V. TREATMENT (FOR UNCOMPLICATED UTI)

A. Single-Dose Regimens
1. Amoxicillin 3 g
2. Sulfisoxazole 2 g
3. Trimethoprim (TMP) 160 mg with sulfamethoxazole (SMZ) 800 mg
4. Nitrofurantoin 100 mg

B. Three-day Regimens

C. Standard Oral Regimens
1. Sulfisoxazole 2 g, then 1 to 2 g q.i.d. for 10 days
2. Nitrofurantoin 50 mg q.i.d. for 7 to 10 days
3. Cephalexin 500 mg q.i.d. for 7 to 10 days
4. TMP 160 mg SMZ 800 mg b.i.d. for 7 to 10 days

a. Acidification of the urine will enhance the action of the aforementioned antibiotics.

b. Long-term treatment is believed to decrease the chance of reinfection though there are little data to substantiate this claim.

c. Treatment of females with frequent uncomplicated infections by allowing the patient to take previously prescribed antibiotics at home with the onset of symptoms is advocated by some. If symptoms persist, increase, or upper tract symptoms are present, the patient is then seen for an office visit.

d. Treatment of recurrent ''honeymoon cystitis'' is a regimen of daily prophylactic antibiotic (one tablet of nitrofurantoin or TMP-SMX), voiding after intercourse, and perineal hygiene. This can be decreased to antibiotic therapy (one tablet) taken with intercourse only).

VI. UTI AND PREGNANCY

A. Four to seven percent incidence of bacteriuria in pregnant females.

B. Thirty percent of infected patients will have symptoms (25% of pregnant women with sterile urine will have symptoms).

C. Twenty to thirty percent if untreated will develop pyelonephritis in the last trimester and treatment will reduce this number.

D. Pyelonephritis is associated with prematurity.

1. The bacteriuric group has a higher incidence of prematurity, hypertension, and bacteriuria after pregnancy, but treatment does *not* improve these statistics.

E. Penicillin, nitrofurantoin, and cephalosporins have been shown to be safe and effective.

1. Sulfonamides should not be used in the last 4 to 6 weeks of pregnancy.

2. Aminoglycosides, tetracyclines, and chloramphenicol should be avoided.

VII. ORGANISMS

A. *E. coli*—75 to 95% of simple UTIs

B. *Klebsiella*—5%

C. *Enterobacter*—2%

D. *Proteus*—2%

E. *Pseudomonas*—hospital acquired

F. *Streptococcus faecalis*

G. *Staphylococcus saprophytious* (? up to 10%)

H. *Candida*

I. Adenovirus 11/21

J. *Chlamydia*

K. *Ureaplasma/Mycoplasma*

APPENDIX: SAMPLE PATIENT INFORMATION GUIDE

1. Cystitis (inflammation of the bladder) is almost always due to germs or bacteria from the bowel. The condition is common in women because of the short female bladder passage (urethra), which ends so close to the bowel opening and which is usually the site of the initial colonization by bacteria. Bacteria can ascend from the skin to the bladder at any time but are particularly liable to do so during sexual intercourse.

2. Means to Help Prevent or Limit Infection
   Bacteria that cause urinary tract infections often establish themselves in the area of the vagina and the skin around the anus. This is especially true in women who suffer from recurrent urinary tract infections. The following recommendations may help to decrease the frequency of infections in women so afflicted.

   a. After a bowel movement, the skin should be cleansed gently only in the direction from front to back.

   b. Underclothes should be changed more frequently than necessary for ordinary social hygiene.

c. A good wash, bath, or shower before intercourse is clearly advisable. This is probably a good idea for the sexual partner as well.

d. The bladder should be emptied immediately after intercourse. This washes out any bacteria that may, in spite of all precautions, have entered the urethra and the bladder.

e. During the day, an effort should be made to void frequently and completely. This prevents the buildup of bacteria in the bladder and symptomatic infection.

BIBLIOGRAPHY

Jenkins RD, Fenn JP, Matsen JM: Review of urine microscopy for bacteriuria. JAMA 255:3397–3403, 1986.

Schröder FH (ed): Recent Advances in the Treatment of Urinary Tract Infections. London: Royal Society of Medicine, International Congress and Symposium Series, no. 97, 1985.

Stamey TA: Pathogenesis and Treatment of Urinary Tract Infections. Baltimore: Williams & Wilkins, 1980.

5

Lower Urinary Tract Infections in Men

Roger E. Schultz

I. INCIDENCE

A. Asymptomatic Infections

Asymptomatic infections are rare: they are estimated to be present in less than 0.6% men under 60 years, 1.5% men aged 60 to 69 years, and 3.6% men over 70 years.

B. Symptomatic Infection

Incidence of symptomatic infection is 10% that of women and usually suggests underlying pathology. Cystitis, per se, is normally secondary to a primary infection of the prostate or kidney. When diagnosed, it should indicate need for further urologic evaluation (unlike cystitis in most women, for whom urologic workup is not rewarding).

C. Recurrent Urinary Infections

Recurrent infections are often seen after urologic instrumentation (i.e., iatrogenic). In the absence of obstruction (e.g., benign prostatic hypertrophy, urethral stricture), urinary stasis (e.g., neuropathic bladder), a foreign body (e.g., urethral catheter), or calculus disease, recurrent urinary infections will usually be traced to bacterial persistence in prostatic fluid.

II. PATHOGENESIS

A. Source

Ascending infection from the urethra is more common than hematogenous/lymphatogenous spread or extension from adjacent organ (e.g., sigmoid diverticulitis).

B. **Pathogens**

Escherichia coli is found in 80% of infections; *Klebsiella, Enterobacter, Proteus, Pseudomonas,* and *Serratia* organisms are also found, and *Streptococcus faecalis* and *Staphlococcus* are occasionally found. More than one bacterium is seen in 15 to 20% of cases of bacterial prostatitis or in presence of foreign body, calculus, or urinary fistula.

C. **Host Resistance**

1. Hydrokinetic clearance of bacteria—washout effect of urine as it passes through urethra.
2. Mucoprotein on mucosal surface of bladder—prevents bacterial adherence.
3. Prostatic Antibacterial Factor (PAF)—Zinc salt isolated 1973 with antimicrobial activity against gram-negative organisms. Prostatic zinc levels are lower in men with chronic bacterial prostatitis; zinc replacement has not been proven to be clinically useful in treatment, however.

III. LOCALIZATION OF LOWER URINARY INFECTION

A. **Segmented Bacteriologic Localization Cultures (Fig. 1)**

Following cleansing of glans, patient initiates urination and physician collects 5 to 10 ml of urine first voided in sterile container close to meatus (VB 1). A sterile midstream urine is obtained after voiding about 200 ml (VB 2). Patient is then asked to stop voiding. Prostatic massage is conducted, following which the expressed prostatic secretion is collected from the meatus (EPS). Gentle proximal to distal pressure exerted on bulbar urethra will help "milk" secretions forward. Immediately following prostatic massage patient voids and specimen (VB 3) is collected in same manner as VB 1. Standard bacteriologic methods used to identify organisms in cultures.

1. Urethral colonization/urethritis—colony count VB 1 > EPS/VB 3
2. Prostatic infection—EPS/VB 3 > VB 1
3. VB 2 positive indicates cystitis. Treat for 4 to 5 days

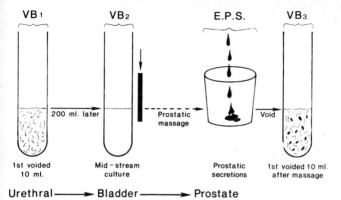

Figure 1. Bacterial localization procedure for male lower tract infection (see text).

with antibiotic that will not diffuse into prostate and then repeat localizing studies.

B. Antibody Coating of Bacteria
This is seen with both infections originating in kidneys and prostate and is not clinically useful.

IV. BACTERIAL CYSTITIS

A. Signs/Symptoms
Urinary frequency, urgency, dysuria, nocturia, suprapubic discomfort, low back pain, and, occasionally, gross hematuria are the principal symptoms of bacterial cystitis. Systemic symptoms of fever, chills, and rigors are absent.

B. Laboratory Results
U/A shows heavy pyuria, bacteriuria. No casts are seen. Urine culture and sensitivity shows more than 10^5 colonies per milliliter.

C. Therapy
Based upon results of urine C&S. Evaluate for renal/prostatic source with IV urography, segmented lo-

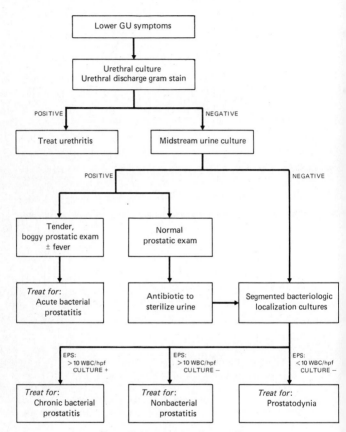

Figure 2. Management of prostatitis.

calization cultures; consider cystoscopy when urine
sterile.

V. PROSTATITIS/PROSTATODYNIA (Fig. 2)

A. General

Inflammatory processes affecting prostate are sub-
categorized into four groups (Table 1). Careful history and

TABLE 1. CLASSIFICATION OF PROSTATITIS

Condition	Pain—Perineum, Groin, Back	Fever, Chills, Rigors	Rectal Exam	EPS— WBC's/Culture	Therapy
Acute Bacterial prostatitis	+	Frequent	Warm, boggy, tender	Massage not advised (Enterobacteriaceae)	Aminoglycoside
Chronic bacterial prostatitis	+	—	Indurated, tender, or normal	>10 WBC/hpf (Enterobacteriaceae)	TMP-SMX: carbenicillin indanyl sodium
Nonbacterial prostatitis	+	—	Normal	>10 WBC/hpf Culture negative	Antiinflammatory Sitz Baths, prostatic massage
Prostatodynia	+	—	Normal	No WBC's Culture negative	Reassurance, occasionally, phenoxybenzamine

physical exam, evaluation of urine, and EPS are critical to evaluation.

B. **Acute Bacterial Prostatitis**
1. *Signs/Symptoms.* Urinary frequency, urgency, dysuria, nocturia, malaise; often with abrupt onset of high fever, chills, low back/perineal pain; occasionally urinary retention. Exquisitely tender, boggy, prostate (do NOT massage—risk of bacteremia).
2. *Laboratory Results.* Leukocytosis, pyuria, bacteriuria. *E. coli* most commonly isolated.
3. *Therapy.* TMP-SMX pending culture results. General toxemia or inability to void warrant hospitalization for IV hydration and antibiotics (e.g., ampicillin and gentamicin pending culture results), antipyretics, analgesics, bed rest, and, occasionally, suprapubic cystotomy tube for urinary retention.
4. *Complications.* Abscess formation that may require transperineal incision and drainage or transurethral drainage.

C. **Chronic Bacterial Prostatitis**
1. *Signs/Symptoms.* Irritative voiding symptoms similar to acute prostatitis but with more insidious onset, absence of systemic illness or fever, persistent perineal/low back pain, and, occasionally, painful ejaculation, hematospermia, and/or arthralgias/myalgias. Prostate is normal to examination.
2. *Laboratory Results.* Localizing cultures (EPS—inflammatory cells and bacteria). Commonly, patients present with recurrent bacteriuria (usually same pathogen) between courses of antibiotic therapy. Needle biopsy of prostate is useless.
3. *Therapy.* Trimethoprim sulfamethoxazole (TMP-SMF) or carbenicilin indanyl sodium for 2 months due to problem of antibiotic access; sitz baths. Failure of therapy may indicate need for parenteral antibiotics (e.g., aminoglycosides for 3 days), followed by resumption of oral antibiotics. It may be necessary to consider chronic prophylaxis (e.g., TMP-SMX qHS) or transurethral prostatectomy (TURP) (cure rate with TURP 30%).

D. Nonbacterial Prostatitis

Prostatosis is the most common form.

1. *Signs/Symptoms.* As for chronic bacterial prostatitis.
2. *Etiology. Chlamydia, Ureaplasma,* herpes simplex, chemical (urinary reflux), and, possibly, prostaglandins.
3. *Laboratory Results.* EPS shows more than 12 inflammatory cells per high power field but NO bacteria.
4. *Therapy.* Prostatic massage, Sitz baths, antiinflammatory agents, sedatives, reassurance, trial of tetracyclines.

E. Prostatodynia (Prostate Pain Without Prostatic Infection or Inflammation)

1. *Signs/Symptoms.* As for chronic bacterial prostatitis.
2. *Laboratory Results.* Absence of inflammatory cells or bacteria in localizing studies.
3. *Therapy.* Reassurance; if symptom complex includes hesitancy and slow stream, consider α-adrenergic blocker (e.g., Prazosin, Phenoxybenzamine) to relax bladder neck.

F. Other Prostatic Infections

Tuberculous, mycotic, viral parasitic, nonspecific granulomatous, allergic granulomatous.

VI. ANTIMICROBIAL THERAPY OF PROSTATITIS

A. General

It is not possible to achieve therapeutic tissue levels of many antimicrobials due to poor passage of drug from plasma into prostatic ducts and acini. Only with acute bacterial prostatitis does the intense inflammatory response allow diffusion of drug into prostate with dramatic recovery.

B. Optimal Characteristics for Diffusion

1. Gram-negative spectrum
2. Limited protein binding
3. Lipid soluble
4. High pK_a—Maximizes trapping of ionized form of

drug within the normally acidic prostatic fluid (pH = 6.4). This is why TMP-SMX, a basic drug, has proved useful. However, recent studies have shown that *infected* prostatic fluid may have pH near to, if not greater than, plasma. A relatively alkaline prostatic fluid would favor ion trapping of an acidic drug, such as carbenicillin. Some investigators feel that the clinical improvement and bacteriologic cure rate are best with carbenicillin. More research and clinical drug trials will be needed to find the optimal therapy for chronic bacterial prostatitis.

VII. SEMINAL VESICULITIS

A. General
Seminal vesiculitis is rarely diagnosed unless there is hard, swollen mass above prostate in presence of UTI.

B. Relation to Infertility
This has never been proven. Studies demonstrating bacteria in ejaculatory cultures of infertile men are invalidated due to probable contamination of these cultures by urethral organisms.

VIII. EPIDIDYMITIS

A. Etiology
1. Sexually transmitted—gonococcal or nongonococcal, urethral discharge common.
2. Nonsexually transmitted
   a. Tuberculous—beading of vas deferens.
   b. Secondary to systemic infection—e.g., *Haemophilus influenza*.
   c. Secondary to GU infection—enteric pathogens.
   d. Following TURP—reflux of urine down vas deferens.

B. Signs/Symptoms
Painful, swollen epididymis, occasionally with high fever and symptoms of cystitis. Tenderness can extend to groin or lower abdominal quadrant of affected side. Boggy epi-

didymis, thickened spermatic cord, reactive hydrocele (common), occasionally with urethral discharge.

C. Laboratory Results
The presence or absence of leukocytosis and pyuria/bacteriuria are determined.

D. Differential Diagnosis
1. Testicular abscess
2. Testis tumor—usually painless
3. Torsion of spermatic cord/appendix testis
4. Testicular trauma
5. Mumps orchitis

E. Therapy
Bed rest, scrotal elevation and support, analgesics, and, occasionally, cord block with bupivicaine are recommended therapies. Antibiotics are given—tetracycline and doxycycline in men under 35 where *Chlamydia* is likely agent and cephalosporin or penicillin in older men to treat probable gram-negative etiology.

IX. URETHRITIS (Fig. 3)

A. General
There are two main groupings, which are readily separated (Table 2).

B. Gonococcal Urethritis
1. *Epidemiology.* Peak group 20 to 24 years, 66% men can be asymptomatic carriers.
2. *Etiology. Neisseria gonorrhea*—intracellular gram-negative diplococci; 98% picked up by GC culture of characteristic discharge.
3. *Pathogenesis.* Three to four day incubation to exudative polymorphonuclear cell response (urethral discharge) to microabscesses beginning in glands of Littre to lymphangitis/inguinal lymphadenitis to denuded epithelium replaced by fibrobasts. Urethral stricture can ultimately develop. Process can extend to vas and globus minor and, if bilateral, can lead to infertility.

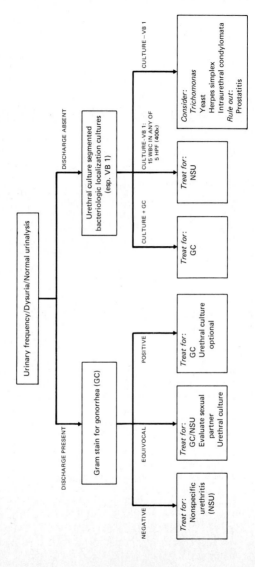

Figure 3. Management of urethritis in men.

142

TABLE 2. CLASSIFICATION OF URETHRITIS

		Gonococcal	Nongonococcal
I.	Epidemiology		
	A. Ethnic group	Mostly black	Mostly white
	B. Socioeconomic group	Lower	Higher
	C. Prevalence among homosexuals	High	Low
II.	Pathogen	*N. gonorrhea*	*C. trachomatis, U. urealyticum* = 80% Other-herpes simplex, *Trichomonas*, warts
III.	Incubation Period	Usually 3 to 10 days	1 to 5 weeks
IV.	Symptoms	Purulent discharge	Thin, mucoid discharge
V.	Gram Stain	Gram-negative diplococci	Negative
VI.	Therapy	Probenecid and penicillin, or tetracycline, for 7 days Treat patient's sexual partner	Tetracycline or Erythromycin for 7 days Treat patient's sexual partner

4. *Laboratory Results.* Gram stain of urethral discharge; chocolate agar culture.
5. *Therapy*
   a. 1 g probenecid (PO)+ 4.8 × 10⁶ procaine PCN (IM)
   b. 1 g probenecid (PO)+ ampicillin 3.5 g (PO) or amoxicillin 3.0 g (PO)
   c. Tetracycline 500 mg PO q.i.d. for 7 days
   d. For penicillinase-producing *N. gonorrhea*—spectinomycin 2 g (IM)
   e. Remember to treat patient's sexual partner

C. Postgonococcal Urethritis

1. *Etiology.* See in 30 to 60% of men about 1 to 3 weeks after treatment of gonococcal urethritis. Only seen in 25% men initially treated with Tetracycline. Fifty percent of cases secondary to *Chlamydia trachomatis*.

2. *Symptoms.* Asymtomatic pyuria, rarely dysuria.
3. *Therapy.* Tetracycline.

D. **Nongonococcal Urethritis**
   1. *Epidemiology.* Sixty-six percent of cases of acute urethritis, more than 80% of cases among college males.
   2. *Etiology.* Eighty percent related to either *C. trachomatis* or *Ureaplasma urealyticum.* Remaining cases possibly related to herpes simplex, *Candida albicans, Trichomonas,* intraurethral condyloma acuminata, or foreign body.
   3. *Therapy.* Tetracycline 500 mg PO q.i.d. for 7 days, or erythromycin 500 mg PO q.i.d. for 7 days. Incomplete or failed response may indicate Tetracycline-resistant *Ureaplasma, Trichomonal* infection, or urethral obstruction. Try erythromycin or doxycycline. If no improvement, consider retrograde urethrography and/or cystoscopy to rule out obstruction (e.g., urethral stricture or condylomata).

E. **Reiter's Syndrome**
   1. *Etiology.* Less than 1% of all cases of urethritis; 30% have chlamydial infection; associated with ankylosing spondylitis, HLA B-27.
   2. *Symptom complex.* Appears 1 to 4 weeks after onset of urethritis.
      a. Ocular. Conjunctivitis/severe anterior uveitis.
      b. Arthritis. Large joints of lower extremities, sacroiliac, Achilles' tendon.
      c. Skin. Circinate balanitis 80%; Hyperkeratotic keratodermia blenorrhagica—especially of soles of feet.
   3. *Therapy.* Tetracycline, which clears only the urethritis.

BIBLIOGRAPHY

Bowie WR: Nongonococcal urethritis. In Berger RE (ed): Urologic Clinics of North America. Sexually Transmitted Diseases. Philadelphia: W.B. Saunders, 1984, pp. 55–64.

Drach GW, Meares EM Jr. et al: Classification of benign diseases associated with prostatic pain: Prostatitis or prostatodynia? J Urol 120:266, 1978.

Fair, WR, Couch J, Wehner N: Prostatic antibacterial factor: Identity and significance. Urology 7:169, 1976.

Jacobs NF Jr, Kraus SJ: Gonococcal and nongonococcal urethritis in men: Clinical and laboratory differentiation. Ann Intern Med 82:7, 1975.

Meares EM Jr: Urinary tract infections in men. In Harrison JH, et al (eds): Campbell's Urology. Philadelphia: W.B. Saunders, 1978, vol 1, chap 13, pp 509–537.

Meares EM Jr, Stamey TA: Bacteriologic localization patterns in bacterial prostatitis and urethritis. Invest Urol 5:492, 1968.

Mobley DF: Bacterial prostatitis: Treatment with carbenicillin indanyl sodium. Invest Urol 19:31, 1981.

Schacter J: Chlamydial infections (3 parts). N Engl J Med 298:428, 490, 540, 1978.

Stamey TA: Urinary infections in males. In: Pathogenesis and Treatment of Urinary Tract Infections. Baltimore: Williams & Wilkins, 1980, chap 7, pp 342–429.

Stamey TA, Meares EM Jr, Winningham DG: Chronic bacterial prostatitis and diffusion of drugs into prostatic fluid. J Urol 103:187, 1970.

6

Pyelonephritis

Jeffrey P. Weiss

I. INTRODUCTION

A. Definition

Pyelonephritis is the term denoting infection of the upper urinary tract, that is, kidney and renal pelvis. There are two forms: acute and chronic.

1. Acute pyelonephritis is characterized by acute suppuration accompanied by fever, flank pain, bacteruria, and pyuria.
2. Repeated attacks of acute pyelonephritis lead to progressive renal scarring, usually asymmetric and irregular, involving both the cortex and pelvic–calyceal system (chronic pyelonephritis).

II. DIAGNOSIS AND CLINICAL CHARACTERISTICS

A. Diagnosis

1. The diagnosis of pyelonephritis is usually made on clinical grounds. The definitive diagnostic method is catheterization of ureters and renal pelvis for urinalysis (revealing pyuria and bacteruria) and culture. This is unnecessarily invasive, however.
2. Routine urinalysis reveals white cell casts.
3. Bacterial antibodies, if present, suggest upper tract infection. There are, however, a significant proportion of false positives using this criterion.
4. The Fairly bladder washout test obtains culture of ureteral urine without ureteral catheterization by

culturing urine in the bladder after residual bladder urine is washed out.

5. Radiographic methods include intravenous urography (more useful in chronic than acute pyelonephritis in defining areas of cortical scarring), radionuclide studies (using iodine-131-labeled hippuran to detect abnormalities in renal blood flow in conjunction with gallium-67 scans to pick up areas of inflammation) and voiding cystourethrography (conventional radiographic or nuclear scanning techniques) to document the presence of vesicoureteral reflux. The latter is a major etiologic factor in pyelonephritis.

6. Renal biopsy with bacterial tissue culture is mentioned only to be condemned not only because of excessive risk to the patient but also due to the focal nature of renal infection which may be easily missed by a random renal biopsy.

7. Because renal concentrating ability is impaired in pyelonephritis, it has been suggested that demonstration of impaired renal concentrating mechanism in the presence of bacteriuria implies pyelonephritis as opposed to lower tract infection. However, this parameter is nonspecific owing to statistical overlap in concentrating abilities between patients with upper and lower urinary tract infections.

B. Clinical Characteristics

1. It is usually sufficient to note that patients with pyelonephritis present with fever, flank pain, costovertebral angle (CVA) tenderness, and infected urine.

2. Bladder and urethral irritation may exist, along with systemic malaise, nausea, and vomiting.

3. Severe cases may cause sepsis, hypotension, and death in a compromised host.

4. Acute pyelonephritis may be self-limited. However, multiple bouts may lead to progressive loss of tubules, thereby impairing renal concentrating ability. This is followed by glomerular damage late in the course (chronic pyelonephritis), producing azotemia and hypertension.

III. ETIOLOGY AND RISK FACTORS

A. **Major Etiologic Factors in the Pathogenesis of Pyelonephritis**
   1. The first, and by far the most common, factor is vesicoureteral reflux (VUR) of infected urine. However, not all patients with reflux of infected urine into the renal pelvis will sustain renal damage. This leads to the concept of intrarenal reflux, or pyelotubular reflux, the absence of which is felt to be protective to the renal tubules and parenchyma.
   2. Obstruction of the urinary tract for any cause contributes to pyelonephritis due to stasis and disabling of the washout mechanisms of urinary clearance of bacteria. Such obstruction may be congenital (e.g., ureteropelvic junction obstruction), acquired (e.g., stone disease) or associated with pregnancy (unilateral, usually right-sided, ureteral obstruction by the gravid uterus).
   3. The third potential mechanism of bacterial invasion of the kidney is hematogenous. However, bacteria are unlikely to seat in the kidney in the absence of urinary obstruction. A fourth possible route of bacterial implantation in the kidney is via lymphatics, although this mechanism has been discounted.

B. **Risk Factors Increasing Vulnerability to Pyelonephritis**
   1. Instrumentation
   2. *Diabetes Mellitus*. Diabetics are more prone to pyelonephritis due to increased substrate availability in the kidney. Increased parenchymal destruction by gas-forming organisms leads to rare complication of diabetes, emphysematous pyelonephritis, treatment of which is nephrectomy.
   3. *Neurogenic Bladder*. This condition provides the urologist with a complex array of problems, among which are urinary retention, high-pressure vesicoureteral reflux, hydronephrosis, and renal calculi.
   4. *Age*. In general, the frequency of bacteriuria increases with age, with accelerated increases due to sexual ac-

tivity in young women and prostatic enlargement with
urinary retention in elderly males.

5. *Sex*. Females are more likely to develop bacteruria due
to the short urethra in close proximity to the GI tract
and favorable milieu for bacterial proliferation compared with the male urethra.

All of these especially promote the severity and persistence of infection in these patients' kidneys.

IV. BACTERIOLOGY

A. Causative Agents

The origin of most bacteria causing pyelonephritis is from
fecal flora. The majority of uncomplicated cases of
pyelonephritis is caused by *E. coli*. Less common
causative agents are

1. *Proteus*
2. *Pseudomonas*
3. *Enterobacter*
4. *Klebsiella*
5. *Enterococcus*
6. *Staphylococcus*

Of interest is infection with *P. mirabilis* and some strains
of *Klebsiella* that contain the enzyme urease, which is
capable of splitting urea with the production of ammonia
and an alkaline environment. The latter is favorable for
precipitation of the salt struvite, or magnesium ammonium phosphate. Struvite tends to settle into branched
calculi that harbor bacteria in their interstices; these calculi are extremely resistant to antibiotic therapy. Thus,
eradication of infection in the presence of struvite calculi
involves both antimicrobial therapy and complete removal
of these "infection stones."

B. Adherence

Since most bacteria contaminating the urinary tract are
washed away before causing infection, it must be that
those bacteria initiating infection somehow become ad-

herent to the urothelium. Adherence is a property of bacteria afforded by fimbriated extensions of the cell wall (pili) that attach to uromucoid or glycolipid receptors of urothelial cells. An additional property of bacteria enabling establishment of infection in the kidney is endotoxin, causing inhibition of ureteral motility, with attendant stasis, ureteral dilatation, and enhancement of low-pressure intrarenal reflux at the level of the renal papilla. Thus, adhesiveness and endotoxins are major weapons of bacteria in causing urothelial infection.

V. CONTRIBUTIONS OF IMMUNE AND INFLAMMATORY RESPONSE

If adhesiveness and endotoxin promote bacterial infection in the urinary tract, the immune response stems the tide against cellular damage.

A. Antibody Response
Bacterial invasion of the kidney brings forth primarily a humoral (antibody) response as opposed to cell-mediated immunity.

B. Inflammatory Response
Activation of the complement cascade attracts polymorphonuclear leukocytes (chemotaxis) that phagocytize bacteria while at the same time causing release of metabolites (known as superoxide radicals, $0_2{}^-$) that damage not only bacteria but also surrounding normal host tissue (e.g., renal tubules).

Thus, renal tissue becomes an ''innocent bystander'' in this subcellular biochemical skirmish, the basis of renal injury in pyelonephritis. There is evidence that suppression of superoxide radicals by administration of the enzyme superoxide dismutase may reduce the inflammatory response and its attendant tissue destruction. A summary of the pathogenesis of pyelonephritis is offered in Figure 1.

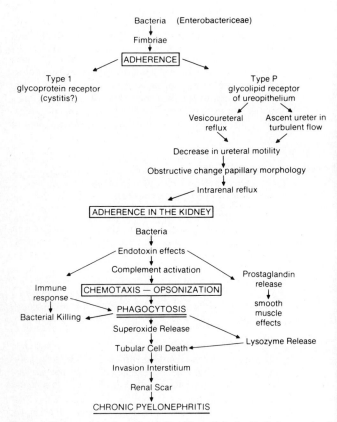

Figure 1. Pathogenesis of pyelonephritis. (*From Roberts JA: Pathogenesis of Pyelonephritis. Houston, TX: American Urological Association, 1983.*)

VI. SPECIAL CASE: XANTHOGRANULOMATOUS PYELONEPHRITIS (XGP)

A. Definition

XGP is an unusual inflammatory lesion of the kidney associated with stones and chronic renal infection.

B. Symptoms and Signs

Aside from the usual symptoms of pyelonephritis, XGP frequently causes nonfunction and often a mass lesion in the kidney. Perirenal fat may be involved with the adjacent subcapsular inflammatory response.

C. Bacteriology

Proteus and *E. coli* comprise the majority of bacterial agents associated with XGP.

D. Pathology

Grossly, these kidneys consist of nodular masses laden with fat. Histopathologic examination reveals a granulomatous type of chronic inflammation.

E. Treatment

The major difficulty with this entity is its distinction from a malignant lesion, notably renal cell carcinoma; radiologic studies may be ambiguous. XGP is usually treated with nephrectomy.

VII. PATHOLOGY

A. Histopathologic Characteristics

Acute pyelonephritis is characterized by the presence of acute inflammation and focal abscess formation in random areas of the kidney (Fig. 2).

B. Pathogenesis

1. *Acute Pyelonephritis.* Infection begins in the interstitium and spreads to destroy tubules, giving rise to white cell casts seen in urinalysis. Gomeruli are characteristically resistant to acute infection. As the cortex is more vascular than the medulla, greater inflammation is present both cortically and in the subcapsular area despite the fact that bacterial invasion may begin in the medulla (Fig. 3). A collection of purulent exudate extending out of the subcapsular area gives rise to a perinephric abscess.

2. *Chronic Pyelonephritis.* As these abscesses in and about the kidney heal they become replaced with contracted scar tissue infiltrated by chronic inflammato-

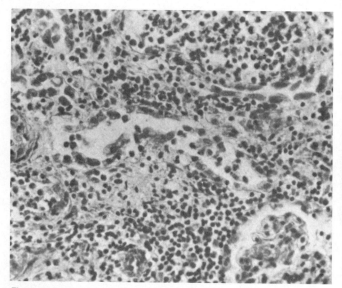

Figure 2. Acute pyelonephritis marked by an acute neutrophilic exudate within the tubules and renal substance. (*From Robbins SL: Pathologic Basis of Disease. Philadelphia: W.B. Saunders, 1974.*)

ry cells (lymphocytes, plasma cells). These form the basis of the distorted cortical and pyelocalyceal anatomy seen in chronic pyelonephritis (Fig. 4). As in acute pyelonephritis, damage to tubules is great while glomeruli tend to be spared.

3. *Thyroidism.* A particular pattern of tubular damage consisting of dilated tubules filled with proteinaceous material is called "thyroidization" (Fig. 5).

4. Collectively, the scarring process in chronic pyelonephritis produces the familiar small, irregularly shaped kidney in its end stage (Fig. 6).

VIII. COMPLICATIONS

A. Renal Insufficiency

The small kidney resulting from chronic pyelonephritis contributes to progressive azotemia and chronic renal

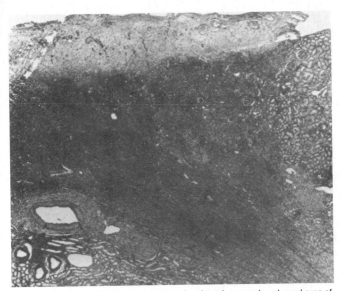

Figure 3. Section (×18) of the renal cortex showing a large wedge-shaped area of the acute and chronic inflammation extending from the medulla to the cortex. The large vessels are not involved with inflammatory reaction. (*From Stamey TA, Pfan A: Invest Urol 1:134, 1963.*)

failure. In particular, 13% of patients with end-stage renal disease have chronic pyelonephritis as its primary etiologic factor.

B. Hypertension

In addition, one-half to three-quarters of patients with chronic pyelonephritis are hypertensive. The mechanism of hypertension in this disease is probably due to fibrosis of the renal parenchyma, with resulting ischemia and secondary activation of the renin–angiotensin system. Although hypertension may accelerate progressive renal failure, the fact that nephrectomy often cures hypertension associated with unilateral chronic pyelonephritis suggests that the renal disease caused the hypertension in these patients and not vice-versa.

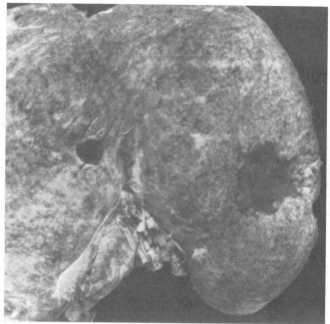

Figure 4. Focal chronic pyelonephritis. A small scar with a dark inflammatory base. (*From Robbins SL: Pathologic Basis of Disease. Philadelphia: W.B. Saunders, 1974.*)

IX. TREATMENT

A. Acute

1. Acute pyelonephritis is managed with intravenous hydration and antibiotic therapy (usually a penicillin and an aminoglycoside) begun after obtaining blood and urine samples for culture.

2. Control of pain and nausea is also helpful. Occasionally patients will respond to oral antibiotics and hydration if nausea is not a limiting factor. This is more common in children than in adults.

3. Exclusion of urinary obstruction should be made with intravenous urography and/or ultrasonography.

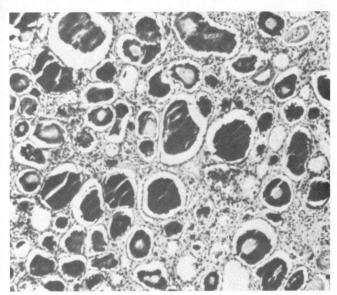

Figure 5. A large area of scarring to illustrate a "thyroid-like" area. (*From Robbins SL: Pathologic Basis of Disease. Philadelphia: W.B. Saunders, 1974.*)

  4. The pediatric patient should be additionally studied with voiding cystourethrography, either radiographically or with nuclear scanning techniques. The disadvantage of the latter is inability to grade the reflux, a consideration in selection of patients for antireflux surgery.

B. Chronic

  In chronic pyelonephritis the physician must search for predisposing risk factors such as obstructive uropathy, reflux, or struvite calculi. These factors should be treated surgically, occasionally in conjunction with the use of chronic suppression with the appropriate urinary antiseptic (e.g., Nitrofurantoin or trimethoprim sulfamethoxisole). Patients with a unilaterally scarred, contracted kidney in addition to hypertension may be candidates for nephrectomy in order to protect the normal kidney from

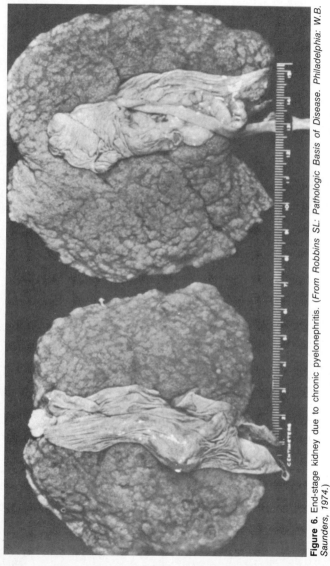

Figure 6. End-stage kidney due to chronic pyelonephritis. (From Robbins SL: Pathologic Basis of Disease. Philadelphia: W.B. Saunders, 1974.)

nephrosclerosis, exacerbation of the hypertension, and progressive renal disease.

X. CONCLUSION

The salient features of this discussion of pyelonephritis include distinction of acute from chronic forms, methods of diagnosis and treatment, and identification of risk factors, causative agents, and underlying mechanisms of tissue damage found in this disease. Pyelonephritis is a clinical diagnosis that may be supported by many other tests. Intravenous urography and voiding cystourethrography remain the mainstay of adjunctive diagnostic methods. Treatment should be aimed at the acute form, with the intent of reducing the incidence of its chronic form and attendant complications. Although the bacteriology and corresponding antimicrobial therapy are straightforward, the discussion of more recent advances in understanding of immunologic and biochemical mechanisms at work in pyelonephritis hold promise for greater success in treatment directed at halting the transformation of acute into chronic pyelonephritis.

BIBLIOGRAPHY

Fridovich I: Superoxide radical: An endogenous toxicant. Annu Rev Pharmacol Toxicol 23:239, 1983.

Harrison JH, Gittes RF, et al (eds): Campbell's Urology. Philadelphia: W.B. Saunders, 1978.

Janson KL, Roberts JA, et al: Noninvasive localization of urinary tract infections clinical investigations and experience. J Urol 130:488, 1983.

Robbins SL: Pathologic Basis of Disease. Philadelphia: W.B. Saunders, 1974.

Roberts JA: Pathogenesis of Pyelonephritis. AUA Update Series, vol II, lesson 8. Houston, TX: American Urological Association, Office of Education, Texas, 1983.

Roberts JA: Pathogenesis of pyelonephritis. J Urol 129:1102, 1983.

Stamey TA: Pathogenesis and Treatment of Urinary Tract Infections. Baltimore: Williams & Wilkins, 1980.

Stamey TA, Pfan A: Some functional, pathologic, bacteriologic, and chemotherapeutic characteristics of unilateral pyelonephritis in man. Invest Urol 1:134, 1963.

7

Urolithiasis

Victor L. Carpiniello

I. INTRODUCTION

A. History
Men who influenced early stone treatment
1. Hippocrates—referred to practice of cutting for stone done by wandering lithotomists.
2. Galen—described renal colic in Book VI of *De Locis Affectis*.
3. Dupuytren—developed instrument for perineal extraction of bladder stones.
4. Bigelow—pioneered methods of lithotripsy still used today.

B. Incidence
1. General
   a. In the United States—annual incidence of stone disease is greater than 1:1000.
   b. Peak age incidence occurs in the third to fifth decades.
   c. Male-to-female ratio of 3:1. However, stones associated with urinary tract infection are more common in females.
   d. Annual patient cost for urolithiasis in the United States is greater than 48 million dollars.
2. Specific stone incidences
   a. Calcium oxalate—33%
   b. Mixed calcium oxalate and phosphate—34%
   c. Magnesium ammonium phosphate—15%
   d. Uric acid—8%
   e. Calcium phosphate—6%
   f. Cystine—3%

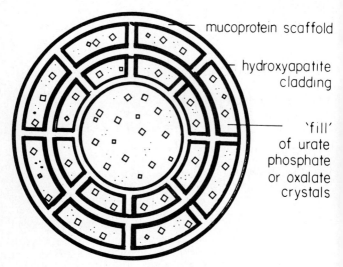

Figure 1. Diagrammatic representation of calculus structure (see text).

C. Structure of Urinary Calculi (Fig. 1)
1. Matrix core called the sperule arranged in layers suggestive of growth rings of a tree.
2. Sperule is supported by an organic scaffold structure filled with crystalline materials (see Etiology).

II. ETIOLOGY

A. Factors Causing Stone Disease
1. Genetic
   a. Enzyme disorders—cystinuria, renal tubular acidosis, decreased renal activity of aldolase, tubular reabsorptive defect of uric acid and ochronosis. All can be associated with urolithiasis.
2. Environmental
   a. Geographic influence related to temperature and humidity—high temperatures causing fluid loss, leading to increase in urinary concentration and decrease in urinary pH.

       (1) Notable occurrences in "stone belt" area of Southeast United States.

    b. Diet—can cause excesses or deficiencies that lead to stone formation, e.g., leafy green vegetables high in oxalate concentration can cause oxalate stones.

  3. Physical and chemical parameters

    a. Supersaturation—can cause stones because beyond this point spontaneous nucleation of crystals begins. Crystal bridging leads to crystal aggregation. Epitaxy is the oriented overgrowth of one type of crystal on the surface of a preexisting crystal of a different type (e.g., uric acid with calcium oxalate overgrowth).

    b. Urinary inhibitors—citrate, urea, pyrophosphate, magnesium, zinc, and alanine all occur in urine and have been proposed as inhibitors of stone formation. A deficiency will lead to stone formation.

    c. Matrix—group of antigenically distinct proteins found in urine and stones of stone formers. It is this noncrystalline derivative of the mucoprotein of urine that appears to bind calcium more readily than the normal mucoprotein of non–stone formers. Can be involved as constituent of urinary stones from as low as 1% to as high as 95% in so-called matrix stones.

B. Specific Stone Types and Their Causes

  1. Calcium stone

    a. Calcium oxalate stones—most common. Calcium carbonate and calcium phosphate are other types usually found in upper tracts. Commonly all caused by supersaturation of urine with calcium.

    b. Causes of urinary supersaturation with calcium

       (1) Intestinal hyperabsorption of calcium—"absorptive type"—seen with vitamin D intoxication, sarcoidosis, large carbohydrate load, and hyperparathyroidism.

       (2) "Bone resorption"—seen in immobilization states and hyperparathyroidism.

       (3) "Renal leak" of calcium—seen with renal tubular acidosis and congenitally.

   c. Hyperoxaluria causing calcium oxalate stone—results from (1) endogenous production (via the glycolic pathway), (2) dietary sources (leafy green vegetables), and (3) in hyperabsorption of oxalates (postoperative morbidity in patients undergoing intestinal bypass for morbid obesity).
   d. Radiopaque on x-ray.
2. Uric acid stone
   a. Results from hyperuricosuria in an acid urine with decreased volume.
   b. Seen in myeloproliferative disorders, idiopathic hyperuricemia, gout and patients with increased dietary intake of purine.
   c. Radiolucent on x-ray.
3. Cystine stone
   a. Results from cystinuria seen in inherited defects of the renal tubule, causing loss of cystine, ornithine, arginine, and lysine.
   b. Faintly radiopaque and with characteristic microscopic appearance of hexagonally shaped crystals on urinalysis.
4. Matrix stone
   a. Coagulated mucoids with little crystalline component.
   b. Associated with *Proteus* urinary tract infections in an alkaline urine.
5. Magnesium ammonium phosphate—"Struvite" stone
   a. Found in urine rendered alkaline by urea-splitting bacteria (such as *Proteus*) which produce urease.
   b. Urea is split by urease into ammonia, which raises the pH, causing a decrease in the solubility of magnesium–ammonium–calcium–phosphate and thus precipitates stone.

III. CLINICAL FEATURES OF STONE DISEASE

A. Renal
1. Calyceal stone
   a. Many asymptomatic and cause no problem—no treatment necessary.
   b. Some impact at neck of calyx and cause obstruc-

tion of calyx with infection behind obstruction. Can cause fever, chills, pain and lead to scarring, atrophy and possible pyocalix. May grow into renal pelvis. Treatment necessary.

2. Renal pelvic stone
   a. Usually arise from calyceal stones.
   b. Sometimes asymptomatic.
   c. Symptoms can include nausea, vomiting, typical renal colic, fever, chills.

B. Ureteral

1. Upper ureteral stone
   a. Colicky pain radiating downward toward the umbilicus and upward toward the flank.
   b. Microscopic or gross hematuria may be present.
2. Midureteral stone and lower ureteral stone
   a. Colicky pain radiating toward ipsilateral scrotum and testicle.
   b. Bladder symptoms of urgency, frequency, and discomfort with voiding as stone nears ureterovesical junction.
   c. Can see microscopic and gross hematuria with any stone in kidney or ureter.

C. Bladder

1. Symptoms include pain referred to penis with voiding symptoms of dysuria, frequency, urgency, and sometimes obstruction.
2. Similar symptoms and signs with urethral stones.

IV. EVALUATION AND WORKUP OF STONE PATIENT

A. History and Physical—see Clinical Features

B. Laboratory Evaluation

1. Urinalysis
   a. Protein seen in urine most likely because of hematuria giving positive reading.
   b. pH greater than 7.6—urease-splitting organisms must be present.
   c. pH lower than 7.6 would favor uric acid and cystine stones.

d. Crystals
   (1) Cystine—hexagonal on microscopic exam.
   (2) Uric acid—amber brown glass sliver type on microscopic exam.
2. Urine testing
   a. Nitroprusside test—used to detect cystinuria and thus cystine stones.
   b. Quantitative 24-hour urine studies—supersaturation can occur above these levels
      (1) Calcium—normal 300 mg.
      (2) Uric acid—normal 600 mg.
      (3) Cystine—normal 50 to 180 mg.
3. X-ray—mainstay of diagnosis
   a. Plain abdominal film (kidneys, ureters, bladder [KUB])—radiopaque stones seen best this way.
   b. Intravenous pyelogram (IVP)—shows degree of obstruction and general architecture of urinary tract.
   c. Retrograde ureterogram and pyelogram—used when there is nonvisualization or poor visualization of collecting system after IVP. Done through cystoscope.
   d. Ultrasonography, computerized axial tomography (CAT), radionuclide renal scanning, and percutaneous nephrography all have recent increasing roles in stone diagnoses.
4. Blood chemistry testing
   a. Serum calcium, uric acid, phosphorous determinations.
   b. Serum protein important because one-half of calcium in body is un-ionized and thus bound to protein. Low protein levels would mean more unbound calcium.
   c. Serum chloride may help in diagnosis of hypercalcemia.
      (1) Elevation above 102 mEq/L in hyperparathyroidism has been reported as a reliable method to support suspected hypercalcemia.
   d. Radioimmunoassay of parathyroid hormone elevation used to diagnose hypercalcemia secondary to hyperparathyroidism.

5. Oral calcium tolerance testing (PAK test)—aids to differentiate between hypercalcuria from hyperparathyroidism (resorbtive type), absorptive type, and "renal leak" type.
   a. May be done on outpatient basis.
   b. Determine dietary effects of calcium loading and abstinence on urinary excretion of calcium. Can then determine type of calcium abnormality and subsequent treatment.
6. Stone analysis
   a. Identifies stone compositions
      (1) Chemical analysis—oldest method
      (2) X-ray diffraction analysis
      (3) Polarizing microscopic analysis

V. MEDICAL TREATMENT OF STONE DISEASE

A. General
Criteria for activity of stone disease
1. Surgical activity—patient has colic, infection, obstruction, necessitating intervention.
2. Metabolic activity—exists if new stone forms, increase in size of preexisting stone or passage of gravel within 1 year.
3. Metabolic inactivity—none of the above has occurred in patient with stones.

B. Medical Therapy
Alters the urine to prevent precipitation by the following:
1. Dilution, pH alteration, increasing urinary inhibitors, decreasing stone forming substances
   a. Mainstay is maintenance of large urine volume by increased fluid intake.
2. Medications
   a. Orthophosphates—decrease urinary calcium, decrease oxalate crystal aggregation. Used to prevent calcium stones.
   b. Alkaline phosphates—increase urinary inhibitors of stone formation in calcium stone formers.
   c. Hydrochlorthiazide—prevents reabsorption of sodium and calcium in loop of Henle, which leads to

increase in proximal tubular reabsorption of sodium and calcium, thus decreasing total urinary calcium excretion.

d. Methylene blue—competes with calcium at matrix site to prevent calcium stone. Not proven completely.

e. Magnesium oxide—promotes solubility of oxalate. Not proven unequivocally.

f. Allopurinol—used in uric acid stones—alters pathway to uric acid by acting as a zanthine oxidase inhibitor. This prevents increase concentration of uric acid.

g. Penicillamine—utilized to dissolve cystine stones by forming cysteine penicillamine, which is more soluble than cystine.

h. Hemiacidrin—efficacious in treatment of residual magnesium, ammonium phosphate stones. Used in irrigation techniques directly onto stone through bladder irrigation or nephrostomy tube irrigation.

VI. SURGICAL TREATMENT OF STONE DISEASE

A. General

1. Surgical—see below.
2. Expectant—careful watching for passage of stone without intervention.
3. Manipulative—use of endoscopic stone basketing or percutaneous extraction through cystoscope or percutaneous nephrostomy.

B. Surgical

1. Renal calculi
   a. Pyelolithotomy—surgical approach through renal pelvis after flank incision.
   b. Nephrolithotomy—incision into kidney parenchyma avoiding major vessels and removing stone. Figure 2 shows anatrophic nephrotomy incision.
   c. Partial nephrectomy—guillotine excision of portion of diseased kidney containing stone.

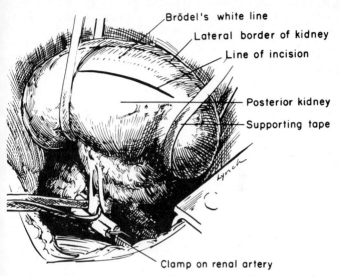

Figure 2. Incision for anatrophic nephrolithotomy to surgically remove staghorn calculi.

    2. Ureteral calculi
        a. Ureterolithotomy—indications
           (1) Stone greater than 1 cm diameter.
           (2) Stone in proximal ureter (accompanied by hydronephrosis) that fails to advance downward over 1-month period.
           (3) Stone associated with sepsis, severe colic, and severe hematuria that is not appropriate for endoscopic manipulation.
        b. Transurethral manipulation—accomplished using stone baskets, loop extractors, ureteral catheters, or ureteroscopic techniques.
    3. Bladder calculi
        a. Suprapubic lithotomy—incision through bladder for stone extraction.
        b. Transurethral litholapaxy—use of lithotrite to crush stone and irrigate transurethrally through endoscope.

    c. Ultrasonic lithotripsy—stone fragmented by ultra-
       sound and removed transurethrally.
    d. Electrohydraulic lithotripsy.

VII. OVERVIEW AND FUTURE OF STONE THERAPY

A. Percutaneous Techniques

Through a flank puncture, a nephrostomy tube is placed
and the stone is manipulated for removal. Ultrasonic
probes can be placed onto stones for fragmentation and
subsequent manipulation.

1. Avoids surgical incisions and complications.
2. Shortens hospital stay.
3. Cost effective in getting patients back to normal life
   style sooner.

B. Laser Therapy

New modality with potential for fragmentation of calculi
into gravel for easy passage. Presently experimental.

C. Extracorporeal Lithotripsy (see Chapter 27)

Shock waves to fragment the stone are passed through
patient while immersed in a water bath.

1. Avoids any surgical or percutaneous intervention.
2. Shortens hospitalization dramatically.
3. Minimal complications reported.
4. Cost effective.
5. Currently in use at specific centers only.

D. Conclusion

1. Future of stone therapy points toward less surgery and
   more medical or noninvasive therapeutic measures for
   stone removal, dissolution and prevention.
2. As of the printing of this book, more than 98% of
   renal, ureteral, and bladder calculi can be managed
   without open surgical techniques. No area of urology
   has made more dramatic advances in the last 5 years
   than management of stone disease.

BIBLIOGRAPHY

Frank M, DeVries A: Prevention of urolithiasis. Arch Environ Health 13:625, 1966.

Furlow WL, Bucchiere, JJ: The surgical fate of ureteral calculi: Review of the Mayo Clinic experience. J Urol 116:559, 1976.

Glenn JF (ed): Urologic Surgery. New York: Harper & Row, 1975, chaps 12, 13, 14, 21, 43.

Glenn JF: Urologic Surgery, ed 3. New York: Harper & Row, 1984.

Harrison JH, et al (eds): Campbell's Urology, ed 5. Philadelphia: W.B. Saunders, 1980.

Malek RS: Renal lithiasis: A practical approach. J Urol 118:893, 1977.

Malek RS, Wilkiemeyer RM, Boyce WH: The stone-forming kidney: A study of functional differences between individual kidneys in idiopathic renal lithiasis. J Urol 116:11, 1976.

Resnick MI (ed): Urol Clin North Am 10(4), 1983.

Roth RA, Finlayson B (eds): Stones—Clinical Management of Urolithiasis. Baltimore: Williams & Wilkins, 1983.

Smith LH: Medical evaluation of urolithiasis. Urol Clin North Am 2(1), 1974.

Stanbury JH, et al (eds): Basis of Inherited Disease. New York: McGraw-Hill, 1972, chaps 9, 62, 65.

8

Emergency Room Urology
Philip M. Hanno

This chapter will consider some common urologic problems that often require decisions to be made in the emergency room setting. Other urologic disorders not covered in this chapter (particularly trauma and infection), may present in casualty departments, and the reader is referred to specific chapters covering these topics.

I. PAIN IN THE URINARY TRACT

A. Types of Pain
1. Local pain—felt in or near the involved organs.
2. Referred pain—originates in a diseased organ but is felt at some distance from that organ, due to common innervation of the target organ and site of perceived pain.

B. Upper Tract Pain (Fig. 1)
1. Caused by distention; severity related to rapidity of development, not to degree (acute vs. chronic distention of ureter, pelvis, calyces).
2. May also be caused by distention of the renal capsule (mild costovertebral angle tenderness) or renal ischemia (mild to moderate flank pain).
3. Colic is caused by intermittent ureteral contraction with a resultant increase in the distention pressure.
4. Visceral afferents from kidney and ureter accompany sympathetics.
5. Spinal cord segments T11, T12 receive sensory fibers from upper ureter and testicle: distention of former may present as testicular pain; similarly, lower ureteral distention may present as scrotal pain.

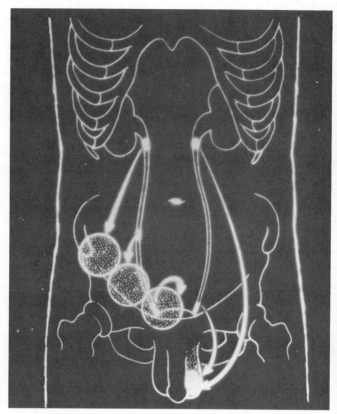

Figure 1. Primary and referred pain sites in the upper urinary tract.

6. Ureteral pain in women may radiate into the vulva.
7. Thus, one may be able to estimate the site of urinary obstruction by the history of pain and the site of referral.
8. Be careful! A stone in the mid right ureter may simulate appendicitis; on the left side it may mimic acute diverticulitis.

  C. **Lower Tract Pain**
1. Visceral afferents from the bladder primarily follow the parasympathetics.
2. Bladder distention causes "fullness," followed by suprapubic pain with desire to urinate.
3. Sensitivity of bladder mucosa is greatly increased by inflammation.
4. Stimulation of the bladder base causes referred pain to the tip of the penis.

II. RENAL COLIC

Although stone disease has been covered in Chapter 7, a few words on emergency room evaluation are in order.

  A. **History**
1. Sudden onset of severe pain; may come in waves; may be constant.
2. Occasionally pain may be associated with nausea and vomiting.
3. Often there is a past history of renal or ureteral colic, stone passage.
4. Beware of the drug addict who has learned how to simulate ureteral colic; beware the Munchausen:
   a. Generally claim to be allergic to contrast.
   b. Usually place blood in urine specimen (obtain voided specimen in your presence or catheterize patient for specimen).
5. Many general surgical intraabdominal emergencies can be confused with renal/ureteral colic:
   a. Acute appendicitis
   b. Small bowel obstruction
   c. Diverticulitis
   d. Ovarian torsion
   e. Rupture of ectopic pregnancy

  B. **Diagnostic Studies**
1. *Urinalysis.* Often positive for red cells; may indicate presence of urinary tract infection; crystals may help identify composition of calculi.

2. *Plain Radiograph.* Care in interpretation required:
   a. Phleboliths may be misleading.
   b. Calcified stone may be hidden by skeletal shadows.
   c. Uric acid stone is radiolucent.
3. Intravenous Urogram
   a. Keystone of diagnosis.
   b. If diagnosis is straightforward and general surgical problem extremely unlikely, study can be postponed until following day when patient has been properly prepared and intravenous urogram will be of optimal quality.
   c. If there is any doubt as to etiology of pain, and the patient is deemed ill enough to require hospital admission, emergency urogram should be done. This will effectively determine whether there is a urologic basis for the problem and allow for appropriate management decisions.

C. Indications for Admission
1. Obstructing calculus in patient with solitary kidney.
2. High-grade upper tract obstruction with calculus that is too large (>1 cm diameter) to pass.
3. Fever and urinary tract infection behind obstructing calculus.
4. Vomiting, intestinal ileus such that patient would be unable to take fluids by mouth.
5. Pain uncontrollable with oral narcotics.

D. Instructions for Patients Discharged from Emergency Room
1. Increased fluid intake is generally recommended (efficacy controversial).
2. Oral narcotics for pain as needed.
3. Strain urine to catch stone for analysis.
4. Regular urologic follow-up.

III. TESTICULAR TORSION

A. Etiology
1. Extravaginal Torsion (Fig. 2)
   a. Rare form, primarily in utero or in neonates and infants.

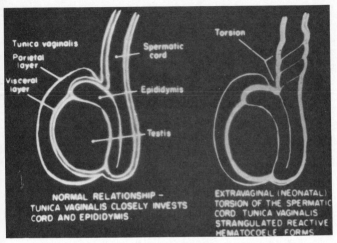

Figure 2. Normal scrotal anatomic relationships/extravaginal torsion.

    b. Caused by loose attachments of tunica vaginalis to surrounding tissue.

    c. Spermatic cord undergoes rotation above the testis.

2. Intravaginal Torsion (Fig. 3)

    a. Most common in adolescents, though may occur through 4th decade.

    b. Related to abnormal anatomy within tunica vaginalis; tunica vaginalis covers the entire epididymis and extends up the cord, attaching above the point of torsion; increased testicular mobility results in free swinging "bell-clapper" deformity—present bilaterally as predisposing factor for torsion in at least 50% of cases.

B. Diagnosis

1. Extravaginal Torsion

    a. Usually presents as firm, hard, enlarged scrotal mass in neonate that does not transilluminate and is nontender.

    b. Differential diagnosis includes hydrocele, incarce-

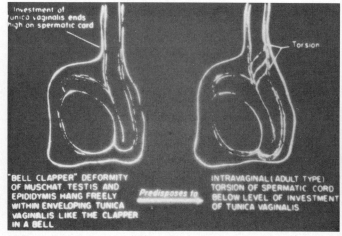

Investment of
tunica vaginalis ends
high on spermatic cord

Torsion

"BELL CLAPPER" DEFORMITY
OF MUSCHAT TESTIS AND
EPIDIDYMIS HANG FREELY
WITHIN ENVELOPING TUNICA
VAGINALIS LIKE THE CLAPPER
IN A BELL

Predisposes to

INTRAVAGINAL (ADULT TYPE)
TORSION OF SPERMATIC CORD
BELOW LEVEL OF INVESTMENT
OF TUNICA VAGINALIS

Figure 3. Scrotal anatomic abnormality predisposing to intravaginal torsion.

rated inguinal hernia, tumor, torsed appendage, hematoma.

c. Testicular salvage is rare in this entity.

2. Intravaginal Torsion

a. Sudden onset of pain in groin, lower abdomen, or scrotum.

b. May occur after exercise or during sleep.

c. Often history of previous similar self-limited attacks.

d. Note: Horizontal position of affected testis; edematous, erythematous scrotum; absence of fever; absence of cells or bacteria on urinalysis; pain increase with elevation of testis (vs. epididymitis); bell-clapper deformity of uninvolved testis.

e. Differential includes epididymitis (see Table 1), testicular tumor, torsion of testicular appendage.

f. Nuclear testicular scans, ultrasound, may be helpful in making diagnosis, but they should not be

TABLE 1. DIAGNOSIS OF TORSION VS. EPIDIDYMITIS

	Torsion	Epididymitis
Age	Puberty to 4th decade, most common age 12–18	Puberty to 8th decade
Onset	Acute	May be gradual
Nausea	Common	None
Pain	Severe	Severe
Pyrexia	Absent	Often present
Urinalysis	Normal	Pyuria common
Manual scrotal elevation	Pain constant	Pain decreased
Testicular position	Elevated	Normal
Opposite testis	Bell clapper	Normal

performed if they will significantly delay diagnosis.

g. When in doubt, surgically explore without delay.

C. Therapy

Immediate surgery to detorse and fix testicle in scrotum, fixation of contralateral testis.

D. Torsion of Testicular Appendages

1. The appendix testis and appendix epididymis may undergo torsion.
2. Clinically, this condition may simulate testicular torsion.
3. If diagnosis is unequivocal, conservative treatment (analgesics) is reasonable.
4. If diagnosis in doubt, exploration is mandatory to rule out testicular torsion. The appendix is surgically excised.

IV. ACUTE URINARY RETENTION

A. History

Age, general health, emotional status, preexistent symptoms, previous episodes, prior urologic manipulation or surgery, medications (sympathomimetics, anticholinergices), and chronic or recent painless or painful overflow retention (paradoxical incontinence).

B. **Etiology**
  1. Anatomic Obstruction
     a. Prostatic hypertrophy or cancer
     b. Urethral stricture
  2. Functional Obstruction
     a. Neurogenic disease
     b. Hysteria, emotional upheaval
     c. Drug or alcohol toxicity
     d. Pain (nocioceptive retention), i.e., postoperative retention after perineal surgery

C. **Management**
  1. Attempt to pass average size Foley catheter (18F).
  2. If above fails, attempt to pass large Foley catheter (22F or 24F) after instilling 8 to 10 ml of lubricating jelly into urethra.
     a. Large catheter will usually push aside obstructing prostatic lobes, if prostate is cause of obstruction. If stricture is etiology, no smaller catheter is likely to pass through a stricture significant enough to cause retention.
  3. If large catheter unsuccessful, someone from the urology service should be called.
  4. A large (22F to 24F) sound should be passed to ascertain point of obstruction. If it passes into bladder, obstruction is secondary to prostate and a large catheter on a catheter guide can usually be passed.
  5. If sound is held up in urethra, obstruction is probably secondary to stricture at that point. An attempt is made to pass a filiform through the stricture. A follower can be threaded onto the filiform and passed into the bladder for drainage.
  6. If above attempts are unsuccessful, the urology team may opt to drain the bladder through placement of a midline suprapubic cystostomy with one of the many commercially available kits designed for use in the emergency room under local anesthesia. Alternatively, panendoscopy in the cystoscopy suite may be per-

formed to try to locate the urethral lumen under direct vision.

7. There is no reason not to allow the bladder to drain rapidly.

8. No patient in retention should be instrumented and drained and then discharged without a urologic consultation.

D. Potential Complications After Relief of Obstruction

1. Postobstructive Diuresis (>200 ml/hr)
   a. Caused by tubular damage as well as by increased BUN and resultant osmotic diuresis.
2. Hypotension
   a. Caused by relief of pelvic venous compression from bladder distention or vasovagal type of response to relief of distention.
3. Hemorrhage Ex Vacuo
   a. Hematuria caused by bladder mucosal disruption following relief of long-standing obstruction.

V. PRIAPISM

A. Definition

Priapism is the pathologic prolongation of a penile erection most often associated with pain but not with sexual excitement or desire.

1. Primary—idiopathic with no obvious predisposing cause (50% of cases).
2. Secondary—trauma, drug ingestion, neoplasm, sickle cell disease.

B. Pathophysiology

1. Primary Priapism
   a. Starts generally with "normal" erection.
   b. Engorgement of corpora cavernosa with full, erect penis, and flaccid glans.
   c. Obstruction of venous drainage; hypoxia of corporal blood and increased carbon dioxide lead to increased blood viscosity and further sludging, impairing drainage.
   d. Eventual vascular thrombosis and tissue fibrosis.

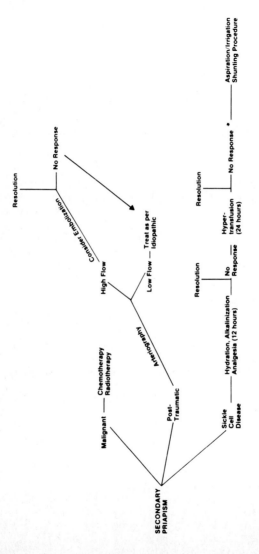

Figure 4. Management plan for secondary priapism.

* In younger (<20 years) patients, many urologists would delay invasive treatment up to 7-14 days

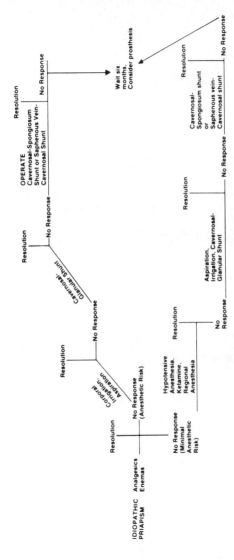

Figure 5. Management plan for idiopathic priapism.

183

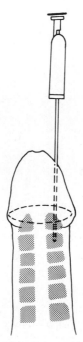

Figure 6. Cavernosal–glanular shunt introduced with biopsy needle (Winter procedure).

2. Secondary Priapism
   a. *Sickle cell* accounts for 20% of all cases of priapism. Decreased blood flow during erection can trigger localized sickling of cells and resultant sludging with decreased venous drainage.
   b. *Trauma* with either disruption of venous drainage or high flow states from arteriovenous fistula formation secondary to arterial injury accounts for 5% of cases.
   c. *Neoplastic disease,* especially leukemia, may infiltrate the corpora, blocking venous outflow.
   d. Many *drugs* including anticoagulants, phe-

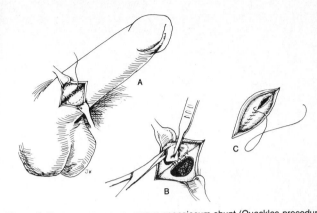

Figure 7. Corpus cavernosum–corpus spongiosum shunt (Quackles procedure).

nothiazines, and alcohol have been implicated in priapism.

C. Treatment (Figs. 4 and 5)
1. Priapism is a urologic emergency and treatment should not be delayed.
2. Therapy is directed towards increasing venous blood flow through one of several surgical shunting procedures if initial medical management as outlined in Figures 4 and 5 is unsuccessful (Figs. 6 and 7).
3. Shunting procedures bypass the obstructed deep venous system, diverting blood through the corpus spongiosum and glans into the more superficial pathways.
4. Overall, priapism portends an impotence rate of up to 50% regardless of treatment modality.

VI. FORESKIN EMERGENCIES

A. Phimosis
1. Inability to retract foreskin over glans penis because of small preputial opening.
2. Treatment is circumcision or dorsal slit of prepuce acutely.

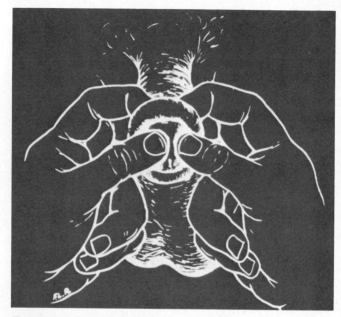

Figure 8. Manual reduction of paraphimosis. (*Reproduced with permission from Marshall VF: Textbook of Urology, ed 2, Hoeber Medical Division, Harper & Row Publishers, New York, 1969.*)

B. Paraphimosis
1. The foreskin, once retracted, cannot be returned to its normal position.
2. The tight opening constricts the venous return of the glans causing edema.
3. Treatment is manual reduction (Fig. 8).

BIBLIOGRAPHY

Hanno, PM: Priapism. AUA Update Series, vol 3, lesson 20. Houston: American Urological Association, Office of Education, 1984.

LaNasa JA, Lang EK: Disorders of the scrotum and its contents. In Resnick

MI, Older RA (eds): Diagnosis of Genitourinary Disease. New York: Thieme-Stratton, 1982, pp 433–483.

O'Flynn JD: Clinical management of ureteral calculi. In Roth RA, Finlayson B (eds): Stones: Clinical Management of Urolithiasis. Baltimore: Williams & Wilkins, 1983, pp 441–452.

9

Upper Urinary Tract Trauma

Robert S. Charles
Philip M. Hanno

I. INCIDENCE

A. **All genitourinary trauma** accounts for only 2 to 3% of total admissions on a major trauma service.

B. **Renal trauma** alone accounts for 46% of all genitourinary trauma.
1. Both kidneys are affected equally.
2. The majority occurs in young males with a male-to-female ratio of 3:1.
3. Blunt renal injury occurs four times more often than penetrating injury overall.
4. Children are particularly prone to renal injury because of the large size of the kidneys relative to overall body size, the underdevelopment of Gerota's fascia and the perirenal fat, and the incomplete ossification of the lower ribs.

C. **The incidence of renal trauma** is increasing directly with increases in transportation and urban violence.

II. ANATOMY

A. **The kidneys are located** within the confines of the lower rib cage in the upper retroperitoneal space and are well cushioned by the paraspinal muscles, Gerota's fascia, and the surrounding soft tissue and bony structures.

    1. This makes renal injury relatively infrequent even in severe accidents.

  B. The close association of the aorta, inferior vena cava, and intraabdominal organs accounts for the high likelihood of associated injury with renal trauma.

  C. The kidney is attached only by the ureter, renal artery, and vein, and avulsion of any of these structures may occur with severe acceleration/deceleration injuries.

III. HEMATURIA

  A. Hematuria is commonly seen with renal trauma.
    1. It may be gross or microscopic.

  B. The degree of hematuria does not correlate well with the severity of renal injury.
    1. The absence of hematuria does not rule out renal injury, as in cases of complete renal pedicle avulsion.

IV. ETIOLOGY OF RENAL INJURIES

  A. Trauma has traditionally been classified as either blunt or penetrating in nature.

  B. Other causes of renal trauma include iatrogenic (ureteral catheterization, closed renal biopsy, percutaneous nephrostomy), foreign bodies, and severe electrical shock.

V. BLUNT RENAL TRAUMA

  A. Accounts for 70 to 90% of all cases of renal trauma.
    1. Motor vehicle accidents account for the majority of cases of blunt renal injury.
    2. Other causes of blunt renal injury include falls, sports injuries, and direct blows to the abdomen or flank.

  B. Eighty percent of patients will have associated injuries to other organs or the skeletal system
    1. Twenty to twenty-five percent will sustain injuries to the intraabdominal organs or intrathoracic structures.

   2. Any patient who has sustained severe trauma to the flank, abdomen, or lower chest should be suspected of having renal trauma whether or not hematuria is present.

C. Careful history and physical exam are extremely important.
   1. Factors such as the speed of the automobile, height of the fall, character of the pain, vital signs, rib tenderness, signs of peritoneal irritation, and flank masses can lead one to suspect renal trauma.

D. Hematuria will be present in 60 to 90% of patients with major renal injury secondary to blunt trauma.
   1. Remember that the most severe renal injury, complete vascular avulsion or thrombosis, may cause minimal or no hematuria.

VI. PENETRATING RENAL INJURY

A. Accounts for approximately 10% of all cases of renal trauma.
   1. In high crime areas, up to 30% of cases of renal trauma may be due to penetrating trauma.
   2. Penetrating renal injuries are rare in children.

B. Seven percent of penetrating wounds to the abdomen will involve renal injury. Conversely, 80% of all penetrating renal injuries will involve injury to other intraabdominal structures.
   1. It is usually these associated injuries that require surgical exploration in these patients.

C. Gunshot wounds may be divided into those occurring from high-velocity and low-velocity weapons.
   1. Wounds caused by high-velocity weapons are usually associated with an entrance and exit wound, and extensive soft tissue injury may be present from the blast effect of a high velocity missile.
   2. Wounds caused by low-velocity weapons usually will not cause significant renal injury unless the missile passes through a major vessel or the collecting system.

D. **Stab wounds** may be divided into those occurring anterior and posterior to the anterior axillary line.
   1. Wounds occurring anterior often involve injuries to other intraabdominal structures. Stab wounds occurring posterior to the anterior axillary line often do not involve associated organ injury.
   2. Puncture wounds may be misleading and one should not be fooled by a small puncture wound, as this may involve serious injury to the kidney.

E. **As with blunt renal trauma,** careful but expedient history and physical examination is very important.
   1. Quickly assess the patient's cardiovascular status and begin resuscitative measures if necessary.
   2. Ascertain the type of weapon used, if possible, to differentiate between high- and low-velocity missiles.
   3. Examine the patient for location of entrance and exit wounds if present.
   4. Signs of peritoneal irritation may be present with associated intraabdominal injuries.
   5. Findings on physical examination do not necessarily correlate with the degree of renal injury.

F. **Hematuria is present** in 70 to 90% of cases of penetrating renal trauma.

VII. PEDICLE INJURIES

A. **Most commonly occur** with penetrating abdominal or back wounds traversing the artery and vein.
   1. Penetrating trauma accounts for 80% of pedicle injury.
   2. The left renal vein is the most commonly injured structure in these wounds because of its long length and the fact that it crosses the midline.
   3. Sixty-five percent of pedicle injuries have damage to greater than one vessel.
   4. The mortality rate for pedicle injuries is 30% overall.
   5. Vein injuries are much more serious than arterial injuries due to greater hemorrhage and the higher percentage of associated major vessel injuries.

B. **Blunt trauma accounts for 20%** of all pedicle injuries.
   1. Usually due to deceleration injuries, with renal artery thrombosis caused by an intimal flap.
   2. Complete vascular avulsion may also occur.

C. **Signs and symptoms** of pedicle injury.
   1. Shock is usually present secondary to blood loss.
   2. An expanding flank mass may be seen.
   3. Hematuria may be absent with complete vascular avulsion.

VIII. CLASSIFICATION OF RENAL INJURY

A. **Injuries** are usually classified as major or minor, with either blunt or penetrating trauma.
   1. Minor renal injuries account for 85% of blunt renal trauma.
      a. Renal contusion—most common renal injury from blunt trauma accounting for 75% of all cases. This is simply a mild injury of the renal parenchyma.
      b. Simple laceration—signifies a shallow cortical laceration that does not communicate with the collecting system.
      c. Subcapsular hematoma—bleeding into the tough, fibrous capsule that surrounds the renal parenchyma.
   2. Major renal injuries account for 15% of blunt renal trauma.
      a. Lacerations through the collecting system and parenchyma (Fig. 1).
      b. Perirenal hematoma—blood collecting outside the renal capsule (Fig. 2).
      c. Renal rupture—portions of renal parenchyma are separated from each other (Fig. 3).
      d. Pedicle injury—may involve the artery, vein, or both.

B. **The kidney may also be classified** by its four major components.
   1. The renal pedicle.

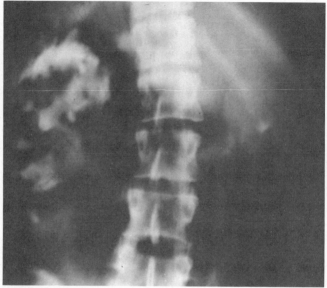

Figure 1. Major renal laceration with extravasation of contrast on IV urogram.

    2. The collecting system.
    3. The renal parenchyma.
    4. The renal capsule and perirenal tissues.

IX. DIAGNOSTIC STUDIES

A. KUB

1. Allows for examination of the soft tissue and bony structures.
2. May show a soft tissue mass or displaced loops of bowel.
3. Loss of the ipsilateral psoas shadow may indicate retroperitoneal blood or urine.
4. Rupture of a hollow viscus with pneumoperitoneum may also be seen.

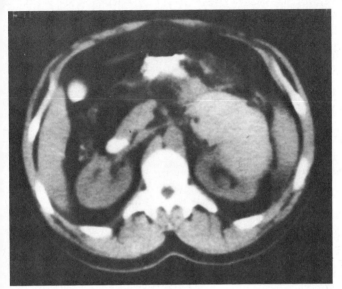

Figure 2. Computed tomography showing perinephric hematoma following left renal trauma.

B. Intravenous Urography (IVU)

1. This remains the most commonly used procedure for the evaluation of renal trauma.
2. If the patient's status does not allow for preoperative studies, an intraoperative IVU may be performed to rule out a significant renal injury and evaluate the function of the contralateral kidney.
3. In a more stable patient, the IVU should be performed with nephrotomography to allow clear visualization of the renal outlines, collecting system, and ureters.
   a. The appearance of the nephrogram on the tomograms is an important radiologic feature as it often indicates the type and severity of injury present.
   b. IVU with nephrotomography will accurately define the renal injury in 85 to 90% of cases.

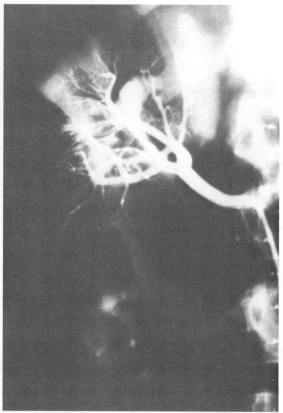

Figure 3. Renal arteriogram of a "shattered" kidney following severe renal trauma.

4. Failure to visualize a kidney, persistence of the nephrographic phase, or visualization of only a portion of a kidney may suggest significant parenchymal or renal pedicle injury.
5. Findings on IVU
   a. Shock—unless the systolic blood pressure is above 80 mm Hg systolic, a faint nephrogram will devel-

op, with delayed excretion simulating renal pedicle injury.

b. Renal contusion—often the IVU is normal; occasionally, however, the nephrogram is diminished in intensity and the pyelographic phase may be less dense than the opposite side.

c. Simple lacerations—appear as small linear densities within the nephrogram.

d. Intrarenal hematoma—appears as circular defect in the nephrogram, with spreading of the calyces and stretching of the infundibuli around the hematoma.

e. Subcapsular hematoma—appears as a large renal outline on plain film, but after contrast is given, the kidney appears compressed with an indented border due to the presence of blood between the kidney and the capsule.

f. Perirenal hematoma—blood will typically obscure a portion of the renal outline and the ipsilateral psoas margin. Loops of bowel may also be displaced by the hematoma as it fills the capacious perirenal space.

g. Lacerations through the collecting system and parenchyma (major laceration)—extravasation will undoubtedly occur with contrast escaping into the supcapsular or perirenal space.

h. Pedicle injuries—the renal parenchyma supplied by the injured vessel(s) will not enhance with contrast, causing either partial or complete absence of the nephrogram.

C. Ultrasonography

1. Often of limited use in the acute setting of renal trauma.

2. Ultrasound is useful for demonstrating fluid collections around the kidney, and in the follow-up of patients managed conservatively to document reabsorbtion of perinephric fluid collections.

D. Computerized Axial Tomography (CAT) Scanning

1. CAT scanning is gaining wide popularity in the evaluation of blunt renal trauma.

   a. Accurately stages renal trauma.

b. Gives information about retroperitoneal and intra-peritoneal involvement that cannot be visualized on IVU.
c. Defines vascular perfusion to the renal parenchyma.
d. Demonstrates urinary extravasation with a high degree of accuracy.
2. Some feel that CAT scanning has surpassed angiography in some respects in the evaluation of renal trauma.

E. Angiography
1. Still considered by many the definitive study in the staging of renal trauma.
2. Indication
a. Nonvisualization of incomplete visualization on IVU suggesting pedicle injury.
b. Expanding or pulsitile flank mass.
c. In suspected arteriovenus (A-V) fistulas, renal infarction, or major vascular injury (if the patient's clinical status permits).

F. Retrograde Pyelography
1. Has limited value in the evaluation of acute renal trauma.
2. It is time consuming and does not supply information regarding the status of the renal parenchyma.
3. Requires urinary tract instrumentation with increased risk of introducing infection.

X. TREATMENT

A. Treatment of renal trauma remains one of the most controversial topics in the field of urology today.

B. Often, the urologist is not consulted until the patient is in the operating room and a large retroperitoneal hematoma is noted.

C. Penetrating Renal Trauma
1. Most authors advocate immediate exploration for all penetrating abdominal injuries except for superficial stab wounds posterior to the anterior axillary line without associated intraabdominal injuries.

2. Following exploration and repair of associated injuries, the renal injury should be explored.
3. The key to safe and successful renal exploration for trauma is early control of the renal pedicle.
   a. Entering Gerota's space without vascular control can lead to exsanguinating hemorrhage, with a high rate of emergency nephrectomy.
4. After vascular control is obtained, Gerota's fascia is entered, and the kidney is carefully inspected.
   a. If brisk bleeding is noted, the renal vessels can be temporarily occluded and the injury repaired.
5. Minor renal injuries may be treated with adequate drainage only.
6. Major renal injuries should always be repaired primarily and renal tissue should be preserved if possible.
   a. In cases of massive renal trauma, extensive pedicle injury, or a shattered kidney, serious consideration should be given to nephrectomy.

D. Blunt Renal Trauma

1. Eighty-five percent of patients with blunt renal trauma have minor renal injuries and can be managed nonsurgically.
2. Approximately 5% of patients with blunt renal trauma will have either injury to the renal pedicle, renal fragmentation, or a shattered kidney.
   a. These patients require immediate exploration, with careful vascular control as discussed with penetrating renal trauma and surgical repair.
3. The remaining 5 to 10% of patients will have an intermediate degree of injury, and the management of these patients may be either surgical or nonsurgical depending on the clinical status of the patient and the need to treat associated injuries.
   a. Exploration only to do a nephrectomy in a stable patient is not indicated in this setting.
   b. Those who favor immediate exploration feel they will conserve more renal parenchyma and therefore more renal function.
      (1) The data to confirm this contention are not clear in the urologic literature.

c. Patients treated nonsurgically may require delayed exploration for persistent bleeding or infected urinoma formation.

XI. COMPLICATIONS OF RENAL TRAUMA

A. Early Complications
1. Shock from massive blood loss.
2. Infected hematoma or urinoma formation.
3. Renal infarction.
4. Abscess formation.

B. Late Complications
1. Hypertension
   a. Usually associated with high renin formation.
   b. Occasionally may resolve spontaneously.
   c. May occur many years after renal trauma.
2. Late nephrectomy
   a. Patients with secondary bleeding or infected hematomas and urinomas have a higher incidence of nephrectomy than those explored earlier.
   b. Ureteral strictures or ureteropelvic junction obstruction may lead to secondary nephrectomy.
   c. Failure of vascular repair of the renal pedicle may result in renal infarction and nephrectomy.

XII. URETERAL TRAUMA—INTRODUCTION

A. **The ureters may be injured** by external violence or iatrogenically during operative procedures.

B. **Ureteral trauma** comprises approximately 4% of all genitourinary trauma.

C. **The majority of ureteral trauma** occurs during the course of pelvic surgery, especially when performing abdominal hysterectomy (Fig. 4).

D. **Successful management of ureteral trauma** is dependent upon early recognition and surgical correction.

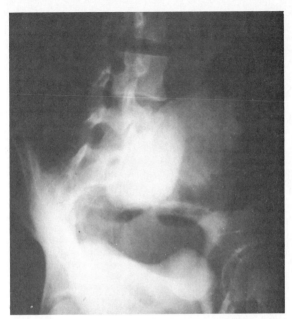

Figure 4. IV urogram following hysterectomy, with urinoma formation posterior to the bladder from ureteral injury.

XIII. EXTERNAL INJURY TO THE URETER

A. **Gunshot wounds** are responsible for approximately 95% of ureteral injuries from external sources.

B. **Rarely, stab wounds** of the abdomen or flank may injure the ureter.

C. **The ureter** is also infrequently injured in blunt abdominal trauma in contrast to renal trauma.

D. **Hematuria (gross or microscopic)** is an unreliable sign of ureteral injury and may be absent in 10 to 35% of cases.

E. **The IVU** will demonstrate the injury in over 90% of cases.

F. **Retrograde pyelography,** as with penetrating renal trauma, is rarely necessary and is time consuming, as these injuries are usually explored for correction of associated injuries.

XIV. SURGICAL INJURY TO THE URETER

A. **Most commonly occurs** during the course of abdominal hysterectomy.

B. **Sites of injury include** the areas adjacent to the uterine vessels and the cardinal and uterosacral ligaments.

C. **The ureters can be injured** in essentially any intraabdominal, retroperitoneal, or pelvic procedure, especially when the normal anatomy is distorted by inflammatory or neoplastic processes (Fig. 5).

D. **Prevention of ureteral injury** includes careful technique and preoperative studies detailing ureteral anatomy [intravenous (IV) urography] when difficult surgical dissection is anticipated.
   1. Placement of ureteral catheters may or may not be helpful as they make the ureters more rigid and possibly easier to injure.
      a. Catheters may also allow the surgeon to drop his guard, as he feels the ureters are safe from injury and therefore does not exercise the proper caution when dissecting in their vicinity.

E. **Diagnosis of intraoperative ureteral injury** may be made by actually seeing the transected ureter dripping urine in the surgical wound or can be suspected when difficult dissection is required in the area of the ureter.
   1. Intravenous dyes such as indigo carmine or methylene blue can be given intraoperatively to look for the typical violet-stained fluid accumulating in the surgical wound.
   2. The ureter should be identified and followed into the area in question to ascertain whether injury has occurred.
   3. A soft, silastic ureteral catheter can be passed through

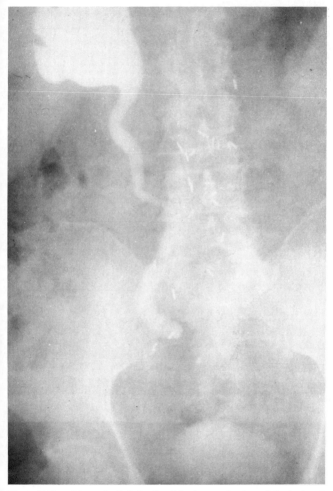

Figure 5. Complete ureteral obstruction following repair of an abdominal aortic aneurysm from surgical clip placed on the distal ureter.

a normal portion of the ureter or through a cystoscope to either confirm or dispel the possibility of ureteral injury.

   a. As the best time to repair ureteral injuries is at the time of diagnosis, every attempt to confirm ureteral injury should be made before the patient leaves the operating room.

4. Postoperatively, ureteral injury presents with abdominal pain and fever with urinary fistula formation.

   a. At this point, the site of injury is best defined with retrograde pyelography.

XV. MANAGEMENT OF URETERAL INJURY

A. **Management of ureteral injury** depends upon the type of injury, the patient's general physical condition, and the time the diagnosis is made.

B. **If the ureter** has been included in a ligature, or clamped with a crushing instrument, it can be released as long as the injury is recognized at the time of surgery.

   1. In these cases, the ureter is stented for 1 to 2 weeks to allow the edema to subside.

C. **If the ureter** is partially transected, it may be primarily repaired if no more than one-half of the circumference is involved and the vascular supply has not been embarrassed.

D. **Injuries to the upper portion of the ureter** are best repaired with an end-to-end anastomosis of the severed ureteral ends (ureteroureterostomy) and urinary diversion with neophrostomy drainage and ureteral stenting.

   1. In cases of upper ureteral injury where the defect is too large to bridge primarily, autotransplantation of the kidney to the iliac vessels or replacement of the ureter with a segment of ileum may be necessary if nephrectomy is to be avoided.

E. **Injuries to the middle third of the ureter** can best be treated with either ureteroureterostomy, or by performing a transureteroureterostomy, whereby the proximal noninjured portion of the ureter is anastomosed to the opposite ureter to provide drainage for both kidneys.

F. Lower ureteral injuries are best managed by reimplanting the ureter above the injury into the bladder in a nonrefluxing fashion.

1. Occasionally, a bladder flap may be needed to reach the ureter proximal to the injury (Boari flap), or the bladder may be sutured to the psoas muscle on the side of injury to correct for loss of ureteral length (psoas hitch).

2. Transureteroureterostomy is another method of managing lower ureteral injury, especially when dealing with associated rectal injury with fecal contamination of the pelvis or previous radiation to the pelvic organs which would make ureteroneocystostomy or ureteroureterostomy less desirable.

   a. Contraindications to transureteroureterostomy include tuberculosis and history of renal calculus disease.

G. Nephrectomy should be reserved for those patients with ureteral injury and noncurable malignancy or associated vascular repair with synthetic grafts to avoid bathing the graft with urine from a nonwatertight repair.

XVI. COMPLICATIONS OF URETERAL INJURY

A. Ureteral fistula.

B. Sepsis.

C. Abscess formation.

D. Ureteral stricture.

BIBLIOGRAPHY

Bernath AS, Schutte H, Fernandex RRD, Addonizio JC: Stab wounds of the kidney: Conservative management in flank penetration. J Urol 129:468–470, 1983.

Bright C: Emergency management of injured ureter. Urol Clin North Am 9(2):285–291, 1982.

Bright TC, Peters PC: Ureteral injuries secondary to operative procedures: Report of 24 cases. Urology 9:68–72, 1977.

Brown MF, Graham JM et al: Renovascular trauma. Am J Surg 140:802–805, 1980.

Carlton CE: Injuries to the ureter. Urol Clin North Am 4(1):33–44, 1977.

Carlton CE, Jr: Injuries of the kidney and ureter. In Harrison JH, Gittes RF, et al (eds): Campbell's Urology. Philadelphia: W.B. Saunders, 1978, vol 1, chap 23, pp 881–905.

Flynn JT, Tiptaft RC et al: The early and aggressive repair of iatrogenic ureteric injuries. Br J Urol 51:454–457, 1979.

Guerriero WG: Penetrating renal injuries and the management of renal pedicle injury. Urol Clin North Am 4(1):3–12, 1977.

Guerriero WG: Trauma to the kidneys, ureters, bladder, and urethra. Surg Clin North Am 62(6):1047–1074, 1982.

Guerriero WG: Injuries to the ureter, Part I: Mechanism, prevention, and diagnosis. AUA Update Ser 2(22):1–7, 1983.

Guerriero, WG: Injuries to the ureter, Part II: Mechanism, prevention, and diagnosis. AUA Update Ser 2(23):1–7, 1983.

Hanno PH, Wein AJ: Urologic trauma. Emerg Med Clin North Am 2(4):823–841, 1984.

McAninch JW: The injured kidney. Monogr Urol 4(2):43–57, 1983.

Peters PC, Bright TC: Blunt renal injuries. Urol Clin North Am 4(1):17–28, 1977.

Scott R, Carlton CE, Goldman M: Penetrating injuries of the kidney: An analysis of 181 patients. J Urol 101:247–253, 1969.

Thompson IM: Expectant management of blunt renal trauma. Urol Clin North Am 4(1):29–32, 1977.

Wein AJ, Arger PH, Murphy JJ: Controversial aspects of blunt renal trauma. J Trauma 17:662–666, 1977.

Wein AJ, Murphy JJ et al: A conservative approach to the management of blunt renal trauma. J Urol 117:425–427, 1977.

10

Lower Urinary Tract Trauma

Philip M. Hanno

I. BACKGROUND INFORMATION

Approximately 10% of injuries seen in the emergency room involve the genitourinary system. Injuries may be classified as renal, ureteral, bladder, urethral, and genital.

The major protection of the urogenital tract against traumatic injury lies in its ability to move. This mobility prolongs the period of deceleration after impact, thus limiting the shock to affected organs. The major exception to this concept is the membranous urethra, immobilized by the urogenital diaphram and subject to shearing injuries in pelvic fractures.

Despite this mobility, however, genitourinary tract injuries are not uncommon. Often in the patient with severe multiple trauma, injuries to the genitourinary tract assume secondary importance. Their definitive management may take place months later.

II. URETHRAL INJURIES

A. General

The least mobile portions of the urethra are the bulbous urethra and membranous urethra. Consequently, these are the areas most susceptible to injury. Bulbar injuries are common following straddle-type falls. Membranous urethral injuries may occur after pelvic fractures.

B. Anatomy

1. Urethral injuries are generally divided into anterior and posterior. The anterior urethra is that part extend-

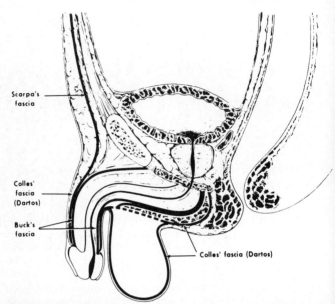

Figure 1. Lateral drawing of the male pelvis showing the critical role that the fascial attachments play in determining the pathology of urinary extravasation. *(From Wyker AW, Gillenwater JY: Method of Urology. Baltimore: Williams & Wilkins, 1975, p 22.)*

ing from the inferior edge of the urogenital diaphram to the external urethral meatus. It includes both the bulbar and penile urethra. The posterior urethra extends from the bladder neck to the inferior edge of the urogenital diaphram. It includes the prostatic and membranous urethra.

2. Fascial anatomy is important when defining urethral injuries (Fig. 1).

   a. The urogenital diaphram separates the pelvis from the perineum. Urine may extravasate into the pelvis in a posterior urethral injury and may extravasate into the perineum after an anterior urethral injury (Fig. 2).

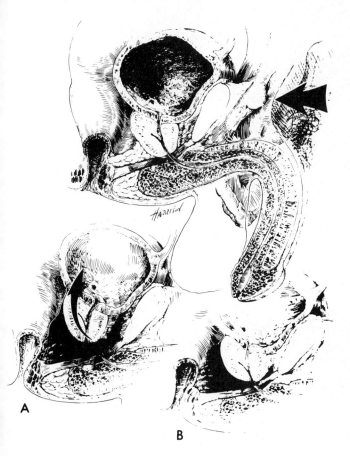

Figure 2. Rupture of urethra superior to urogenital diaphram showing normal anatomy; arrow represents vector through which the force is applied. **A.** Complete rupture of the urethra with elevated prostate and large pelvic hematoma. **B.** Incomplete rupture of urethra. *(From Harrison JH, Gittes RF, et al (eds): Campbell's Urology, ed 4. Philadelphia: W.B. Saunders, 1978, p 913.)*

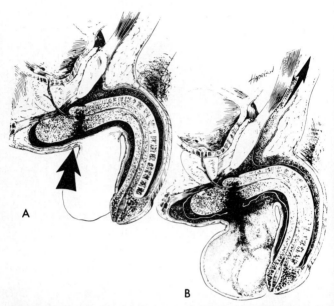

Figure 3. Rupture of urethra inferior to urogenital diaphram. **A.** Rupture of urethra with Buck's fascia intact, showing limitation of urine and blood extravasation. **B.** Rupture of urethra through Buck's fascia, showing path of extravasation of blood and urine from Colle's fascial attachments at the perineal body into the scrotum and extending on to the abdominal wall deep to Scarpa's fascia. *(From Harrison JH, Gittes RF, et al (eds): Campbell's Urology, ed 4. Philadelphia: W.B. Saunders, 1978, p 24.)*

    b. If Buck's fascia remains intact, urinary and blood extravasation will be contained within the penis. Disruption of Buck's fascia allows extravasation to the fascia lata of the thighs, the perineum, and anteriorly to the clavicles or neck. This is because of the attachments of the superficial fascia of the abdominal wall, penis, scrotum, and perineum (Fig. 3).

    c. This contiguous superficial fascial plane is called Scarpa's over the abdominal wall and Colle's or

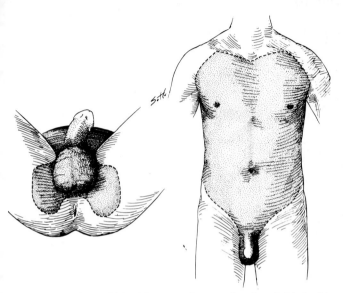

Figure 4. Areas of potential fascial extravasation extending along Colle's fascial attachments. *(From Harrison JH, Gittes, RF, et al (eds): Campbell's Urology, ed 4. Philadelphia: W.B. Saunders, 1978, p 11.)*

Dartos in the penis, scrotum, and perineum. The fascia is attached at the urogenital diaphram and fascia lata below the inguinal ligaments. There is no superior attachment (Fig. 4).

C. Anterior Urethral Injury

1. Indications for Urologic Consultation

   a. There is often a history of a fall and, in some cases, a history of instrumentation. There may be bleeding from the urethral meatus. The patient may have difficulty voiding or be unable to void. There may be pain localized to the perineum. If voiding has occurred and extravasation is noted, sudden swelling in regions outlined by the fascial plains may be noted. If diagnosis has been delayed, sepsis and local evidence of infection may be evident.

     b. On physical examination a pendulous urethral injury may be manifest by a penile hematoma. A bulbar urethral injury may be evidenced by a perineal hematoma. Delayed presentation may present with massive urinary extravasation and infection.

2. Diagnostic Procedures
     a. Voiding should be discouraged so as to prevent urinary extravasation. A retrograde urethrogram with installation of 15 to 20 ml of contrast material will demonstrate extravasation and the location of injury. With urethral contusion alone, no extravasation will be seen.
     b. Catheterization should be discouraged prior to x-ray studies, as instrumentation might convert a partial tear into a complete urethral disruption.

3. Emergency Management
     a. Urethral contusion accompanied by an inability to void secondary to pain (nocioceptive retention) can be treated with catheter drainage. If the patient can void and the urine is relatively clear, no catheter or additional treatment is necessary.
     b. A minimal urethral tear with no extravasation can be treated with a small 14F to 16F Silastic indwelling catheter for 7 to 10 days. Alternatively, a suprapubic tube can be placed for drainage. Partial urethral ruptures may heal without the need for further procedures. Complete urethral disruption can be handled by reconstruction at a later date if a suprapubic tube is placed. Almost any urethral injury can be managed with a suprapubic tube until definitive management is provided.
     c. Many urologists advocate surgical exploration of all significant anterior urethral injuries and debridement of devitalized tissue, with primary realignment of the spatulated urethral ends, along with appropriate drainage. As most of these patients do not have serious, life-threatening injuries elsewhere, immediate reconstruction is not unreasonable.
     d. Penetrating injuries should be debrided and

cleansed and may be managed with either immediate reconstruction or suprapubic cystotomy drainage.

e. Urethral injuries are rare in women, but may be manifest by marked perineal bleeding, which can often be controlled endoscopically. Associated urinary retention is common.

D. Posterior Urethral Injuries

1. Mechanism of Injury
   a. These injuries usually occur in association with fractures of the bony pelvis. There is a shearing effect at the rigid attachment of the apex of the prostate to the fixed, muscular urogenital diaphram. The prostatic urethra is rarely ruptured. The injury is almost always at the level of the membranous urethra.
   b. Five percent of patients with pelvic fractures will have partial or complete ruptures of the posterior urethra.
2. Indications for Urologic Consultation
   a. Classic triad—blood at the urethral meatus, inability to void, distended bladder.
   b. Findings of a pelvic fracture or wide separation of the symphysis pubis.
   c. Rectal examination consistent with a prostate gland displaced upward and posteriorly, with a soft boggy mass in its place.
   d. The perineum and genitalia usually show no sign of bleeding, as blood collects above the urogenital diaphram in the pelvis.
3. Diagnostic Procedures
   a. The "diagnostic catheter" is to be condemned. Attempted passage of a catheter may convert a partial laceration into a full-thickness tear or complete rupture, thus changing a minor problem into a potentially major one.
   b. An initial retrograde urethrogram forms the keystone for diagnosis. Forty milliliters of water-soluble contrast material are injected into the urethra.

A loss of continuity implies rupture. If some contrast finds its way to the bladder, there may be a partial tear in the urethra.
c. If there is no loss of continuity, a catheter is passed and a cystogram is done. Cystography and intravenous urography may demonstrate elevation of the bladder base. The latter study is essential to demonstrate the condition of the upper tracts.

4. Emergency Management
   a. The ideal management approach to posterior urethral injury is a subject of controversy. Several methods have evolved to deal with this serious injury.
      (1) Suprapubic cystostomy and urethral manipulation. The bladder is opened and interlocking sounds are placed, one through the penile urethra and one through the bladder, in order to establish urethral continuity and place an indwelling catheter. A suprapubic tube is left in place and a silastic urethral retention catheter is placed on traction to approximate the severed ends of the urethra. Some urologists advocate placement of perineal traction sutures through the prostatic capsule rather than balloon catheter traction for urethral approximation.
      (2) Primary anastomosis. Immediate dissection of the severed urethral ends is undertaken at the initial surgical procedure, with a primary closure of the urethra end to end and placement of a urethral catheter as a stent.
      (3) Suprapubic cystostomy alone. This is the most conservative and probably the most popular approach at the present time. A suprapubic cystostomy catheter is placed at the time of injury, with a delayed elective urethral reconstruction several months later. The pelvic hematoma is not evacuated, perivesical drains are not placed, and the retropubic space is not explored. The goal is to prevent the hematoma

from becoming infected so that it will be reabsorbed with minimal scar formation.
   b. Advantages of conservative approach
      (1) Reduced blood loss.
      (2) No need for urologic specialists.
      (3) Speed in patient who may have serious associ-
          ated injuries.
      (4) Possibility of spontaneous urethral closure if
          rupture is only partial.
5. Complications of Posterior Urethral Injuries
   a. Fifty to ninety percent incidence of urethral
      stricture.
   b. Fifty percent incidence of impotence.
   c. With conservative approach of suprapubic
      cystostomy, impotence occurs in approximately
      10% of cases.

III. BLADDER INJURIES

A. Mechanisms of Injury
1. Direct injury from a bone fracture.
2. Injury via an explosive hydraulic effect after blunt
   trauma.
3. Injury secondary to penetrating trauma.

B. Indications for Urologic Consultation
1. Five to ten percent of patients with a fractured pelvis
   will have an associated bladder rupture.
2. When both public rami are fractured, the incidence of
   bladder rupture rises to 20%.
3. Fifty to eighty percent of bladder ruptures secondary to
   pelvic fracture are extraperitoneal.
4. Blunt trauma to a distended bladder generally results
   in rupture of the dome of the bladder into the peritoneal cavity. The peritoneal covering over the dome
   prevents the muscle from stretching and thus the least
   elastic portion of the bladder wall will tear.
5. Bladder injury should be suspected in patients with
   lower abdominal pain and/or hematuria, with a history
   of trauma. Some patients will be unable to void.

6. If diagnosis has been delayed, the presentation may be that of an acute abdomen.
7. Rectal examination may suggest a pelvic hematoma with the lack of discernible landmarks.
8. Any penetrating pelvic or lower abdominal wound should be investigated for bladder injury. Penetrating trauma accounts for up to 25% of incidents of bladder rupture.

C. **Diagnostic Procedures**
1. Abdominal plain films are ordered to look for pelvic fractures and soft tissue masses.
2. Intravenous urography will rule out upper tract lesions and show bladder configuration.
   a. Fifteen percent of bladder ruptures may be noted on urography.
   b. A normal cystogram phase of an intravenous (IV) urogram does not rule out a bladder perforation.
3. Urethral injury must be excluded primarily with a retrograde urethrogram.
   a. If urethral injury is present, definitive examination of bladder integrity awaits either safe establishment of urinary drainage or open exploration, if that is necessary to treat urethral injury.
4. Three-phase cystogram is performed.
   a. Fifty milliliters of contrast are instilled in the bladder and may show a massive rupture.
   b. If extravasation is not seen, an additional 300 ml are instilled to distend the bladder fully and x-rays are taken.
   c. The bladder is then emptied to allow postevacuation films, which may reveal small amounts of contrast outside the bladder previously obscured by the opaque bladder image, generally implying a small posterior tear.
5. Women with a bladder rupture need a careful pelvic examination to exclude the possibility of a urethral tear or vaginal injury.

D. **Classification of Bladder Injuries**
1. "Tear Drop Bladder" (Fig. 5)
   a. This is not strictly a traumatic injury of the blad-

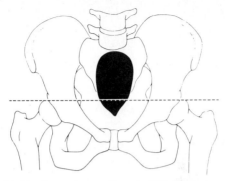

Figure 5. Pelvic bleeding produces a "tear drop" bladder by compressing the bladder from all sides and lifting it out of the pelvis. *(From Wyker AW, Gillenwater JY: Method of Urology. Baltimore: Williams & Wilkins, 1975, p 119.)*

der, but the result of a laceration of pelvic vessels and muscles from fracturing of the pelvis. Pelvic hematoma causes bilateral compression, and the bladder appears elongated and pyriform in shape and lifted out of the pelvis.

2. Bladder Contusion
   a. This is a diagnosis of exclusion after an IV urogram and cystourethrography have demon-

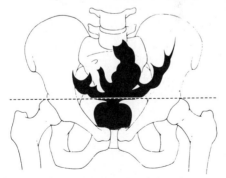

Figure 6. Intraperitoneal extravasation showing contrast medium in the peritoneal cavity extending along the pericolic gutters. *(From Wyker AW, Gillenwater JY: Method of Urology. Baltimore: Williams & Wilkins, 1975, p 119.)*

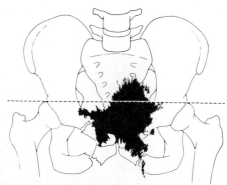

Figure 7. Extraperitoneal extravasation occurs below the line across the roof of the acetabular cavities into the prevesical space and pelvic tissues. *(From Wyker AW, Gillenwater JY: Method of Urology. Baltimore: Williams & Wilkins, 1975, p. 120.)*

strated an intact urinary tract. It is usually secondary to nonpenetrating trauma and manifested by hematuria secondary to a partial thickness tear of the bladder.
3. Intraperitoneal Rupture (Fig. 6)
   a. Contrast is visible in the peritoneal cavity, above the level of the acetabular cavities, and may outline bowel loops.
4. Extraperitoneal Rupture (Fig. 7)
   a. This usually occurs on the anterolateral walls and is associated with pelvic fracture.
   b. A "sunburst" appearance of contrast is seen, with extravasation visible below a line drawn across the roof of acetabular cavities.

E. **Treatment**
   1. Penetrating Bladder Injuries
      a. These injuries can be very lethal because of the high incidence of associated rectal injury.
      b. Exploration and debridement of the injury with two-layer closure and suprapubic drainage is recommended.

   c. The peritoneal cavity should be inspected for associated injury. Injury to the vas deferens, adnexa, and iliac vessels is searched for.
2. Blunt Bladder Injury
   a. Blunt injuries with evidence of intraabdominal trauma (positive peritoneal lavage and those with intraperitoneal bladder rupture) are managed similarly to penetrating injuries.
   b. Although a suprapubic tube is used for vesical drainage in males, females may be managed with a large Foley catheter per urethra.
   c. The perivesical space should be drained.
   d. Patients with extraperitoneal bladder rupture after pelvic fracture can be surgically explored through a purely extraperitoneal approach.
   e. Extraperitoneal ruptures can be managed with urethral catheter drainage alone when the following conditions are met: (1) no reason to suspect a complicating injury requiring exploration; (2) diagnosis is made within 12 hours; and (3) no evidence of urinary tract infection.
3. "Tear Drop" Bladder and Bladder Contusion
   a. These can be managed with catheter drainage alone until the patient is able to void and bleeding has stopped.

IV. GENITAL TRAUMA

The relative mobility of the genitalia tend to protect them from serious injury in civilian life.

A. Nonpenetrating Trauma
1. These wounds of the penis and scrotum may be associated with marked edema of the tissues because of the elastic nature of the skin and fascia layers.
2. Cold packs, rest, elevation, and occasionally pressure dressings are indicated when damage to the testes and corpora cavernosa is not suspected.
3. Persistent hemorrhage requires open surgical hemostasis and drainage.

4. Crush injuries where rupture of the testes or corporal tissue is suspected require immediate surgical exploration and repair.

B. Penetrating Trauma
1. These injuries are treated similarly to penetrating trauma elsewhere on the body.
2. Retrograde urethrography may be important to document urethral integrity.
3. Lavage, debridement, removal of foreign bodies, attainment of hemostasis, repair of underlying structures, and primary wound closure (unless gross contamination is present) are the mainstays of therapy.

C. Avulsion Injuries
1. Avulsions of the penile and scrotal skin are usually secondary to machinery accidents.
2. Skin separation occurs along relatively bloodless planes superficial to Buck's fascia in the penile shaft and just beneath the Dartos fascia of the scrotum.
3. Immediate treatment consists of analgesics, application of sterile moist saline packs, broad spectrum antibiotics, tetanus and gas gangrene antitoxins, and emergency surgical repair within hours of the injury.
4. Split thickness skin grafts are used to cover the denuded penile shaft. Skin distal to the avulsion should be debrided to the area of the glans (leaving a small cuff on which to anchor the graft) to prevent marked lymphedema.
5. An indwelling urethral catheter and pressure dressings are usually necessary.
6. If scrotal skin is lost, the testicles should be covered with whatever scrotal skin remains.
   a. Scrotal tissue will return to normal size and consistency in a period of months.
   b. If skin is insufficient to provide testicular housing, the testes may be implanted immediately beneath the thigh.

BIBLIOGRAPHY
Cockett: Symposium on urological trauma. Contemp Surg 14:95–125, 1979.
Guerriero WG: Trauma to the kidneys, ureters, bladder and urethra. Surg Clin North Am 62:1047–1074, 1982.

Hanno PM, Wein AJ: Urologic trauma. Emerg Med Clin North Am 2:823–841, 1984.

Kessler R: Diagnosis and treatment of genitourinary emergencies. Urol Dig October:12–28, 1976.

Kulp DA: Genital injuries: Etiology and initial management. Urol Clin North Am 54:143–156, 1977.

McAninch JW: Trauma to the bladder and urethra. Infect Surg February:134–148, 1983.

McConnell JD, Wilkerson MD, Peters PC: Rupture of the bladder. Urol Clin North Am 9:293–296, 1982.

Montie J: Bladder injuries. Urol Clin North Am 54:59–68, 1977.

Morehouse DD: Emergency management of urethral trauma. Urol Clin North Am 9:2, 1982.

11

Bladder Outlet Obstruction

Kathleen Murphy
Terrence R. Malloy

I. GENERAL CONSIDERATIONS

A. Definition
Inability to completely empty the bladder due to anatomic obstruction.

B. Incidence
Incidence increases with age in the male from the fifth to the ninth decade. Obstruction can be seen in the female from childbearing years to the seventh and eighth decades.

C. Common Causes of Bladder Obstruction in the Male
1. Benign prostatic hyperplasia
2. Carcinoma of the prostate
3. Urethral stricture
4. Bladder neck contracture
5. Bladder calculi
6. Prostatitis—acute and chronic

D. Common Causes of Bladder Obstruction in the Female
1. Urethral stenosis
2. Urethral trauma
3. Urethral diverticula—sac-like dilatations that are separate from but communicate with the urethra
4. Bladder decensus with cystourethroceles—bladder protrusion into the urethra

II. SYMPTOMS OF BLADDER OUTLET OBSTRUCTION

A. Obstructive Symptoms
1. Decreased force of urinary stream
2. Hesitancy of urinary stream
3. Double voiding (patient voids and is able to void again within 5 to 10 minutes)
4. Postmicturition dribbling
5. Interrupted urinary stream
6. Urinary retention
7. Overflow urinary incontinence (the bladder is always full and overflows with coughing or straining)

B. Irritative Symptoms
1. Dysuria
2. Frequency
3. Nocturia
4. Urgency and urgency incontinence

III. DIAGNOSIS OF BLADDER OUTLET OBSTRUCTION

A. Physical Examination
1. Abdominal examination—bladder percussible or visibly distended
2. Penile examination
   a. Meatal stenosis
   b. Inability to pass urethral sound or catheter
3. Female pelvic examination
   a. Urethral diverticulum—may be palpable on examining urethra
   b. Bladder descensus with cystourethrocele
   c. Meatal stenosis obvious on urethral calibration (measurement of urethral meatal diameter with special sounds)
4. Rectal examination
   a. Prostate exam
      (1) Enlarged, benign-feeling prostate
      (2) Enlarged, boggy, tender prostate suggestive of prostatitis

(3) Enlarged hard prostate suggestive of carcinoma
b. Perianal/rectal fistulae

B. Laboratory Studies
1. Urinalysis
2. Microscopic examination of the prostatic fluid and/or urethral secretions
3. Blood laboratory examination
   a. Blood urea nitrogen
   b. Serum creatinine
   c. Serum electrolytes

C. Radiographic Examinations
1. Intravenous urography—indicated in all patients who have obstruction and hematuria; may reveal upper tract changes or bladder changes secondary to obstruction (hydronephrosis, bladder trabeculation, bladder diverticula)
2. Voiding cystourethrogram—contrast placed in the bladder and voided during fluoroscopic examination; may demonstrate functional (failure of bladder neck to open normally during bladder contraction) as well as anatomic outlet obstruction
3. Urethrogram—indicated in patients suspected of having urethral stricture (Fig. 1)
4. Ultrasound studies of kidneys, ureter, and bladder (may reveal obstruction of upper tracts, chronic urinary retention)

D. Urodynamic Evaluation of Patient (See Chapter 16)
1. Cystometrogram
   a. May combine with urecholine supersensitivity testing in patients suspected of having neurogenic bladder dysfunction
2. Urine flowmetry
3. Urethral pressure profile
4. Combined cine–urinary flow studies with electromyographic studies of the perineum (video urodynamics for complicated cases of obstruction where etiology is in doubt)

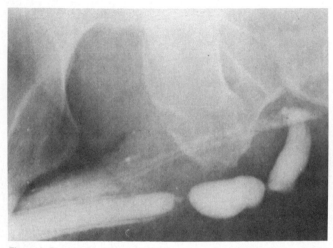

Figure 1. Retrograde urethrogram showing two areas of significant narrowing due to stricture disease.

E. Endoscopic Examination of the Urethra and Bladder
1. Urethroscopy—direct examination of the urethra
2. Cystoscopy
   a. Examination of the prostatic urethra and bladder with both 30- and 70-degree lens systems
   b. One must not make the diagnosis of obstruction secondary to prostatic enlargement solely on the basis of cystoscopic appearance of the prostatic lobes

F. Diagnosis
It is important to base a diagnosis of obstruction on a combination of study results. One must evaluate the patient's symptoms in conjunction with the results of urodynamics and endoscopic procedures.

IV. BLADDER OUTLET OBSTRUCTION DUE TO THE PROSTATE
A. Functions of the Prostate
1. The prostate produces 1 ml of cloudy fluid daily, carried out in the urine.

  2. It is responsible for about half of the semen volume of ejaculation.
  3. Prostatic fluid facilitates fertilization by acting as a vehicle for spermatozoa and as an aid to semen liquefication through the enzyme fibrinolysin.

B. Prostatic Growth
  1. There is a slow increase in prostatic size from birth until puberty.
  2. For the prostate to reach the adult size of 20 to 25 g, two factors are necessary—time and testes.
  3. There is a rapid increase in the size of the prostate from puberty to age 20. It then remains constant until about age 45.
  4. Above the age of 45 the prostate will either atrophy, with progressive decrease in size, or undergo benign prostatic hyperplasia (BPH).

C. Factors Associated with BPH
  1. No BPH occurs in men castrated prior to puberty.
  2. Regression has been reported after castration in adults.
  3. BPH can be produced by hormones in animal models.
  4. BPH is associated with abnormal accumulation of dihydrotestosterone.
  5. There is no relation between BPH and cancer.

D. Prostatism
Prostatism is the term used to designate obstruction to urinary flow due to enlarged prostate. It may be benign, inflammatory, or malignant in etiology (Fig. 2).

E. Upper Tract Decompensation—Pathophysiology
  1. For urine to pass from the ureter to the bladder, ureteral contraction pressure must exceed intravesical pressure.
  2. If intravesical pressure is increased, urine passes only when ureteral pressure increases and decompensation of the upper tracts is possible.
  3. This can lead to chronic renal failure ("postrenal failure").
  4. "Silent protatism" occurs in up to 5% of patients with BPH. Patients present with weakness and

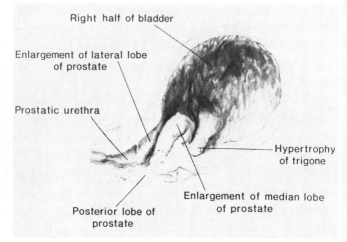

Figure 2. Sagittal view of prostatic urethra and bladder illustrating prostatic hypertrophy.

azotemia due to unrecognized and long-standing outlet obstruction with renal failure.

F. Treatment
1. Cystoscopy with biopsy—cystoscopy evaluates the amount of obstruction and needle biopsy may be used to determine the pathology of the prostate.
2. Prostatectomy for benign disease
   a. Indications—signs of significant bladder outlet obstruction on intravenous pyelogram (IVP) or endoscopy and/or significant symptoms such that a surgical procedure would improve the quality of life with a low and acceptable risk.
   b. Types of procedures
      (1) Transurethral incision of bladder neck and prostate—used in young men who have decreased flow rates without an anatomically enlarged prostate; also used in men who have

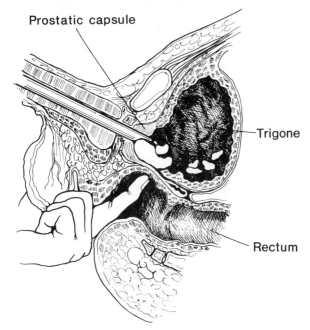

Figure 3. Transurethral prostatectomy.

bladder neck contractures or bladder neck hypertrophy.

(2) Transurethral resection of the prostate (Fig. 3)—used in men who have enlarged prostates and in whom the ureteral orifices can be clearly seen.

(3) Suprapubic (open) prostatectomy—removal of prostatic adenoma by opening the bladder so as to visualize the ureteral orifices that may be obscured by a large prostate; also useful if a simultaneous procedure on the bladder is necessary.

(4) Retropubic (open) prostatectomy—an abdominal approach to removing the prostatic ade-

noma for glands larger than 60 g. The prostatic capsule is visualized directly underneath the pubic bone and opened to remove the growth.

(5) Perineal prostatectomy—removal of prostatic adenoma through an incision between the scrotum and anus.

G. **Early Perioperative and Postoperative Complications of Prostatic Surgery**

1. Hematuria—can have excessive blood loss during the surgery or immediately afterwards.
2. Extravasation of urine due to damage to bladder or urethra.
3. Damage to urethral sphincteric mechanism with incontinence (approximately 0.5% of cases).
4. Urinary sepsis (avoid prostatic surgery in the presence of infected urine).
5. Posttransurethral resection (TUR) syndrome—hypertension, bradycardia, and change in mental status in patient undergoing transurethral prostatectomy. This is due to absorption of irrigation fluid through open venous sinuses. Treat with saline infusion and diuretics.
6. Postoperative epididymitis or orchitis secondary to reflux of infected urine through ejaculatory ducts.
7. Pulmonary emboli.

H. **Late Complications of Prostatectomy**

1. Bladder neck contracture (up to 10% of cases).
2. Urethral stricture (3 to 15% of cases).
3. Urinary incontinence.
4. Impotence
   a. Six percent incidence in literature following transurethral resection prostatectomy (TURP).
   b. Up to 30% incidence following perineal prostatectomy
   c. Five percent incidence with suprapubic and retropubic prostatectomy
5. Retrograde ejaculation occurs in up to 90% of patients after prostatic surgery. The bladder neck is surgically resected and cannot reflexly close at the time of emis-

sion and ejaculation. Semen goes backwards into the bladder and is voided out with urination.

I. Results of Prostatectomy
1. The overall success rate using modern surgical techniques is greater than 90%. Complications are minimal and morbidity is low, especially with transurethral resection.

V. URETHRAL OBSTRUCTION

A. Meatal Stenosis
1. Can be dilated or surgically corrected in males and females
2. Generally excellent results from surgical therapy
3. Minimal complications to therapy

B. Urethral Strictures
1. Etiology
   a. Congenital
   b. Infectious agents—especially sexually transmitted diseases such as gonorrhea can give long-term urethral strictures
   c. Trauma—especially pelvic crush injuries which can result in posterior urethral strictures or perineal injuries which can result in bulbar urethral strictures (see Chapter 10)
   d. Iatrogenic causes
      (1) Most common cause of urethral stricture
      (2) May be secondary to indwelling urethral catheters, transurethral surgery, or transurethral diagnostic procedures
   e. Neoplasms
      (1) Carcinoma of the urethra
      (2) Venereal warts (condyloma accuminata)
      (3) Benign urethral polyps
2. Treatment of Urethral Strictures
   a. Dilation of strictures
      (1) Dilatation with urethral sounds or filiforms and followers

           (2) Intermittent self-catheterization by the patient
- b. Internal optical urethrotomy
  - (1) Incision of the strictured area under direct vision through a specially designed endoscope
  - (2) One-year follow-up reveals 59% success rate—higher when patient catheterizes himself on a regular basis to keep scar from reforming
- c. Urethroplasty (reconstruction of urethra)
  - (1) One-stage urethroplasty with or without patch graft—excision of stricture with primary reanastomosis
  - (2) Two-stage urethroplasty—generally two-stage urethroplasties have the greatest historical success rate. The area of stricture is marsupialized and allowed to heal. At a second stage 6 months later the tissue is retubularized to form a new urethra.
- d. Neodymium Yag Laser photoradiation for treatment of urethral strictures—newest therapy with mixed results. Long-term place in stricture treatment is unknown at this time.

VI. BLADDER NECK CONTRACTURE

A. Definition
Concentrically narrowed bladder neck without concomitant prostatic enlargement.

B. Etiology
1. Congenital
2. Secondary to previous prostatic surgery
3. Secondary to trauma either external or surgical

C. Treatment
1. Dilatation
2. Transurethral incision of bladder neck contracture
3. Transurethral resection of bladder neck
4. Open surgical correction with Y-V plasty of bladder neck

VII. BLADDER OBSTRUCTION IN FEMALES

A. Meatal Stenosis
1. Etiology
   a. Congenital
   b. Secondary to infection
   c. Secondary to trauma (vaginal deliveries)
2. Treatment
   a. Dilatation with sounds or catheters
   b. Antibiotic therapy to relieve infection
   c. Urethroplasty
3. Results of Treatment
   a. Surgical therapy corrects condition in more than 95% of cases.
   b. Follow-up is essential to prevent further recurrence of meatal stenosis.
   c. Elimination of infection and trauma to the urethra is essential for long-term good results.

B. Urethral Diverticula
1. Etiology
   a. Infection of periurethral glands
   b. Trauma secondary to vaginal delivery
   c. Previous vaginal surgery
2. Treatment
   a. Incision and drainage—may temporarily relieve acute obstruction
   b. Urethral diverticulectomy with urethroplasty—excision of urethral diverticulum through vaginal incision and primary closure of urethra
   c. Spence–Duckett procedure—opening up the urethra from the meatus through to the area of the diverticulum (useful primarily for distal diverticula)

C. Bladder Decensus with Cystourethrocele
1. Etiology
   a. Postmenopausal pelvic relaxation.
   b. Increased incidence with multiple vaginal deliveries.

2. Treatment—a variety of operative approaches have evolved to deal with this problem. As the condition may be associated with stress urinary incontinence, the reader is referred to Chapter 16.

BIBLIOGRAPHY

Benson M, Olson CA: The bladder. In Paulson DF (ed): Genitourinary Surgery. New York: Churchill Livingston, 1984, p 209.

Flocks RH, Scott WW (eds): The prostate. Urol Clin North Am 2:1975.

Kendall AR, Karafin L: Obstructive uropathy—Prostatism. In Lapides J (ed): Fundamental of Urology Philadelphia: W.B. Saunders, 1976, p 317.

O'Connor VJ, Nanninga JB: Benign disease of the prostate Müllerian duct reminants. In Devine CJ, Stucker JF (eds): Urology in Practice. Boston: Little, Brown, 1978, p 853.

Paulson DF: The prostate. In Paulson DF (ed): Genitourinary Surgery New York: Churchill Livingston, 1984, p 313.

Turner-Warwick R, Whiteside CG, et al: The urodynamic view of prostatic obstruction and the results of prostatectomy. Br J Urol 45:631, 1973.

12

Acute Renal Failure: Recognition and Management

Robert A. Grossman

I. NORMAL RENAL ANATOMY AND PHYSIOLOGY

A. Anatomy

Each kidney contains about 1 million nephrons. The nephron consists of a glomerulus, a capillary tuft that serves as a filter, and a tubule lined with epithelial cells that acts upon the filtrate.

B. Physiology

The kidneys receive about 20% of the resting cardiac output or about 1 liter/min of blood. With a hematocrit of about 40%, the renal *plasma* flow is about 600 ml/min. Normally, 20% of this plasma is filtered at the glomeruli giving a glomerular filtration rate (GFR) of 120 ml/min or about 170 liters/day. The filtrate is acted upon by the renal tubule such that over 99% is reabsorbed leaving a urine output of 1.0 to 1.5 liters/day. The tubule consists of three parts.

1. *The proximal tubule.* Here 70% of the filtrate is absorbed isosmotically, i.e. without substantial change in its sodium, potassium, or bicarbonate concentrations.

2. *The Loop of Henle.* In this region 20% of the filtrate's solute, mainly chloride with its cation, sodium, is removed. Solute is removed in greater amounts than

water so that the filtrate leaving the loop is *hypo-
osmolar* compared with plasma. The solute so removed is concentrated in the medulla by a countercurrent mechanism rendering the medulla hyperosmolar
to plasma. This allows for concentration of the urine as
the collecting duct swings back through the medulla on
its way to the renal pelvis.

3. *The Distal Convoluted Tubule and Collecting Ducts.*
Here, the final composition of the urine is attained.
Water may be absorbed through the action of vasopressin yielding a urine with an osmolality as great as
four times that of plasma. Conversely, in the absence
of vasopressin, and with continued removal of solute,
the urine may be diluted to an osmolality one-fourth
that of plasma. Potassium and hydrogen ions are actively and passively secreted; the final adjustment of
sodium excretion is made.

C. Clearance

If there were a substance y present in the blood at a stable
level, freely filtered at the glomerulus, and neither absorbed nor secreted by the tubule, such a substance could
be used to estimate the GFR by the following formula.

$$\text{GFR} \times P_y = U_y \times V \text{ (urine flow rate)}$$
$$\text{or}$$

The amount of "y" filtered = the amount of "y"
excreted

Rearranging the formula gives:

$$\text{GFR} = \frac{U_y \times V}{P_y}$$

This is the clearance equation, which can be used not only
to estimate GFR but to assess the manner in which the
kidney handles a multitude of substances.

Clearance: The theoretical amount of plasma from
which a substance is completely removed by the action of
the kidney in a defined period of time. It is usually expressed as milliliters per minute.

The creatinine clearance (C_{cr}) is used clinically to measure GFR. Creatinine for practical purposes has all the characteristics of "y" mentioned in the previous equation.

$$C_{cr} = U_{cr} \frac{(mg/dl \times V(ml/min)}{P_{cr}(mg/dl)}$$

A more practical method for calculating creatinine clearances which is valid *only* for 24-hour collections follows:

$$C_{cr} = \frac{24\text{-hour urinary creatinine in grams} \times 70}{\text{serum creatinine in milligrams per deciliter}}$$

The number "70" is not a "fudge factor"; rather, it results from the factoring of all the units used.

D. Fractional Excretion

Many substances are acted upon by the renal tubular cells. Substances that are predominately secreted by the tubules may have a clearance greater than C_{cr}. Many drugs fall into this category. In contrast, substances that are predominately reabsorbed by the renal tubule may have clearances much slower than C_{cr}. The renal handling of sodium is an example. At a GFR of 120 ml/min and a serum sodium concentration of 140 mEq/liter the normal kidneys filter about 24,000 mEq of sodium daily. Of the amount filtered, only about 120 to 240 mEq is excreted in the urine, a fractional excretion of 0.5 to 1.0%. The fractional excretion of any substance may be considered a measure of tubular function for that substance. The fractional excretion of sodium $(F.E._{Na})$ has many useful clinical applications. Clinically, the fractional excretion of a substance is measured by dividing the clearance of that substance by the clearance of creatinine (the amount excreted/amount filtered). The quotient is multiplied by 100 to give the fractional excretion as a percent. For sodium the expression would be:

$$F.E._{Na} = (C_{Na}/C_{cr}) \times 100$$

Writing out the expression fully:

$$F.E._{Na} = \frac{U_{Na}V/P_{Na}}{U_{cr}V/P_{cr}} \times 100$$

In the preceding equation the Vs cancel, yielding:

$$F.E._{Na} = \frac{U_{Na} \times P_{cr}}{U_{cr} \times P_{Na}} \times 100$$

Since the Vs cancel, a fractional excretion can be performed on any volume of urine, a 24-hour collection is not required. The clinical use of the $F.E._{Na}$ in differentiating different types of renal failure will be explained as we proceed.

E. **Concentration, Dilution, and Oliguria**

Through the countercurrent mechanism, the activity of the loop of Henle, and the action of vasopressin, the urine in a normal person can be concentrated to an osmolality of 1200 mOsm/kg H_2O (four times that of plasma). In the opposite direction, urine can be diluted to about 75 mOsm/kg H_2O, one-fourth that of plasma. The normal adult eating a standard diet is obligated to excrete about 500 mOsm of solute per day; half of this is sodium, potassium, and their anions and the other half is urea, the end-product of protein catabolism. If these 500 mOsm can be excreted in a urine concentrated to 1200 mOsm/kg (or liter) H_2O, it will require a volume of urine slightly greater than 400 ml. By this definition, a urine output of less than 400 ml/day is considered oliguria. However, in almost any disease state, the kidneys lose concentrating ability; additionally, in catabolic states, the obligatory solute load may far exceed 500 mOsm/day. Both of these conditions would increase the volume of urine required. Nonetheless, the convention stands: a urine output of less than 400 ml/day is considered oliguria.

II. PRERENAL AZOTEMIA (Table 1)

A. **Pathophysiology**

In prerenal azotemia, the kidneys, by definition, are normal but are being poorly perfused because of decreased plasma volume or an "ineffective" plasma volume caused by vasodilatation or severely depressed plasma protein levels. Alternatively, the kidneys may be poorly

TABLE 1. CAUSES OF PRERENAL AZOTEMIA

Volume Depletion	*Volume Shifts*
Hemorrhage	"Third space losses"
GI losses	Vasodilating drugs
Vomiting	Gram-negative sepsis or
Diarrhea	"warm shock"
Renal losses	
Excessive diuretics	*Volume Expansion*
"Salt losing nephritis"	Congestive heart failure
Addison's disease	Nephrotic syndrome
Burns	Cirrhosis with ascites
Heat prostration	

perfused because of poor contractility of the heart. Because the kidneys are intrinsically normal, one would expect the urine produced to be concentrated with a low urinary sodium level and $F.E._{Na}$. The microscopic sediment should be benign.

B. History

1. Fluid losses—vomiting or diarrhea are usually evident; however, excessive use of diuretics or high insensible losses may be more subtle.
2. Recent surgery or fevers.
3. Drug history—many blood pressure medications, particularly combination drugs, contain thiazide diuretics.
4. The degree of congestive heart failure or cirrhosis necessary to cause prerenal azotemia is usually obvious in the uncomplicated patient.

C. Physical Examination

1. Low or relatively low blood pressure.
2. Decreased skin turgor—the inner aspect of the thighs is a good place to check.
3. Dry mouth and axillae.
4. Orthostatic changes in pulse or blood pressure. This is an overly emphasized physical finding; substantial volume depletion may exist without orthostatic changes.
5. The edematous states are usually self-evident.
6. In complicated cases, measurement of central pres-

TABLE 2. URINALYSIS IN ACUTE RENAL FAILURE

	Prerenal	AGN	ATN	Obstruction
Urine osmolality (mOsm/kg H_2O)	>350	>350	<350	<350
Urine sodium (mEq/L)	<30	<30	>30	>30
Qualitative urine protein	- To trace	3+-4+	1+-2+	- To trace
Urinary sediment	Normal	Red cells and red cell casts	"Dirty"[a]	Normal
Fractional excretion of sodium	<1%	<1%	>>1%	>1%

[a]Sediment contains RBC's, WBC's, renal tubular cells, casts of all types, and broad dirty brown casts.

sures and/or cardiac output may be necessary to define pre-renal azotemia.

D. Laboratory Data (see Table 2):
1. Urinary sodium concentration less than 20 mEq/L *prior to administration of diuretics.*
2. F.E.$_{Na}$ less than 1%, again in the absence of diuretics.
3. Urine osmolality greater than 110% of plasma osmolality.
4. Little or no proteinuria.
5. Benign microscopic urinary sediment.
6. BUN–creatinine ratio often greater than 20.

E. Therapy
1. Volume depletion or shifts: expand plasma volume with *isotonic* fluids, i.e., 0.9% saline, lactated Ringer's solution, albumin solutions, or blood.
2. Edematous states: correct the underlying condition if possible.

III. OBSTRUCTIVE UROPATHY (Table 3)

A. Pathophysiology
In obstructive uropathy there is not an inflammatory process within the renal parenchyma; instead, there is in-

ACUTE RENAL FAILURE

ACUTE RENAL FAILURE 241

TABLE 3. CAUSES OF OBSTRUCTIVE UROPATHY

Bladder Outlet
  Prostatic hyperplasia
Bilateral Ureteral Obstruction
  Tumor invasion
  Retroperitoneal fibrosis
  Calculi
  Surgical accident
Renal Pelvic and Intrarenal Obstruction
  Staghorn calculi
  Papillary necrosis
  Acute uric acid nephropathy (tumor lysis syndrome)

creased back-pressure on the renal tubules causing tubular dysfunction. Almost all tubular functions are compromised: concentration of urine, reabsorption of sodium and water, and secretion of hydrogen and potassium ions. Therefore the urine produced is usually not concentrated and has a high sodium concentration and $F.E._{Na}$. The microscopic sediment is usually benign.

B. History
1. The history is of little value, particularly when the site of obstruction is above the bladder neck. The process of obstruction of the ureters is often asynchronous; one kidney is lost silently, then the process affects the remaining kidney.
2. Bladder outlet obstruction—hesitancy, dribbling, frequency of urination, decrease in urinary stream.
3. Obstruction above the bladder—the only historical fact, occasionally found, is a change in voiding pattern. Remember, a partially obstructed kidney is *polyuric;* frequency and nocturia may be noted. Rarely a pattern of complete anuria alternating with polyuria may be found.

C. Physical Examination
1. Bladder outlet obstruction—palpable bladder after voiding, enlarged prostate on rectal examination.
2. Obstruction above the bladder usually cannot be determined by physical examination.

D. Laboratory Data

1. *Urine Analysis* (see Table 2). The urine is usually bland microscopically with little or no protein present. Because of tubular defects, the urine is usually isosmolar with plasma. It contains a high sodium concentration and a high $F.E._{Na}$, usually greater than 3%.

2. *Diagnosis*. Bladder outlet obstruction can often be determined by the placement of a Foley catheter. Above the bladder diagnosis is almost exclusively radiologic.

   a. Renal ultrasound examination

   b. Radionuclide scanning

   c. Computerized tomography

   d. Intravenous urography

E. Treatment

1. Mechanical Relief of Obstruction

   a. Foley catheterization

   b. Percutaneous nephrostomy placement

   c. Retrograde ureteral catheterization

2. Postobstructive Diuresis

   a. Following relief of the obstruction there may be a diuresis of many liters per day. The diuresis is due to the tubular defects mentioned above; in addition, at the time of the relief of the obstruction, the patient usually is hypertensive, edematous, and has a high BUN level, all of which enhance the diuresis. The urine produced may be grossly bloody. During obstruction with high pressures within the collecting system, small blood vessels may be torn. However, the high pressure within the system tamponades these vessels. On release of the pressure, bleeding occurs.

   b. The urine usually contains 70 to 80 mEq/L of sodium with its anion. It usually contains only a small amount of potassium. Replace the urine with 0.45% saline with or without dextrose. Potassium chloride and sodium bicarbonate may be added depending on the serum levels of the patient and measured urinary losses.

   c. If the patient is edematous and/or hypertensive at the start of the diuresis, do not replace the full

TABLE 4. CAUSES OF RENAL PARENCHYMAL DISEASE

Acute Glomerulonephritis	*Acute Tubular Necrosis*
Isolated	Ischemic injury (see Table 1)
Post-strep	Toxic injury
Idiopathic	Endogenous toxins
In systemic disease	Heme pigments
Lupus	Gram-negative endotoxemia
Chronic bacteremia (SBE)	Exogenous toxins
Microvascular disease	*Aminoglycoside antibiotics*
Vasculitis	*X-ray contrast dyes*
Malignant hypertension	Heavy metals
Scleroderma	Organic solvents
	Ethylene glycol
Large-Vessel Occlusion	Insecticides
Atherosclerosis	Herbicides
Tumor invasion	
Trauma	*Allergic Interstitial Nephritis*
Renal arterial emboli	Antibiotics
Renal vein thrombosis	Penicillins and cephalosporins
	Nonsteroidal antiinflammatory drugs
	Thiazide diuretics including furosemide
	Allopurinol
	Antiseizure medications

urine output until the patient becomes euvolemic; then replace the urine output fully until the BUN and creatinine levels have become normal or reached a plateau. At that point replace less than the urine flow so that the urine output is not being driven by the replacement fluids.

IV. RENAL PARENCHYMAL DISEASE (Table 4)

A. Acute Glomerulonephritis (AGN)

1. *Pathophysiology.* In AGN the principal abnormality is inflammation of the glomeruli with relative sparing of the tubules. As a result, the GRF is low, the urine contains large amounts of protein, red cells, and red cell casts. Because the tubules are relatively intact, the urine has a low U_{Na} and $F.E._{Na}$.

2. *History.* Often not terribly helpful. An antecedent strep infection of the pharynx or *skin* can sometimes be found. Symptoms of serosal inflammation with joint

pain, pleural or pericardial pain, rashes, fever, or weight loss may point toward a systemic vasculitis or lupus.

3. *Physical Examination.* Edema and hypertension are very common; changes in the optic fundi may suggest the latter. Skin lesions, arthritis, pleural or pericardial rubs may suggest vasculitis. A new or changing murmur can suggest the diagnosis of bacterial endocarditis.

4. *Laboratory Data* (see Table 2). The urinalysis is the key for diagnosis. It is usually concentrated, with a low sodium concentration and low $F.E._{Na}$ and usually contains a large amount of protein. Microscopic exam shows red cells, white cells, coarse and fine granular casts. The presence of red blood cell casts is the hallmark of AGN.

Further tests are beyond the scope of this chapter but include blood cultures for endocarditis and serologic tests for recent streptococcal infections, lupus or vasculitis. Diagnosis is often confirmed by a renal biopsy.

5. *Treatment.* Details of treatment of AGN are also beyond the scope of this chapter but include no treatment for poststreptococcal AGN, proper antibiotics for chronic bacteremia, lowering of blood pressure in malignant hypertension, and corticosteroids and/or immunosuppressive drugs for lupus or vasculitis.

B. Allergic Interstitial Nephritis (AIN)

1. *Pathophysiology.* In recent years it has been recognized that a wide variety of drugs (see Table 4) are associated with the development of an acute decrement in renal function in sensitive individuals. Histologically, the kidneys show an intense interstitial infiltrate with mononuclear cells and eosinophils. This reaction is often accompanied by systemic symptoms listed below. The composition of the urine in this condition is not well defined but over half of the patients will have eosinophils present in the urine.

2. History
   a. Almost any drug can cause AIN; the list grows longer by the month. It may be a new drug or a drug the patient has taken for years.
   b. An unexplained fever, a maculopapular eruption, and arthralgias occur in a majority of patients but are not necessary for the diagnosis.
3. *Physical Examination.* The presence of fever and/or rash are the only clues from examining the patient.
4. Laboratory Data
   a. Eosinophilia is found in a majority of patients.
   b. Eosinophils in the urine are found in about half of patients with AIN. Urine sediment is difficult to stain with Wright's or Giemsa's stain, as the cells in the urine disintegrate. Spin the urine, pour off the supernate, and mix the "button" with a few drops of the patient's serum, then stain. The protein in the serum stabilizes the cells in the sediment so that they accept the stain without disintegration.
   c. Renal biopsy may be necessary for diagnosis.
5. Treatment
   a. Cessation of offending or presumed offending drug.
   b. It is unclear whether corticosteroids change the course of the disease.

C. Large Vessel Occlusion

1. *Pathophysiology.* In arterial occlusion by tumor invasion or atherosclerosis, one kidney is lost with little or no symptoms; only when the second kidney is involved do signs or symptoms appear. With renal ischemia, there is usually activation of the renin–angiotensin system, resulting in severe hypertension. In addition, a single functioning kidney with impaired blood flow is "prerenal" by definition. If the occlusion of arterial supply is gradual, collateral circulation opens from capsular, adrenal, ureteral, and lumbar vessels. In sudden arterial occlusion from trauma or emboli there may be infarction of the kidney and no hypertension.

Renal vein thrombosis is a rare cause of renal insufficiency. If the thrombosis is gradual, collateral venous circulation may appear. If is it rapid, the kidney sometimes undergoes venous infarction. There is a high degree of association between renal vein thrombosis and membranous glomerulonephritis; which of the two conditions is primary is still unresolved.

2. *History.* The classic history of flank pain and hematuria is almost never found in gradual arterial occlusion. With traumatic or embolic arterial occlusion these symptoms are more common but not universally found. Nausea, vomiting, and symptoms suggesting ileus are sometimes found in sudden renal infarction. Pulmonary emboli are the main concern in renal vein thrombosis.

3. Physical Examination
   a. Severe hypertension is very common in gradual arterial occlusion.
   b. Flank mass and tenderness are rare.
   c. In sudden arterial occlusion with renal infarction blood pressure may be normal; however, flank tenderness, nausea, vomiting and ileus may be present.

4. Laboratory Data
   a. In gradual arterial occlusion, the urinalysis is usually benign with a high osmolality, low U_{Na} and low F.E.$_{Na}$.
   b. In slowly occurring renal vein thrombosis there may be heavy proteinuria.
   c. In sudden arterial or venous occlusion, gross or microscopic hematuria may be found. High serum LDH levels are also found but are very nonspecific.
   d. Radiographic studies
      (1) Radionuclide scans give crude information in arterial thrombosis. There are no good data on their usefulness in renal vein thrombosis.
      (2) Angiographic studies are the ''gold standard'' for definitive diagnosis of both arterial and venous occlusion.

5. Treatment
   a. Gradual arterial occlusion. Collateral circulation may maintain viability of the kidney even though it appears to be nonfunctional, particularly if the kidney has not shrunk in size. Surgical or angiographic (transluminal angioplasty) revascularization may restore renal function.
   b. Sudden arterial occlusion. Even in sudden arterial occlusion from emboli, the kidney may remain viable for days because of capsular colateral circulation. Interestingly, there are no good data to support surgical revascularization; success in salvage of kidney function appears to be just as good with anticoagulation. Whether surgical or medical therapy should be used for traumatic occlusion of the renal arteries depends on the individual situation.
   c. Renal vein thrombosis
      (1) Surgical thrombectomy is usually futile because the clot propogates in a retrograde fashion well into the renal parenchyma.
      (2) The major risk of gradual renal vein thrombosis is pulmonary emboli, which occurs in as many as 50% of untreated patients. Anticoagulation is instituted to reduce the risk of emboli; there is little to suggest that it enhances recanalization of occluded veins.

D. Acute Tubular Necrosis (ATN)

1. Pathophysiology
   a. Mechanism of ATN. The intimate pathophysiology maintaining ATN remains unclear although it has been studied for over 30 years. Four theories have been proposed, no one of which entirely fits the data that are available.
      (1) Restriction of blood flow to filtering glomeruli at a glomerular or regional level within the kidney.
      (2) Decreased permeability of the filtering basement membrane of the glomeruli following injury.

      (3) Tubular plugging with a mixture of necrotic cellular debris and protein.

      (4) Disruption of the renal tubules allowing glomerular filtrate to pass directly back into the blood stream.

  b. Inciting events for ATN. The event causing ATN may be ischemic as listed in Table 1 or toxic as shown in Table 4. Why an ischemic event that causes prerenal azotemia in one individual leads to ATN in another is a mystery. There are several conditions that seem to predispose to the development of ATN of either ischemic or toxic cause.

      (1) Advanced age

      (2) Preexisting renal disease

      (3) Hypovolemia

      (4) Recent administration of a nephrotoxic agent

      (5) Right upper quadrant surgery

      (6) ?Acidosis?

  c. Oliguric versus nonoliguric ATN. With the inciting event, either toxic or ischemic, both GFR and renal plasma flow fall dramatically to a few percent (or less) of normal. Over the next several hours renal plasma flow returns to 20 to 30% of normal but GFR remains severely depressed. At this point the patient may be oliguric, or nonoliguric with a urine flow as great as several liters per day. In either case, however, BUN and creatinine levels rise. How can a patient be polyuric yet still have a rising BUN–creatinine? As noted in Section I-B, the normal fractional excretion of *urine*, (GFR/urine flow) $\times$ 100, is less than 1%. With any decrement in renal function fractional excretion of urine rises, often to levels of 20 to 50%, that is, 20 to 50% of the glomerular filtrate comes out as urine. A couple of examples may illustrate the point: (1) Following a renal insult, a patient excretes 2.8 to 3.0 liters of urine per day and yet BUN and creatinine levels rise. This can be explained by proposing a GFR of 4 ml/min with a fractional excretion of urine of 50%. The total

GFR per *day* is 5760 ml; of this 50% is excreted as urine or 2880 ml. Nonetheless, the GFR is still only 4 ml/min, i.e., severe renal insufficiency. (2) This patient suffers a renal insult that reduces his GFR to 1 ml/min with a 20% fractional excretion of urine; his urine output will be less than 300 ml/day. Clinically, the difference between a GFR of 1 and a GFR of 4 is slight and yet urine outputs differ dramatically.

    d. Urinary findings. ATN behaves as a predominant tubular injury. Because of this the urine is usually isosmolar with plasma, contains a modest amount of protein, and has a high sodium level. The sediment contains signs of tubular injury with cells and all types of casts, especially broad, "dirty brown" casts; red cell casts are almost *never* found in ATN.

2. *History.* A careful history will uncover an inciting event for ATN, as listed in Tables 1 and 4, in about 70% of cases. However, in as many as 30% of cases no cause can be found.

3. *Physical Examination.* There are no specific physical findings in ATN. The exam is necessary to determine the volume status of the patient. Signs of volume depletion should be checked. In the opposite direction, signs of volume expansion with hypertension and/or congestive heart failure in the presence of oliguria may hasten or necessitate dialysis.

4. *Laboratory Examination.* Short of renal biopsy, which is often nonspecific in the face of certain ATN, the diagnosis is one of exclusion.

    a. Urine (see Table 2)

        (1) Osmolality of urine within 10% that of plasma

        (2) Trace—2+ protein

        (3) U_{Na} >30 mEq/l, F.E.$_{Na}$ >1%

        (4) White cells, red cells, renal tubular epithelial cells, fine and coarse granular casts, white cell casts, and broad "dirty brown" casts are usually found in the urine sediment.

        (5) If the patient is nonoliguric or a few days have

passed since the insult, the urine microscopic sediment may be bland.
  b. Radiologic investigation
     (1) Ultrasound examination to exclude obstruction and to measure the size and "density" of the kidneys
     (2) Radionuclide scan to ensure renal blood flow
5. *Treatment.* The treatment of ATN, including dialysis, when necessary, is beyond the scope of this chapter. The text will be confined to early treatment, potential reversibility, and indications for dialysis.
  a. MAKE SURE THAT THE CIRCULATING PLASMA VOLUME IS ADEQUATE.
     (1) Careful physical examination
     (2) In complicated cases, measurement of central pressures and/or cardiac output by means of a Swan–Ganz catheter may be necessary.
  b. Correct
     (1) Volume depletion
     (2) Congestive heart failure
     (3) Severe plasma protein deficiency
  c. Having done the above, at the time of the insult or within a few hours try mannitol, one or two 50-ml ampules of 25% solution by rapid IV infusion. Hazard of treatment: Each ampule of mannitol acutely expands the plasma volume by 250 ml; congestive heart failure may occur in predisposed individuals.
  d. If mannitol fails to cause a diuresis or more than a few hours have passed since the insult, try furosemide. Initially give 100 mg by IV infusion. If there is no increase in urine flow after 2 hours, give 200 mg of furosemide IV; if there is again no response, give 400 mg. At any dose if there is a brisk diuresis that gradually declines, that dose may be repeated as necessary. There is probably no advantage in using doses of furosemide greater than 400 mg. *Hazard of treatment:* The hazards of high-dose IV furosemide are very small if the drug is properly administered. Infuse furosemide at a

rate no greater than 1000 mg/hr, i.e., give 200 mg over 10 to 15 minutes, 400 mg over 20 to 30 minutes. Do *not* use IV ethacrynic acid. There is a 1 to 3% incidence of permanent neural deafness following the administration of IV ethacrynic acid in the presence of renal insufficiency. There is no evidence that it is superior to equivalent doses of furosemide. If the patient is allergic to furosemide, bumetanide (Bumex, Roche) may usually be substituted at equivalent doseage.

There is no proof that the use of furosemide changes the course of the renal failure. However, there are many anecdotal reports where the use of furosemide has converted an oliguric patient to polyuria.

e. Indications for dialysis
   (1) Uremia or impending uremia
   (2) Volume overload with congestive heart failure or hypertension
   (3) Severe electrolyte abnormalities, usually hyperkalemia or hyponatremia
   (4) Severe acidosis
   (5) ?Bleeding diathesis?

f. Outcome
   (1) ATN of any form resolves by the development of a diuresis. During the early diuretic phase of ATN the BUN and creatinine levels may continue to rise until the diuresis reaches a peak. During the diuretic phase electrolytes are lost in the urine in an unregulated fashion leading to volume depletion; during the diuresis the patient may become overtly uremic with all the attendant complications of that condition. Fully 25% of the deaths from ATN occur during the diuretic phase.
   (2) If the patient survives, 50% will undergo a diuresis in about 2 weeks, 90% by about 4 weeks; of the remaining 10%, half will require more than 4 weeks to resolve and the other half will never resolve.

(3) The resolution of ATN is usually complete from a clinical point of view. However, if careful studies are performed on patients who have recently recovered from ATN, it will be found that they have GFRs of about 80% of that expected and will show defects in concentrating ability and acid and potassium excretion. These defects resolve completely in a period of time measured in months to years.

(4) Mortality of ATN: ATN is a serious disease; an estimate of death rates follows:

Polyuric ATN	25%–35%
Oliguric ATN	
Surgical causes	50%–70%
Medical causes	30%–50%

(5) Causes of death in ATN: With the advent of dialysis, patients die *with* renal failure, not *of* renal failure. Common causes of death include:
   (a) The disease causing renal failure
   (b) Infections
   (c) Hemorrhage
   (d) Electrolyte imbalance
   (e) Cardiovascular disease

V. RECOGNITION OF ACUTE VERSUS CHRONIC RENAL FAILURE

Patients will often be found to have renal insufficiency without prior history of renal disease or without prior laboratory evaluation. The differentiation of acute renal failure from "acute discovery of chronic renal failure" is often important and difficult. Short of a renal biopsy, which is often impractical, there are clues that point in the direction of chronic disease:

• Small or "dense" kidneys on ultrasound examination
• Anemia without other cause
• Elevated phosphate level with a normal or near normal calcium level

- Evidence of chronic hypertension
- Stable renal insufficiency; acute renal failure gets better or worse

BIBLIOGRAPHY

Brenner BM, Lazarus JM: Acute Renal Failure, Philadelphia: W.B. Saunders, 1983.

Knox FG (ed): Textbook of Renal Pathophysiology, Hagerstown, MD: Harper & Row, 1978.

Linton AL, Clark WF, et al: Acute allergic interstitial nephritis due to drugs. Ann. Intern Med 80:735–741, 1980.

Schrier RW: Acute renal failure: Pathogenesis, diagnosis, and management, Hosp Prac 16(3):93–112, 1981.

13

Chemotherapy of Urologic Malignancies

Donna Glover

I. INTRODUCTION TO CHEMOTHERAPY

A. General Comments

In the last 3 decades major advances have been made in identifying many antineoplastic agents with significant antitumor activity in urologic malignancies. The major difference between these chemotherapeutic agents and other commonly used medications is that a minor increase in drug dose could markedly increase toxicity and not necessarily improve therapeutic efficacy.

B. Toxicity

The dose-limiting factors for most forms of chemotherapy are their adverse effects on normal tissues. Side effects frequently occur in rapidly proliferating cells, such as bone marrow, skin, mucosa, and gut epithelium. However, these tissues also have the capacity to reproduce rapidly. Although hematologic toxicity, hair loss, nausea, vomiting, and mucositis are possible side effects with many drugs, some drugs have the potential to damage other organs. When cyclophosphamide is administered without adequate hydration, hemorrhagic cystitis may result. Damage to the bladder epithelium is significantly reduced when the patient voids frequently and receives adequate hydration, which ensures that the irritating metabolites of cyclophosphamide are well diluted in the urine. Cis-platinum's nephrotoxicity was originally the dose-limiting factor, until renal toxicity was reduced with

TABLE 1. CLASSIFICATION OF CHEMOTHERAPEUTIC AGENTS ACCORDING TO THEIR MECHANISM OF ACTION

Alkylating agents	Antimetabolites
Cyclophosphamide	5-Fluorouracil
Nitrogen mustard	Cytosine Arabinoside
Melphalan	Methotrexate
Cis-platinum	6-Thioguanine
Carmustine (BCNU)	6-Mercaptopurine
Lomustine (CCNU)	
Antitumor Antibiotics	Vinca Alkaloids
Adriamycin	Vincristine
Daunomycin	Vinblastine
Mitomycin	VP-16
Bleomycin	VM-26
Actinomycin	

intensive intravenous hydration, mannitol diuresis, and hypertonic saline. Renal dysfunction may also result with methotrexate and mitomycin. Peripheral neuropathy is observed with vincristine, vinblastine, and cis-platinum. The incidence of pulmonary toxicity increases with higher cumulative doses of bleomycin and the nitrosoureas. Adriamycin's cardiotoxicity is definitely dose related and may be avoided by monitoring monthly cardiac ejection fractions once a cumulative adriamycin dose of 450 mg/m^2 is reached.

C. Mechanism of Action

Most anticancer drugs exert their major tumorcidal effects by altering DNA synthesis in actively dividing cells. Chemotherapeutic drugs are generally subdivided according to their mechanism of action. Table 1 lists commonly used chemotherapeutic agents according to their mechanism of cytotoxicity. The cytotoxicity of alkylating agents (e.g., cyclophosphamide, cis-platinum, nitrogen mustard, thiotepa) appears to be in part related to free radical formation in DNA and associated proteins. Antitumor antibiotics (e.g., adriamycin, mitomycin) damage DNA by both intercalation and free radical formation. Essential intracellular metabolic pathways are interrupted by antimetabolites [e.g., methotrexate, 5-fluorouracil (5-FU)]. The cytotoxicity of vinca alkaloids (vincristine, vinblastine) and the epipodollotoxins (e.g., VP-16) are a function of their binding to the microtubular structures in the mitotic spindles.

Each drug may have its maximal effect at a different phase of the cell cycle, while certain drugs appear to be cell-cycle nonspecific. In choosing a combination chemotherapy regimen, one would like to include active drugs with different dose-limiting toxicities, different mechanisms of action, and maximal cytotoxicity throughout the cell cycle. This should allow higher drug doses with acceptable host toxicity and maximal therapeutic benefit.

D. Evaluating Antitumor Responses

1. *General Comments.* In evaluating the antitumor effects of single agent or combination chemotherapy regimens, standard terminology should be employed to define response rates, duration of reponse, and survival. Unfortunately, many clinical trials have used their own response criteria, which makes it impossible to compare different regimens. Response rates will also vary depending on the patient characteristics (e.g., performance status, prior therapy, and extent of disease).

2. Clinical Response Rates

   a. Measurable disease. A lesion is considered measuable if two perpendicular diameters can be determined on physical examination or radiographically. Hepatomegaly due to multiple metastases is accepted and a measurable lesion, if it extends at least 5 cm below the right costal margin at the midclavicular line or below the tip of the xiphoid. Masses that can be measured in two dimensions on serial ultrasounds or computed tomography (CT) scans are also considered measurable.

   b. Complete response is defined as complete disappearance of all clinically measurable tumor.

   c. Partial response is defined as a 50% or greater decrease in the sum of the products of major diam-

eters of all measurable lesions with no increase in
size of any lesion or appearance of new lesions. If
malignant hepatomegaly is the primary indicator,
there must be a reduction of the sum of the liver
measurements below the costal margin at the midclavicular line or xiphoid process of at least 30%.

d. Stable disease. Less than 50% decrease or less than
25% increase in the sum of the products of the
diameters of all measurable lesions.

e. Progression. Appearance of new metastases or a
25% or greater increase over pretreatment tumor
measurements.

f. Evaluable disease is defined as disease that cannot
be measured in the conventional fashion, but can
be evaluated for tumor response if gross changes in
the lesions occur (e.g., pleural effusions, ascites
and pelvic or abdominal masses with ill-defined
borders).

II. RENAL CELL CANCER

A. General Comments

Disseminated renal cell cancer is refractory to most chemotherapeutic drugs. In Harris' extensive review of the
literature neither a single agent nor a combination of
agents could be identified that produced consistent response rates.[1] Although the most widely used drugs have
not been tested thoroughly in careful systematic clinical
trials, investigators have not been encouraged to initiate
these studies due to the low objective remission rates reported in previous pilot studies. At present, no single
chemotherapeutic agent or drug combination has produced
over a 10% objective response rate in a large clinical
trial.[2]

B. Single Agents

1. *Vinblastine.* Vinblastine is the only chemotherapeutic
agent that has been studied in a large number of patients.[2] As a single agent, vinblastine has been used in
135 patients with metastatic renal cell cancer. Howev-

er, vinblastine's antineoplastic activity appears to decrease when it is given in lower doses, either as a single agent or in combination with other agents. In 39 patients who were treated with higher weekly doses 31% responded. However, only 15% of 96 patients receiving low vinblastine doses responded.[2]

2. *Alkylating Agents.* In several small series of patients with advanced renal cell cancer, alkylating agents such as cyclophosphamide, dibromodulcitol, chlorambucil, and nitrogen mustard, have been reported to have response rates of 10 to 21, 17, 14, and 10%, respectively. With hydroxyurea, responses were seen in 5 of 39 patients. However, preliminary data from these small studies must be substantiated in large prospective clinical trials using objective criteria.[2]

3. *Other Agents.* Table 2 lists the antitumor responses observed with a variety of single agents. No significant responses were noted with either antimetabolites, such as 5-fluorouracil, methotrexate, 6-mercaptopurine, or antitumor antibiotics, including adriamycin, bleomycin, DTIC, mitomycin, or actinomycin.[2]

C. Combination Chemotherapy

Unfortunately, antitumor effects have not been augmented when lower doses of potentially active chemotherapeutic agents are used in combination. Currently, all new investigational agents are being tested for activity in this resistant neoplasm, but response rates have generally been very low.[2] Other older, commercially available agents, which have not received adequate clinical trials, must also be evaluated.

D. Immunotherapy

New therapeutic approaches may involve augmenting the patient's immune response against his or her own tumor. Several in vitro studies have demonstrated that patients have immunologic reactivity directed against their malignant cells. Based on these laboratory investigations, patients with metastatic renal cell cancer have been treated with an autologous polymerized vaccine with promising preliminary results. Eight of 30 patients with advanced

**TABLE 2. CHEMOTHERAPY
RESPONSE RATES IN
ADENOCARCINOMA OF THE KIDNEY**

Drug	Response Rates
Alkylating Agents	
Cyclophosphamide	21
Chlorambucil	14
CCNU	12
Dibromodulcitol	21
Antimetabolites	
5-Fluorouracil	0
Hydroxyurea	13
5-Floxuridine (5-FUDR)	5
Methotrexate	6
6-Mercaptopurine	13
Dacarbazine (DTIC)	3
Antimitotic Agents	
Vinblastine	24
Vindesine	0
Antitumor Antibiotics	
Adriamycin	5
Actinomycin	26
Mitomycin C	7

(From Harris DT: Semin Oncol 10:422–430, 1980.)

hypernephroma had regression of their lung metastases.
The immunotherapy group's 5-year survival rate of 24%
also compared favorably to the 4.3% 5-year survival rate
of a concurrent control group.

E. Interferon

Investigators have reported that renal cell cancer is one of
the most sensitive tumor types to α-interferon. Sixty-nine
percent ($^{11}/_{16}$) of tumors tested by clonogenic assay had at
least 60% decrease in colony formation following exposure to interferon. In vitro sensitivity testing to α-inter-
feron may identify the small subset of responders, as
clinical antitumor responses with α-interferon were observed in four of four patients with positive in vitro results, while three of three patients without antitumor effects in the in vitro test system had progressive disease.

Preliminary results from two other recent studies have demonstrated partial response rates from 10 to 18% with α-interferon or human lymphoblastoid interferon. However, in one series, moderate toxicity was noted, with 30% of patients experiencing significant fatigue, 50% mild to moderate hepatotoxicity, and 30% moderate leukopenia.

III. BLADDER CANCER

A. Systemic Chemotherapy

1. *General Comments.* Systemic chemotherapy for metastatic bladder cancer had not been carefully evaluated in prospective clinical trials prior to 1975. Many patients with advanced disease had only pelvic or intra-abdominal recurrences, which made it difficult to evaluate antitumor responses prior to ultrasonography and computerized axial tomography. Patients were also excluded from Phase II chemotherapy studies due to compromised renal function secondary to advanced age, obstructive uropathy, and complications from prior cystectomy, urinary diversion, and pelvic radiation. Nevertheless, several active antitumor agents have recently been identified. Subsequently, combinations of active drugs have been tested to determine whether antitumor efficacy and response duration are improved.

2. Single Agent Chemotherapy

   a. Cis-platinum. Among the active chemotherapeutic drugs listed in Table 3, cis-platinum may be the most effective single agent. In the first Phase II study of cis-platinum, Yagoda reported that 35% of all patients obtained objective antitumor responses, while the response rate was 57% among previously untreated patients.[3] These data have been confirmed by other investigators, who used varying cis-platinum doses and administration schedules.[3–5] Objective response rates range from 26 to 57% depending on the patient population under study. Higher response rates are observed in previously untreated patients with ambulatory per-

TABLE 3. SINGLE AGENT RESPONSE RATES IN DISSEMINATED BLADDER CANCER

Drug	Percent Response
Cis-platinum	36
	47
	47
	26
Methotrexate	38
	26
	31
	7
Adriamycin	17
	16
Cyclophosphamide	31
Vinblastine	20
	18
5-Fluorouracil	35
	27
Mitomycin	14

formance status. Most responders will have rapid tumor shrinkage after their first treatment.

The median response duration with single agent cis-platinum is 5 months. However, occasional patients have long-term complete remissions for over 24 to 48 months. Although controlled trials have not been performed, most patients will relapse within 3 to 4 months if cis-platinum is discontinued.

The most common toxicities of cis-platinum are nausea, emesis, bone marrow suppression, renal dysfunction, and, rarely, ototoxicity and periphral neuropathy. The incidence of nephrotoxicity can be decreased with appropriate intravenous hydration and mannitol diuresis, which are especially important in patients with suboptimal renal function. Nephrotoxicity is frequently the dose-limiting factor in patients with bladder cancer, due to the relatively high incidence of preexisting renal dysfunction secondary to ureteral obstruction, infection, and advanced age. Hematologic toxicity is mild to moderate even in patients heavily pretreated with pelvic radiotherapy. Prior to effective antiemetic regimens, patients would often refuse further treatment due to severe nausea, emesis, and prolonged anorexia. However, with metoclopropramide and corticosteroid pretreatment, gastrointestinal toxicity is generally mild to moderate.

b. Adriamycin. Adriamycin produces 15 to 20% objective response rates. Although controlled studies are lacking, antitumor response rates appear to increase as the adriamycin dose is escalated from 30, 45, 60, to 75 mg/m^2. Higher response rates occur in patients who have not been previously treated with other chemotherapeutic agents. However, even with high adriamycin doses, the duration of response is brief, lasting only 4 to 6 months.[3,6]

c. Methotrexate. Methotrexate is an effective antitumor agent in both local-regional and metastatic bladder cancer. Higher response rates were observed in previously untreated patients with good functional status. Further randomized clinical trials are necessary to define the optimal methotrexate dose and method of administration. Since methotrexate is excreted by the kidney, appropriate dose modifications are necessary with even mild renal insufficiency.[3,6]

d. Cyclophosphamide. Early series reported high response rates with cyclophosphamide, but when strict objective response criteria are employed response rates dropped to 7.4%. Other active agents are listed in Table 3.

3. Combination Chemotherapy

a. General comments. Although there are numerous reports of enhanced therapeutic responses in small groups treated with a variety of combination chemotherapy regimes, significant improvement in response rates, duration of response, and survival can only be confirmed in randomized Phase III clinical trials. In the murine bladder cancer model,

**TABLE 4. COMBINATION CHEMOTHERAPY RESPONSE
IN DISSEMINATED BLADDER CANCER**

Drug	Percent Response
Cyclophosphamide, adriamycin, cis-platinum (CISCA)	50
Cyclophosphamide, adriamycin, cis-platinum (ECOG)	22
Adriamycin, cis-platinum	55
Vinblastine, methotrexate	44
Vinblastine, methotrexate, cis-platinum	57
Methotrexate, vinblastine, cis-platinum, adriamycin	67

synergistic effects were noted with combinations of adriamycin, cis-platinum, cyclophosphamide, and 5-fluorouracil.[7] At present, however, there are no large controlled clinical trials that confirm a statistically significant improvement with combination chemotherapy over single agents.

b. Combination regimens containing cis-platinum, cyclophosphamide, adriamycin, and/or 5-fluorouracil (Table 4). Initially, investigators reported a 90% response rate in ten patients treated with moderately high doses of cis-platinum, adriamycin, and cyclophosphamide (CISCA). However, when additional patients were treated with CISCA, the response rate decreased to 50%. The Eastern Cooperative Oncology Group conducted a randomized controlled trial comparing cis-platinum to cytoxan, adriamycin, and cis-platinum (CAD). There was no significant difference in overall response rate between the two regimens, but the complete response rate of 22% with CAD was significantly higher than the complete response rate of 2% with cis-platinum alone.

With higher monthly doses of adriamycin and cis-platinum, a 55% response rate and 27% complete response rate was observed among 29 patients with metastatic disease. The median duration of response was 19 months with a complete response and 7 months with a partial remission. Similar response rates ranging from 30 to 65% have been reported with two or three drug regimens containing cytoxan, adriamycin, 5-fluorouracil, and platinum.

   c. Vinblastine–methotrexate combinations. Initial clinical trials produced a 44% objective response rate with weekly vinblastine and methotrexate. Since then, several trials have been conducted combining vinblastine, methotrexate, and cis-platinum. With this combination, 35% ($^{13}\!/_{17}$) complete responses and 22% ($^8\!/_{37}$) partial responses have been reported. Complete responses were seen in all sites, including bone and liver. Several complete responders are long-term, disease-free survivors. Similarly, with methotrexate, vinblastine, adriamycin, and cis-platinum, Sloan-Kettering reported a 67% response rate and 42% complete response rate in metastatic transitional cell carcinoma. These encouraging data must be confirmed in large multiinstitutional trials.

4. Adjuvant Chemotherapy

   a. General comments. Despite radical surgery and/or pelvic radiotherapy, 40 to 65% of patients with stage B_2 or C bladder cancer will develop recurrent local or distant metastases. Virtually all patients with stage D_1 disease develop distant metastases, usually within 1 to 2 years of diagnosis. The major factor that determines the survival of patients with locally advanced disease is the development of distant metastases rather than local recurrence. In an attempt to improve disease-free survival, several centers have initiated clinical trials combining systemic chemotherapy with definitive local treatment. Although preliminary results compare favorably to retrospective series, randomized controlled trials will be necessary to establish the degree of clinical benefit and toxicity of adjuvant therapy. At present, there are no convincing data to recommend adjuvant chemotherapy in patients with Stage B_2, C, or D_1 bladder cancer.

b. Cis-platinum. Only one large randomized trial of adjuvant therapy has been initiated. The National Bladder Cancer Collaborative Group initiated a randomized controlled trial of cis-platinum 70 mg/m^2 every 3 weeks for eight courses following standard radiotherapy and radical cystectomy. Unfortunately, most patients randomized to receive postoperative chemotherapy refused to continue the program due to severe gastrointestinal toxicity. This study demonstrated the difficulties encountered in treated patients with adjuvant cis-platinum. The disease-free survival data were inconclusive due to patient noncompliance.

c. Other adjuvant regimens. Using adjuvant adriamycin in Stage D_1 bladder cancer, one trial reported a mean survival of 23 months, which compared favorably to previous series with radiation and surgery alone. Preliminary results with adjuvant cis-platinum and adriamycin are also encouraging with 90% of patients with stage C or D_1 bladder cancer free of disease after a median follow-up of 15 months.

d. Preoperative chemotherapy for locally advanced disease. The prognosis of patients with unresectable transitional cell carcinoma is similar to patients with pelvic lymph node metastases. Over 75% will die of disseminated disease within 1 year of diagnosis. Investigators at Memorial Sloan-Kettering reported a 64% response rate and 37% complete remission rate among 27 patients with locally advanced, unresectable bladder cancer treated with combined intraarterial and intravenous chemotherapy with cytoxan, adriamycin, and cis-platinum. The median duration of complete response was 37 weeks (range 11+ to 92+ weeks). However, these results must also be confirmed in controlled studies with larger numbers of patients to determine the potential for improved survival.

Several pilot studies with neo-adjuvant or postoperative cis-platinum have been initiated. To improve the 5-year survival rate of 20 to 35% for invasive T_3 and T_4 bladder cancer, Raghaven et al. initiated a clinical trial combining two cycles of cis-platinum 100 mg/m², followed by radiotherapy and/or surgery.[8] After chemotherapy, there was a 70% objective response rate at repeat cystoscopy. The actuarial survival at 12 months and 24 months are 88 and 82%, respectively.

Based on the radiosensitizing and chemotherapeutic responses with cis-platinum, investigators at Sloan-Kettering treated 31 patients with T_3 or T_4 bladder cancer with 2000 rads of preoperative whole pelvic radiotherapy and neoadjuvant cisplatinum. At surgery, only 6 of 31 were nonresectable and 7 of 31 had pelvic lymph node metastases. With a median follow-up of 35 months, 55% of all patients and 68% of the cystectomy group had no evidence of recurrent disease. These results are superior to historical controls treated with radiotherapy and surgery alone.

B. Intravesical Chemotherapy

Superficial transitional cell carcinomas are generally treated with surgical transurethral resection. Several courses of intravesical chemotherapy are employed to reduce the high incidence of local recurrence. With intravesical chemotherapy, high drug concentrations are presented to the superficial tumor surface. Intravesical thiotepa, administered weekly for 4 weeks and then monthly for approximately 4 months, is the agent most commonly used. Treatment response is evaluated by check cystoscopy. Thiotepa provides long-term control in approximately one-third of patients with early stage, noninvasive cancer and decreases recurrence rates in two-thirds of patients. However, thiotepa is relatively ineffective in controlling multifocal carcinoma in situ.[9]

Other agents, such as mitomycin, adriamycin, bleomycin, BCG, and interferon have been used for intravesical therapy. Intravesical adriamycin is extremely well tolerated and effective in localized superficial bladder cancer.[9] However, carcinoma in situ is rarely controlled with intravesical adriamycin. Complete responses in 6 to 8 patients with carcinoma in situ have been observed with intravesical interferon.

The combination of intradermal and intravesical BCG decreased the number of tumors and prolonged the time to recurrence in patients with multiple recurrent superficial bladder tumors. Preliminary results with intravesical BCG alone from an Eastern Cooperative Oncology Group pilot trial suggest that the intradermal BCG may not be necessary.

IV. PROSTATE CANCER

A. General Comments

1. *Response Criteria*. Chemotherapy trials in advanced prostate cancer are limited by small numbers of patients with measurable or evaluable disease. The majority of patients have extensive osteoblastic bone metastases or retroperitoneal adenopathy long before they develop measurable metastatic disease. In an attempt to evaluate objective antitumor efficacy, the National Prostatic Cancer Project (NPCP) established parameters to measure response in patients with or without bidimensional measurable disease. These criteria are listed in Table 5. It is important to remember that many past series used different response criteria in evaluating antineoplastic effects.

2. *Prognostic Factors*. It is unclear whether the improved survival of patients with "stable" disease is due to meaningful antineoplastic responses to chemotherapy or due to more indolent disease within this subgroup.[10] However, response to chemotherapy and survival are decreased in patients with the following poor prognostic factors: elevated acid and alkaline phosphatase; elevated prolactin, LDH, and SGOT; poor performance status; anemia; bone pain; age greater than 65; hypoalbuminemia; and liver, lung, or subcutaneous metastases.

3. *Dose Modification*. Chemotherapy dose modification

TABLE 5. RESPONSE CRITERIA IN METASTATIC PROSTATE CANCER[a]

Complete Remission
    The absence of any clinically detectable soft tissue masses
    A normal acid phosphatase
    Recalcification of all osteolytic lesions
    Absence of progressive osteoblastic lesions
    Complete reduction in liver size and normalization of liver function
    Absence of new metastases
    No significant weight loss ($>$ 10%) or deterioration in performance status

Partial Responses
    At least a 50% reduction in measurable soft tissue masses
    A normal acid phosphatase
    Recalcification of some osteolytic bone metastases
    At least a 30% reduction in liver size and abnormal liver functions if liver
    metastases were present prior to treatment
    The absence of new metastases, significant weight loss, or deterioration in
    performance status

Stable Disease
    Less than 50% regression or less than 25% increase in size of measurable
    lesions
    Persistent elevation in acid phosphatase
    Absence of significant weight loss, new metastases, or a deterioration in
    performance status

Progressive Disease
    A significant weight loss or deterioration in performance status
    A new site of metastatic disease
    A $\geq$ 25% increase in a measurable lesion
    An increase in acid or alkaline phosphatase alone is not indicative of
    progression, unless associated with other signs suggestive of tumor
    progression.[a]

[a]*Chabner BA, Myers CE: Clinical pharmacology of cancer chemotherapy. In
DeVita VT, Hellman S, Rosenberg SA (eds): Cancer Principles and Practice
of Oncology. Philadelphia: J.B. Lippincott, 1982.*

is frequently necessary with advanced disease due to
decreased bone marrow reserve from advanced age,
prior pelvic radiotherapy, and extensive bone marrow
metastases. Potentially effective drugs, such as cis-
platinum, may be contraindicated due to renal dysfunction from obstructive uropathy.

B. Single Active Agents

Due to past problems in objectively evaluating antitumor
response, the treatment of hormone-unresponsive metastatic prostate cancer is investigational at the present time.

Adriamycin may be one of the most active agents;[11] however, response rates may vary from 33% when measurable disease is assessed to 86% when NPCP criteria are utilized. Other potentially active agents include cyclophosphamide, cis-platinum, and 5-fluorouracil.[11] However, there is a definite need to identify other active agents in this disease.

1. *Adriamycin.* Adriamycin is an active drug in prostatic cancer. The Eastern Cooperative Oncology Group reported a 24% objective response rate with 60 mg/m^2 of adriamycin every 3 weeks. With weekly adriamycin (20 mg/m^2), investigators at Sloan-Kettering observed an 83% response rate using NPCP criteria and a 30% objective response rate in endocrine-unresponsive carcinoma of the prostate.

2. *Cis-Platinum.* There was a great deal of enthusiasm when Merrin reported a 29% objective response rate with weekly cis-platinum in advanced prostate cancer. Cis-platinum (1 mg/kg) was initially administered as weekly infusions for the first 6 weeks and then every 3 weeks. Responses were observed in liver, nodal, and bone metastases, pleural effusions, and local disease. However, using every-3-week dosage schedules, less impressive objective response rates of 19 and 12% were reported by the Southwest Oncology Group and Yagoda,[12] respectively.

3. *Alkylating Agents.* Alkylating agents were among the first chemotherapeutic drugs used in advanced prostate cancer. In Carter's literature review response rates for nitrogen mustard and cyclophosphamide were 39 and 14%, respectively.[13] The first randomized trial of the National Prostatic Cancer Project (NPCP) randomized patients between cyclophosphamide, 5-FU, or only supportive therapy. Their data showed that cyclophosphamide (1 g/m^2 every 3 weeks) provided significant clinical benefit in terms of both survival and response. Other alkylating agents, such as alkeran, have been shown to have minimal activity in prostate cancer.[13]

4. *5-Fluorouracil.* In early reviews 5-fluorouracil (5-FU)

had been reported to have response rates as high as 36% in hormone-resistant prostate cancer when NPCP criteria were used.[13] However, when objective response rates were considered, only 8% responded. The NPCP trial demonstrated that 5-FU was superior to standard supportive therapy, but more toxic and perhaps less effective than cyclophosphamide.

5. Other Potentially Active Chemotherapeutic Agents
   a. DTIC may have significant antitumor efficacy. The National Prostatic Cancer Project reported that the response rate for DTIC (including partial responses and stable disease) was 48%, with an average response duration of 50 weeks.
   b. Several institutions have reported impressive objective response rates for hydroxyurea and CCNU of 50 and 40%, respectively. However, a recent controlled series demonstrated only a 4% objective response rate to hydroxyurea emphasizing the necessity of adequate patient numbers.
   c. With a 5-day continuous infusion of vinblastine, objective partial responses were seen with minimal toxicity in 26% of 39 advanced heavily pretreated patients refractory to hormonal therapy.
   d. Investigators at Sloan-Kettering observed a 24% objective response rate when weekly MGBG was given to patients with Stage D_2 prostate cancer. Since this drug has minimal myelosuppression, it may be beneficial in combination with drugs with hematologic toxicity.

C. **Combination Chemotherapy**
   1. *Cyclophosphamide, Adriamycin, and Cis-Platinum (CAP).* Ihde at the National Cancer Institute has reported favorable results in previously untreated D_2 patients treated with cyclophosphamide 600 mg/m², adriamycin 50 mg/m², and cis-platinum 50 mg/m² every 3 to 4 weeks.[14] Thirty-nine percent of previously untreated patients had a partial response with a median response duration of 9+ months (range: 3 to 18 months) and 28% had stable disease for a median

TABLE 6. COMBINATION CHEMOTHERAPY IN ADVANCED PROSTATE CANCER

Drugs	Response Rate
Cyclophosphamide, 5-fluorouracil	6%
Cyclophosphamide, adriamycin	6%
Adriamycin, cis-platinum	48%
Cyclophosphamide, adriamycin, cis-platinum	41%
5-Fluorouracil, adriamycin, mitomycin	8%

duration of 10 months (range: 5 to 12 months). Although most patients had bone marrow involvement, hematologic toxicity was not generally dose limiting. Initial CAP chemotherapy did not appear to adversely effect subsequent hormonal responses, as over 80% responded to hormonal therapy after CAP failure. The response rate decreased to 23% in patients with endocrine unresponsive tumors. Similar objective response rates to cyclophosphamide and adriamycin alone or combined with BCNU have been reported.

2. *Other Combination Chemotherapy Regimens.* Table 6 lists response rates to combination chemotherapy in several small series. Although initial results often appear promising, these data must be confirmed in a larger series. At present, there is no convincing evidence from a large randomized trial that combination chemotherapy is superior to single agents in advanced prostate cancer.

D. **Chemohormonal Therapy**

1. *General Comments.* Combining chemotherapy and hormonal therapy, which have different antitumor activity and toxicities, may be superior to sequential therapy.[15]

2. *Estramustine.* Estramustine, which is a complex of estradiol and nitrogen mustard, has been reported to provide responses in 35% of patients refractory to hormonal therapy.

3. *Adriamycin and Stilphosterol.* Citrin et al.[16] recently

reported that 63% of patients failing initial hormonal therapy experienced clinical improvement and a reduction in acid phosphatase, with adriamycin and stilphosterol. The Eastern Cooperative Oncology Group is currently determining the objective response rate in a large patient population with measurable or evaluable disease.

E. Adjuvant Chemotherapy

Once an effective chemotherapy regimen is found, adjuvant chemotherapy may improve disease-free survival of patients with locally advanced, high grade tumors. However, without a randomized controlled study, there are no data to support the use of adjuvant chemotherapy in locally advanced, nonmetastatic disease.

V. TESTICULAR CANCER

A. Nonseminomatous Germ Cell Tumors

1. *Historical Perspective.* Today, with advances in combination chemotherapy, the majority of patients with disseminated nonseminomatous germ cell tumors are cured.[17] In 1960, Li et al. first reported a 30% complete response rate in metastatic testicular cancer.[18] Subsequently, other investigators reported encouraging complete remission rates with a variety of cytotoxic drugs. Most of these early regimens contained an alkylating agent (e.g., cyclophosphamide, chlorambucil); an antibiotic (mithramycin or dactinomycin); and an antimetabolite (e.g., methotrexate). In 1975, Samuels et al. reported a 39% complete response rate with vinblastine and bleomycin. Possibly, the most important advancement was the addition of cis-platinum to regimes containing velban and bleomycin. As a single agent, cis-platinum was reported to produce complete remissions in 20 to 50% of patients refractory to other drug combinations.[17] In 1977, Einhorn[17] reported a 70% complete response rate with velban, bleomycin, and cis-platinum. An additional 10% of patients were in complete remission after surgical re-

section. Now, with VP-16 and cis-platinum salvage therapy, a significant number of relapsed or refractory patients can be cured.[17]

2. *Combination Chemotherapy.* Major advances leading to increased cure rates have come from studies conducted at Indiana University and Memorial Sloan-Kettering Cancer Center.

a. The Einhorn regimen. Several cooperative groups have confirmed that the Einhorn regimen, cis-platinum, vinblastine, and bleomycin (PVB), produces 70% complete remission rate, with an additional 10% of patients rendered disease free after surgical resection of residual masses.[17,19,20] Nephrotoxicity is rarely encountered with appropriate intravenous hydration. The most serious side effects were originally due to vinblastine. However, the incidence and severity of granulocytopenia, sepsis, ileus, and myalgias have been significantly decreased with a minor vinblastine dose reduction. There has been no difference in response rate or duration with the lower vinblastine dose of 0.3 mg/kg compared with 0.4 mg/kg.[19] Nausea and emesis are decreased with metoclopramide and corticosteroid pretreatment.

b. VAB regimens. A series of protocols employing vinblastine, actinomycin, and bleomycin (VAB) were initiated in 1972 at Memorial Sloan-Kettering Cancer Center. These regimens are summarized in Table 7.

(1) VAB I: The first regimen (VAB I), which included vinblastine, actinomycin, and bleomycin, produced an overall response rate of 47%, a complete response rate of 22%, and a cure rate of 13%.[19]

(2) VAB II: In 1974 platinum was added to the original three-drug regimen and bleomycin was administered as a continuous infusion. The modified protocol increased the complete response rates to 50%, but only 24% of patients now remain free of disease.[19]

TABLE 7. VAB PROGRAMS FROM MEMORIAL SLOAN-KETTERING CANCER CENTER

Protocol	Drug Regimen	CR	NED with Surgery	Percent Overall CR	Presently NED
VAB-I[5,7]	Vinblastine Actinomycin Bleomycin	14	—	14	12
VAB-II[5,7]	Vinblastine Actinomycin Bleomycin[a] Cis-platinum	46	4	50	24
VAB-III[5,7]	Vinblastine Actinomycin Bleomycin[a] Cis-platinum Cyclophosophamide Chlorambucil	54	7	61	45
VAB-IV[5,7,8]	Same drugs as VAB-III, but different schedule of administration	61	19	80	68
VAB-VI	More frequent cis-platinum decreased treatment duration (1 year)	64	28	92	84

[a]Continuous infusion

    (3) VAB III: VAB III added high-dose cis-platinum with mannitol diuresis and cyclophosphamide during the initial induction period. These modifications improved the potential cure rate to 54%.[19]

    (4) VAB IV: In 1976, all patients at Sloan-Kettering were treated with VAB IV, a complicated program employing three cycles of high-dose cis-platinum, bleomycin infusions, vinblastine, cyclophosphamide, and adriamycin, alternating with four cycles of consolidation therapy with vinblastine, adriamycin, chlorambucil, and actinomycin. Complete response

and long-term, disease-free survival rates appear to be comparable to those obtained with the less complex Einhorn regimen.[20]

(5) VAB VI: The highest cure rates have been achieved with the VAB VI regimen. Cis-platinum, the most active single agent, was used every 3 to 4 weeks instead of every 4 months. Toxicity was decreased by reducing the treatment duration from 2½ years to 1 year. With these modifications, complete response and cure rates appear to be comparable to the Einhorn regimen.[19-22]

3. *More Aggressive Chemotherapy Regimens.* Despite the high cure rates with PVB and VAB VI, several subgroups have inferior response rates. Poor prognosis is associated with bulky abdominal disease (≥ 10 cm), extensive lung disease, extragonadal primaries, liver metastases, and serum human chorionic gonadotropin (hCG) $> 10,000$ mIU or AFP > 2000 mg/ml. These patients may benefit from more aggressive initial chemotherapy.

Several more aggressive chemotherapy regimens employing high-dose cis-platinum (40 mg/m²/day for 5 days) with hypertonic saline have been tried in patients with the poor prognostic features. Although complete remission rates appear improved, randomized controlled studies are necessary to determine superiority over standard PVB, followed by salvage therapy. The National Cancer Institute has instituted a randomized trial for patients with poor prognostic factors to compare PVB to high-dose cis-platinum with hypertonic saline, vinblastine, VP-16, and bleomycin. Their preliminary data suggest improved disease-free survival in poor prognostic patients with the more aggressive regimen. Although patient numbers are small and follow-up short, only 30% of PVB-treated patients are free of disease versus 68% with more intensive treatment.

4. *Salvage Therapy.* Approximately 30% of patients with disseminated disease will not be cured after standard

first-line chemotherapy and surgical resection of residual disease.[19,20] VP-16, an epipodophyllotoxin, appears to produce higher response rates than vinblastine, and may be synergistic with cis-platinum therapy. With single agent VP-16, 33% of patients refractory to standard treatment responded.[23] Based on these data, Einhorn et al. devised a salvage regimen containing VP-16 and cis-platinum, with or without bleomycin and adriamycin depending on prior therapy. With chemotherapy alone, 24% of refractory patients achieved a complete remission and an additional 30% were free of disease after surgical resection.[24]

Now, several cancer centers have reported that over 30% of patients treated with VP-16 and platinum-containing chemotherapy appear to be free of disease from 15 to 24 months following salvage therapy.[19,20,23,24]

5. *Maintenance Chemotherapy.* Although past series employed maintenance chemotherapy after a complete remission was achieved with induction chemotherapy, it is now evident that prolonged treatment is unnecessary. In a randomized trial, performed by the Southeast Cancer Study Group, there appeared to be no benefit for maintenance vinblastine.

6. *Adjuvant Chemotherapy.* A randomized national Intergroup study was conducted to determine if there is any benefit to adjuvant chemotherapy in patients with pathological Stage II disease completely resected at retroperitoneal node dissection. With careful monthly patient follow-up, essentially all patients who have relapsed with minimal disease have obtained complete remissions. At present, there is no obvious benefit to adjuvant treatment.

There is now interest in conducting a randomized study in patients with clinical Stage I nonseminomatous disease to establish the role of retroperitoneal node dissection. This study would be based on preliminary data from four major cancer centers who carefully follow their patients after orchiectomy without node dissection. With a median follow-up of 24 months, 80% of 165 patients are free of disease. Of the 28 relapsed patients who completed chemotherapy, 27 had complete responses to chemotherapy and remain free of disease. Patients with clinical Stage I disease would be randomized to observation or node dissection. All patients would be followed carefully to assure early treatment when there is minimal disease.

7. *Surgery After Chemotherapy.* Patients with bulky retroperitoneal disease often require retroperitoneal node dissection following four courses of chemotherapy. Despite the location following chemotherapy, any residual masses should be surgically resected. Resected specimens may contain a combination of hemorrhage, inflammation, calcification, fibrosis, necrosis, cystic changes, immature teratoma, mature teratoma, and frank cancer. Although in many cases benign disease (e.g., mature teratoma or fibrous tissue) will be found, removal of viable tumor clearly increases the chances for cure. Patients with persistent tumor in the resected specimen require further chemotherapy, usually with a VP-16 or more intensive platinum-containing regimen.

B. Seminoma

The majority of patients with pure seminoma present with localized disease that has a high cure with radiotherapy. Patients who later develop metastases may convert to a different histology. Because of the relatively small number of patients with metastatic seminoma in any medical center, the optimal treatment regimen is not known.[25]

The group at Indiana have shown that 63% of patients have complete responses with PVB and 58% of patients will remain free of disease from over 12 to 36 months.[25] High complete response rates in metastatic seminoma have also been achieved with intensive weekly cis-platinum and combination chemotherapy with vinblastine, actinomycin D, cyclophosphamide, bleomycin, and cis-platinum. From these data, it appears complete remission and cure rates with metastatic seminoma are comparable to those achieved with nonseminomatous disease.[25]

VI. CARCINOMA OF THE PENIS

Carcinoma of the penis, like other squamous cell tumors, appears to be responsive to cis-platinum, methotrexate, and bleomycin.[26,27] Unfortunately, all series include small numbers of patients, so that valid response rates are difficult to determine. With standard-dose methotrexate, response rates have approached 50%. However, Garnick et al.[26] reported 100% response rates and 50% complete response rates with high-dose methotrexate with leukovorin rescue. Platinum also has produced a 50% response rate in small numbers of patients. However, many patients have poor tolerance to chemotherapy due to previous pelvic radiotherapy, obstructive uropathy, and chronic local infections.

VII. TRANSITIONAL CELL CARCINOMAS OF THE RENAL PELVIS AND URETERS

Due to the small numbers of patients with carcinoma of the renal pelvis or ureters, even at major cancer centers, response rates are difficult to determine. Most oncologists have used regimens active in transitional cell carcinoma of the bladder.[28]

REFERENCES

1. Chabner BA, Myers CE: Clinical pharmacology of cancer chemotherapy. In DeVita VT Jr, Hellman S, Rosenberg SA (eds): Cancer Principles and Practice of Oncology. Philadelphia: J.B. Lippincott, 1982.
2. Harris DT: Hormonal therapy and chemotherapy of renal cell carcinoma. Semin Oncol 10:422–430, 1983.
3. Yagoda A: Chemotherapy of metastatic bladder cancer. Cancer 45:1879–1888, 1980.
4. Merrin C: Treatment of advanced bladder cancer with cis-diammine-dichloroplatinum (II): A pilot study. J Urol 119:493–495, 1978.
5. Oliver RTD, Newlands ES, et al: A phase II study of cis-platinum in patients with recurrent bladder carcinoma. Br J Urol 53:444–447, 1981.
6. Carter SK, Wasserman TH: The chemotherapy of urologic cancer. Cancer 36:729–747, 1975.
7. Soloway MS, Murphy WM: Experimental chemotherapy of bladder cancer: Systemic and intravesical. Semin Oncol 6:166–183, 1979.
8. Raghaven D, Hedley D, et al: Fifty patients treated with first-line intravenous cis-platinum for deeply invasive ($T_{3-4}N_xM_o$) bladder cancer: Response rate, survival, and flow cytometry. Proc ACSO 3:C-613, 1984.
9. Anderson T: Developmental concepts: Effective chemotherapy for bladder cancer. Semin Oncol 6:240–248, 1979.

10. Schmidt JD, Gibbons RP, et al: Chemotherapy of advanced prostate cancer: Evaluation of response parameters. Urology 7:602–610, 1976.

11. Torti FM, Carter SK: The chemotherapy of prostatic adenocarcinoma. Ann Intern Med 92:681, 1980.

12. Yagoda A, Watson RC, et al: A critical analysis of response criteria in patients with prostatic cancer treated with cis-diamminedichloroplatinum (II). Cancer 44:1553–1562, 1979.

13. Carter SK, Wasserman TH: The chemotherapy of urologic cancer. Cancer 36:729–747, 1975.

14. Ihde DC, Bunn PA, et al: Combination chemotherapy as initial treatment for stage D-2 prostatic cancer: Response rate and results of subsequent hormonal therapy. Proc ASCO 22:648, 1981.

15. Capizzi RL, Keiser LW, Santorelli AC: Combination chemotherapy— Theory and practice. Semin Onocl 4:227–253, 1977.

16. Citrin DL, Hogan TF, Davis TE: Chemohormonal therapy of metastatic prostate cancer. A pilot study. Cancer 52:410–414, 1984.

17. Einhorn LH, Williams SD: Chemotherapy of disseminated testicular cancer. Cancer 46:1339–1344, 1980.

18. Li MC, Whitmore WF, et al: Effects of combined drug therapy for metastatic cancer of the testis. JAMA 175:1291–1299, 1960.

19. Drasga RE, Einhorn LH, Williams SD: The chemotherapy of testicular cancer. Ca Cancer J Clin 32:66–77, 1982.

20. Einhorn LH: Testicular cancer as a model for a curable neoplasm: The Richard and Hinda Rosenthal Foundation Award Lecture. Cancer Res 41:3275–3280, 1981.

21. Golbey RB, Reynolds TF, Vugrin D: Chemotherapy of metastatic germ cell tumors. Semin Oncol 6:82–85, 1979.

22. Vugrin D, Herr HW, et al: VAB-6 combination chemotherapy in disseminated cancer of the testis. Ann Intern Med 95:59–61, 1981.

23. Lederman GS, Garnick MB, et al: Chemotherapy of refractory germ cell cancer with etoposide. J Clin Oncol 1:706–709, 1983.

24. Wiliams SD, Einhorn LH: Etopside salvage therapy for refractory germ cell tumors: An update. Cancer Treat Rev 9:67–71, 1982.

25. Donohue JP, Roth LM, et al: Cytoreductive surgery for metastatic testis cancer: Tissue analysis of retroperitoneal masses after chemotherapy. J Urol 127:1111–1114, 1982.

26. Garnick MD, Skarin AT, Steele GD Jr: Metastatic carcinoma of the penis: Complete remission after high dose methotrexate chemotherapy. J Urol 122:202, 1979.

27. Ichikawa T: Chemotherapy of penis carcinoma. Recent results. Cancer Res 60:140, 1977.

28. Paulson DF, Perez CA, Anderson T: Genitourinary malignancies. In DeVita VT Jr, Hellman S, Rosenberg SA (eds): Cancer Principles and Practice of Oncology. Philadelphia: J.B. Lippincott, 1982.

14

Carcinoma of the Genitourinary Tract

Alan J. Wein
Philip M. Hanno

I. CARCINOMA OF THE KIDNEY

A. General Considerations

Renal cell carcinoma is one of the most challenging tumors faced by the urologist. It has been called the "internist's tumor" because of its diverse and often obscure presenting signs and symptoms. Because of its relatively hidden anatomic location and its unpredictable clinical course and response to treatment, the differential diagnosis and management of renal cell carcinoma requires a multidisciplinary medical and surgical approach. It has been classed with syphilis and tuberculosis as among the great mimics encountered in clinical medicine.

B. Incidence

1. Relatively uncommon, accounting for 3% of adult malignancies
2. U.S. incidence—7.5 per 100,000 population per year
3. 2.1% male cancer deaths and 1.6% female cancer deaths
4. Renal parenchymal tumors account for 85 to 90% of all renal tumors
5. Adenocarcinoma accounts for 85 to 90% of renal parenchymal tumors

C. Epidemiology

Renal cell carcinoma usually affects those over 40 years of age, with the incidence increasing steadily between the fourth and eighth decades. It is twice as common among men as among women. Incidence among blacks and whites is similar. Iceland and Scandinavia have relatively high rates, with low rates in Japan and intermediate incidence statistics in Western Europe and the United States. It occurs more commonly in urban than in rural areas.

D. Etiology

Tobacco use is probably the only environmental factor that can be considered to be etiologically related to cancer of the kidney. The higher incidence of the disease in males and the lower incidence in Mormons may be related to this variable. With the exception of an unusually high risk among coke-oven workers, occupational studies have not identified any high-risk groups. Familial aggregation, though rare, occurs with peculiar disease characteristics that may predict similar cancers in the proband's relatives with a high degree of accuracy. In 40 to 60% of patients with von Hippel–Lindau disease renal cell carcinoma is found at autopsy, and in 25% a renal cancer is diagnosed clinically. The majority of these patients have bilateral involvement if they live 50 years or more. All phakomatoses have a significantly increased incidence of renal abnormalities.

E. Pathology

1. *Renal Hamartoma (Angiomyolipoma).* These are benign lesions that can usually be differentiated from renal cell carcinoma on the basis of the computed tomography (CT) scan and ultrasound pattern, as their high fat content shows a distinctive pattern. They may occur as an isolated phenomenon, but more often are seen in conjunction with the syndrome associated with tuberous sclerosis. Patients in the latter group often have multiple and bilateral hamartomas and the triad of mental retardation, seizure disorder, and miscellaneous cutaneous lesions including ''adenoma sebaceum.'' The isolated angiomyolipomas are single, unilateral, and most common in middle-aged women. The first indication of a problem is usually sudden, spontaneous perirenal hemorrhage. Isolated lesions

can be treated with partial or total nephrectomy, but conservative management is indicated in the tuberous sclerosis group because of the multiplicity of lesions.

2. *Cortical Adenoma.* Tumors indistinguishable from low-grade renal carcinomas that are less than 3 cm in diameter have been referred to by some as benign adenomas. Symptoms are unusual and the lesions are generally found at autopsy or incidentally. Pathologically, small adenomas are indistinguishable from small renal cell carcinomas; each originates from proximal tubular epithelium. In the past, benign tumors were differentiated from malignant tumors primarily on the basis of size (metastases are rare in tumors with diameters less than 3 cm); it is now generally conceded, however, that this distinction is somewhat artificial and that these tumors can reasonably be considered as small adenocarcinomas.

3. *Renal Cell Carcinoma.* Adenocarcinomas vary in size from a few centimeters to tumors that fill the abdomen. They are usually unilateral. They tend to grow toward the medullary portion of the kidney and toward the pelvis, which they seldom penetrate. Infiltrating tumors usually enlarge the kidney and may penetrate the capsule and extend to the perinephric fat. On section they are often yellow, may have cystic areas, and often show evidence of hemorrhage and necrosis. Electron microscopy has confirmed their origin to be the cells of the proximal convoluted tubules. They can be divided light microscopically into three groups—papillary, granular cell, and clear cell types.

4. *Sarcoma.* Sarcomas constitute 2 to 3% of malignant tumors of the kidney. Differentiation from adenocarcinoma preoperatively is usually difficult or impossible. Sixty percent of these tumors are leiomyosarcomas. Treatment of sarcomas is radical nephrectomy.

5. *Hemangiopericytoma.* These tumors are usually small, benign, and renin secreting. They may produce severe hypertension. They are profusely vascular tumors and may have local or distant metastases in up to 15% of cases.

6. *Lymphoblastoma.* Reticulum cell sarcoma, lympho-
   sarcoma, and leukemia are uncommon and generally
   occur in the kidney as only one manifestation of the
   systemic disease.
7. *Oncocytoma.* Renal oncocytomas are well-circum-
   scribed parenchymal masses composed of densely
   acidophilic cells, which on electron microscopy show
   multiple mitochondria. At times they may be difficult
   to differentiate from granular cell carcinoma. Grossly
   they are usually tan in color, encapsulated, and contain
   a central dense fibrous band or scar with fibrous tra-
   beculae extending out in a stellate pattern. Angiographically there is often a "spoke-wheel" appearance of the vessels. Clinically they behave as
   benign lesions and thus may merit more conservative
   surgical techniques than renal cell carcinoma. The
   problems lie in the unreliability of the preoperative
   diagnosis vis-à-vis renal cell carcinoma, the difficulty
   in making the diagnosis on a frozen section, and the
   possibility of malignant elements and oncocytoma
   cells in the same tumor. Radical nephrectomy is still
   the safest method of therapy unless other factors argue
   for a more conservative approach.
8. *Metastases.* The most common primary tumors metastasizing to the kidney are carcinomas of lung, breast,
   and uterus. Radiologically, metastases have ill-defined
   borders and are poorly vascularized.

F. Clinical Presentation

1. *Classic Triad.* Only 11% of renal cell carcinomas present with the classic triad of hematuria, flank pain, and
   a palpable mass, and these patients generally have far-
   advanced disease. Most patients do have one or two
   parts of the triad, with about 60% demonstrating
   hematuria, 50% flank pain, and 34% palpable lesions.
2. *Systemic Syndromes.* Fever occurs in 15% of renal
   carcinomas. Unexplained anemia is found in one-third
   of patients. Stauffer's syndrome (reversible hepatic
   dysfunction) refers to reversible abnormal liver function studies with hepatomegaly. These revert to nor-

mal upon removal of the primary tumor. This has been estimated to occur in 10 to 40% of patients. The incidence of amyloidosis in renal cell carcinoma (3 to 5%) is higher than with other cancers. Neuromyopathy may occur in 1 to 5% of patients. Other associated findings include erythrocytosis, hypercalcemia, protein-losing enteropathy, and gonadotropin production.

3. *Other Presentations.* Weight loss, fever, and night sweats are not uncommon. The tumor may present by virtue of its metastases. Growth along the renal vein may block the testicular vein, producing a varicocele. Thus the sudden appearance of a varicocele, especially one which does not disappear on recumbency, in a man over 40 warrants an investigation. Bone or brain metastases may lead to presenting symptoms.

G. Diagnosis and Staging

As about 50% of patients over the age of 55 have at least one renal mass, and over 90% of renal masses are benign cysts, radiologic evaluation is essential in preventing the morbidity of unnecessary surgery or the mortality resultant from undiagnosed malignancy.

1. Diagnostic Studies
   a. Plain abdominal film. The "scout film" may give information as to the position, size, and outline of the kidneys, but its primary use is in demonstrating the presence of calcifications. Mottled central calcifications indicate a solid mass (usually a carcinoma) with over 90% specificity. Peripheral calcifications are associated with a renal carcinoma in at least 10 to 20% of cases.
   b. Intravenous urogram. Despite the many recent advances in imaging techniques, the intravenous urogram remains the paramount preliminary investigation. With it one can discover lesions of the urothelium as well as mass lesions of the parenchyma. Nephrotomography—a combination of tomography done during the excretory phase of concentrated contrast medium—adds further important information.

Findings in a renal mass include enlargement of the kidney, elongation, displacement, compression, or amputation of a calyx, displacement of the renal pelvis, and indistinct or irregular renal borders. Nephrotomography may indicate a mass to be a malignancy by revealing irregular calcification, a density greater than, the same as, or slightly less than the adjacent renal cortex, a thick irregular wall, and margins that are poorly defined, fading almost imperceptibly into the normal renal parenchyma.

c. Renal sonography. Ultrasound and percutaneous cyst puncture with fluid analysis and cystography when necessary can differentiate a benign cyst from a malignant growth with close to 100% accuracy. Thus exploration of benign renal masses can be avoided in the wide majority of cases. Ultrasound is primarily employed to distinguish cystic from solid masses. A classic cyst will have the absence of internal echogenicity, smooth and sharply defined borders, acoustic enhancement beyond the posterior wall, and narrow bands of acoustic shadowing often visualized just beyond the outer margins of the cyst. Cyst puncture is advocated when all criteria of a simple cyst are not met. Fluid is sent for cytology and contrast material is injected into the cyst to determine its internal architecture.

d. Computed tomography. CT examinations evaluate the renal parenchyma both with and without the injection of IV contrast material. Not only does CT accurately distinguish renal cysts from carcinoma, but it also allows intraabdominal staging of renal carcinoma. Perinephric extension, lymph node involvement, and renal vein and vena caval extension can be determined, as well as possible liver involvement.

e. Radionuclide imaging. Renal nuclear scanning is primarily helpful in defining "pseudo-masses." A normal variant such as a hypertrophied column of

Bertin can be distinguished from a tumor by the uniform distribution of radioisotope uptake. Both benign cysts and tumors will appear as photon-deficient areas of uptake.

f. Angiography. Prior to the availability of the CT scan, renal angiography was the time-honored method of evaluating a renal mass lesion. Carcinoma is indicated by a vascular mass, abnormal tumor vessels within a mass, arteriovenous fistulas, and microaneurysms. Hypovascular tumors pose the major diagnostic problem. With the availability of newer diagnostic modalities, the place of angiography at this time is uncertain. It provides a "road map" for the operating surgeon, and for this reason is essential when a parenchyma-sparing procedure is to be carried out, as, for example, in a patient with a tumor in a solitary kidney. Hypervascular tumors can be embolized preoperatively with the aid of angiography, thus making the surgery safer in some cases. Angiography is also indicated in the patient with an equivocal finding on a CT scan wherein the finding of tumor vessels would make the surgeon perform a radical nephrectomy rather than an open exploration and biopsy of the lesion, thus minimizing the potential for intraoperative dissemination of the lesion.

g. Magnetic resonance imaging. The value of this study is currently being examined in many medical centers.

2. Evaluation of the Renal Mass. The intravenous urogram is the primary modality for the detection of renal masses. An indeterminate mass can be evaluated as either a true mass lesion or varient of normal tissue with the aid of a nuclear renal scan. True masses are next evaluated with ultrasonography to determine if they meet all criteria for a simple cyst. Cystic lesions not meeting all diagnostic criteria for the end point of "benign cyst" are punctured and contrast material is injected. Clear fluid, negative cytology, and a smooth

inner architecture are indications that the lesion is benign and evaluation can end. Any solid lesion, calcified lesion, or lesion indeterminant after ultrasound and cyst puncture should at least undergo CT scanning. The place of angiography is primarily to deliniate the vascular anatomy prior to surgery, or as a prelude to embolization of the tumor. Lesions that appear to be malignant on these studies are resected using en bloc technique without open biopsy and frozen section. Equivocal lesions can be evaluated further with percutaneous "skinny needle" aspiration biopsies. A diagnosis of malignancy allows for radical resection with a "no touch" technique. A negative percutaneous aspiration is not helpful, and open exploration and biopsy of all renal lesions not meeting the strict criteria of a benign cyst is indicated.

3. Staging
  a. Robson modification of system of Flocks and Kadesky
    (1) Stage 1: Tumor confined to the kidney; perinephric fat, renal vein, and regional nodes without tumor
    (2) Stage 2: Tumor involves the perinephric fat but is confined within Gerota's fascia; renal vein and regional nodes have no evidence of malignancy
    (3) Stage 3: Tumor involves the renal vein or regional nodes, with or without involvement of the vena cava or perinephric fat
    (4) Stage 4: Distant metastases or contiguous histologic tumor involvement of visceral structures
  b. TNM classification
    (1) T0: No evidence of primary tumor
    (2) T1: Small tumor without enlargement of kidney
    (3) T2: Large tumor with deformity of renal architecture, cortex intact
    (4) T3: Involvement of perinephric fat, peripelvic fat, or hilar vessels

      (5) T4: Involvement of neighboring organs or abdominal wall

      (6) N0: No involvement of regional nodes

      (7) N1: Single homolateral node involved

      (8) N2: Contralateral or bilateral multiple regional nodes involved

      (9) N3: Fixed regional nodes

     (10) N4: Juxtaregional node involvement

     (11) M0: No distant metastases

     (12) M1: Distant metastases

  c. Staging evaluation

      (1) Chest x-ray with tomograms or computed tomography of the lungs

      (2) Liver function studies

      (3) Computed tomography of abdomen and retroperitoneum

      (4) Bone scan with plain films as indicated

      (5) Brain scan (if central nervous system symptoms)

      (6) Barium enema (left-sided tumors with possible colonic extension)

      (7) Inferior vena cavagram (optional, CT scan will show involvement)

H. Natural History: Routes of Dissemination

1. *Lymphatic Spread.* The incidence of regional lymph node metastases varies between 9 and 23% in reported series. The presence of regional lymph node metastases in the retroperitoneal space correlates significantly with the existence of lymph node metastases above the diaphragm. Distant nodes may contain tumor without involvement of regional nodes. Lymphatics have been demonstrated running directly from the kidney to the thoracic duct without first passing through regional nodes. Thus lymph node dissection in conjunction with radical nephrectomy is generally considered prognostic rather than therapeutic, although this is still a somewhat controversial point.

2. *Venous Spread.* When not associated with involvement of perinephric fat or regional lymph nodes, renal

vein involvement or extension into the vena cava does not significantly alter the prognosis from that of tumors confined to the kidney unless the tumor thrombus extends well above the diaphragm.

3. *Metastatic Disease.* About 25% of patients present with metastatic disease. Common sites include lung, lymph nodes, bone, adrenal, liver, opposite kidney, and brain. Many unusual sites, including the iris, gallbladder, urinary bladder, vagina, and epididymis, have been reported.

4. Survival
   a. Stage 1 (after radical nephrectomy): 60 to 80% 5-year survival
   b. Stage 2 (after radical nephrectomy): 47 to 80% 5-year survival
   c. Stage 3 (after radical nephrectomy): 35 to 51% 5-year survival
   d. Stage 4: 53% at 6 months, 34% at 18 months, 3% at 5 years
   e. Solitary metastasis. The incidence of apparently solitary metastasis is 1 to 3%. Aggressive surgical management (radical nephrectomy and excision of a true solitary metastatic lesion) can result in a 5-year survival rate of up to 35%.

5. *Bilateral Tumors.* The incidence of bilateral renal cell carcinoma is approximately 1 to 2%, some synchronous and some asynchronous. The patient with synchronous bilateral renal cell carcinomas seems to be a ''special case'' in that the prognosis, if surgical removal can be achieved (generally with a radical nephrectomy on one side and a partial nephrectomy on the other), is equal to that of a circumscribed single renal cell carcinoma. However, if the occurrence is asynchronous, this patient has a significantly poorer prognosis even if a partial nephrectomy is technically possible to remove just the tumor in that remaining kidney. The implication is that the latter may actually represent a metastatic lesion.

6. *Late Recurrence.* As with breast cancer, long dormancy is a notable feature of renal carcinoma and a 5-year

survival without evidence of disease does not necessarily indicate a cure. In one series of over 500 patients, 11% of the 158 who survived over 10 years had late recurrence. Metastatic lesions have been reported to occur up to 31 years after nephrectomy.

7. *Idiopathic Regression.* Idiopathic regression of renal tumors has been described and is probably a rare phenomenon. A recent report stated that 3.4% of 235 clinically unrecognized renal tumors showed evidence of at least some regression on postmortem examination. None were associated with metastases. Metastases have been known to regress, with pulmonary lesions the most commonly reported. Unfortunately, histologic confirmation is lacking in many cases.

I. Treatment

1. *Localized Disease.* Total surgical extirpation is the only effective method of treatment of primary renal carcinoma. Prior to the 1960s, a standard simple nephrectomy was the procedure of choice. This has been supplanted by the ''radical'' nephrectomy, which is presumed, but not proven, to improve the surgical cure rate. Radical nephrectomy implies early ligation of the renal artery and vein and en bloc removal of the kidney, surrounding Gerota's fascia, ipsilateral adrenal, and upper ureter. Very large, vascular tumors are sometimes embolized angiographically preoperatively to make the operative procedure technically easier. Transabdominal, thoracoabdominal, and lower interspace incisions have all been employed for radical nephrectomy. At our institution, a 10th interspace extrapleural incision has proven satisfactory for even the largest carcinomas. Involvement of the regional lymphatics and periaortic lymph nodes has been noted in almost 25% of patients with renal cell carcinoma. Thus, a rationale for regional lymphadenectomy exists. Although helpful prognostically, the therapeutic value of lymphadenectomy remains to be conclusively proven. Spread of renal cell carcinoma does not necessarily proceed in an orderly manner, and distant nodal

and/or bloodborne metastases may be present even with negative regional nodes. If successful adjuvant therapy becomes a reality, the importance of the status of regional nodes will increase, as the 5-year survival in patients with regional node involvement is substantially less than that in patients with stages I and II tumors.

2. *Inferior Vena Caval Extension.* Five percent of patients with renal cell carcinoma have inferior vena caval involvement. Tumor can extend into the renal vein, vena cava, and reach the right heart chambers. This usually occurs as a well-vascularized thrombus covered with its own intimal surface. Aggressive surgery to remove the tumor thrombus at the time of radical nephrectomy is indicated, as the prospect for cure is excellent if there is no other regional or distant disease. Survival of patients with actual invasion of the wall of the vena cava (as opposed to tumor thrombus alone) is poor.

3. *Locally Invasive Renal Cell Carcinoma.* Less than 5% of patients with tumor extension into adjacent viscera survive 5 years after surgery. As surgical therapy is the only potentially curative treatment for renal carcinoma, extended operations are sometimes indicated if it is felt, on the basis of the staging evaluation, that all disease can be resected. Postoperative radiotherapy may be appropriate in cases where tumor is known to have been left behind.

4. *Tumors in the Solitary Kidney or Bilateral Simultaneous Tumors.* Bilateral carcinoma occurs synchronously or asynchronously in 3% of cases. When no metastases are found, there are several options for managing bilateral renal carcinoma or carcinoma in a solitary kidney. These include radical nephrectomy and dialysis (with possible later renal transplantation), standard partial nephrectomy for polar lesions, in situ tumor excision with local hypothermia and laser photoirradiation of the tumor bed, and ex vivo "bench surgery" and subsequent autotransplantation of the tu-

mor-free kidney. Stage for stage, survival rates approximate those for radical nephrectomy for unilateral disease when the contralateral kidney is present.

5. *Metastatic Renal Cell Carcinoma.* Nephrectomy is of doubtful value in patients with disseminated disease who have no local or systemic symptoms. Although spontaneous regression of metastases following nephrectomy has been reported, the occurrence is rare (0.8%)—less than the morbidity and mortality rate of the operation.

Nephrectomy is considered of value in patients with solitary metastatic lesions when the kidney and metastatic lesion can be excised. Five-year survival rates of up to 34% have been reported. Patients with asynchronous presentation of a solitary metastatic lesion do better than those who present with the metastatic lesion at the time of initial diagnosis.

Management of metastatic disease with hormonal and cytotoxic chemotherapy is discussed in Chapter 13.

II. UROTHELIAL TUMORS OF THE RENAL PELVIS AND URETER

A. General Considerations

The urothelium can be considered as a single continuous membrane that lines the urinary tract from the kidneys to the urethra. In this section we concern ourselves with tumors of the renal collecting system and ureter, but much of the information is related to malignancies of the bladder and urethra as well. The part of the urinary tract lined by transitional epithelium (urothelium) extends from the most proximal calyces to the proximal urethra, and in a sense, like the skin, this can be viewed as a single organ system. Knowledge of the natural history of urothelial cancers, including the sites, patterns of growth, and methods of spread, is critical in determining the most appropriate treatment for each individual patient.

B. Incidence

About 1 case of renal pelvic carcinoma occurs for every 64 cases of bladder carcinoma. This accounts for 7% of all renal cancers. One ureteral carcinoma can be expected for every 51 cases of bladder carcinoma. Overall anatomic distribution of uroepithelial tumors shows 90% involving the bladder, 7% involving the urethra, and 3% involving the renal pelvis or ureter. Patients with an upper tract urothelial tumor have a 15 to 50% likelihood of ultimately developing transitional cell carcinoma of the bladder. Patients with an upper tract transitional cell tumor have a 2 to 4% chance of developing a contralateral upper tract tumor. Likewise, patients with a urothelial bladder cancer have a 2 to 3% incidence of developing an upper tract tumor. Thus, the entire urothelium must be routinely surveyed for the development of cancer once any part has undergone malignant change.

C. Pathology

Upper urinary tract tumors include the same pathologic types as those of the bladder. Tumors may be papillary (exophytic) or nonpapillary (endophytic), invasive or noninvasive. One pathologic staging system for both pelvic and ureteral tumors is as follows:

1. Stage A—tumor infiltration into the subepithelial connective tissue stroma
2. Stage B—muscular invasion without extension through the muscle layer
3. Stage C—invasion into the renal parenchyma or the peripelvic or periureteral fat
4. Stage D—extension outside the kidney or ureter into adjacent organs, regional lymph nodes, or distant metastases

D. Epidemiology

1. *Transitional Cell Carcinoma.* This cell type accounts for up to 85% of renal pelvic tumors and the vast majority of ureteral carcinomas. The male-to-female ratio is 3:1.
2. *Squamous Carcinoma.* The male-to-female ratio is 1:1. These tumors are usually associated with calculus

disease and chronic irritation. Lesions often have associated metaplastic changes and leukoplakia. They are often flat and very extensive with invasion at the time of diagnosis. Squamous carcinoma accounts for 15 to 20% of renal pelvic tumors and a much smaller percentage of ureteral carcinomas.

3. *Adenocarcinoma.* Adenocarcinoma of the upper tract is very rare, comprising only 1% of renal pelvic tumors. This tumor occurs predominantly in females, is associated with chronic infection or irritation, and is often seen in conjunction with pyelitis cystica and pyelitis glandularis.

E. Etiology and Natural History

Chemical carcinogens have been implicated in upper tract transitional cell carcinoma in a manner similar to bladder cancer (see Bladder Carcinoma). It may be that rapid transit time through the upper tracts as opposed to exposure to the bladder accounts for the relative rarity of these tumors. Balkan nephropathy is a slowly progressive inflammation of the renal interstitium affecting inhabitants of Greece, Yugoslavia, Rumania, and Bulgaria. It has been associated with tumors of the renal pelvis and ureters. Phenacetin abuse and cigarette smoking are also considered etiologic factors.

Papillary tumors tend to be of low grade and, conversely, solid or flat tumors tend to be of high grade. Five-year survival for high-grade tumors (grade 3) of the renal pelvis is 20%, compared to a 90% 5-year survival for grade 2 lesions and a 100% 5-year survival for well-differentiated lesions. Corresponding 5-year survivals for ureteral tumors are similar.

F. Clinical Presentation

From 60 to 90% of patients have hematuria as a presenting symptom. About one-third of patients with a renal pelvic tumor have flank pain and one-sixth of patients with ureteral carcinoma complain of pain. About 10% of cases are found serendipitously while being evaluated for unrelated problems.

G. Diagnosis
  1. Radiologic Studies
     a. Intravenous urogram
        (1) Nonvisualization of all or part of collecting system
        (2) Radiolucent defects
        (3) Mottled calcifications
     b. Retrograde pyelography: demonstrates filling defects in 75% of cases
     c. Computer tomography: may differentiate between renal and transitional cell tumors
     d. Renal angiography
        (1) Tumors are avascular and poorly demonstrated
        (2) May delineate invasion of the renal parenchyma
     e. Ultrasound: distinguishes nonopaque calculi from soft tissue filling defects
  2. Ureteroscopy
     a. Direct vision and biopsy helpful if diagnosis in doubt
     b. Risk of ureteral perforation and tumor spillage
  3. Cytology
     a. Eighty percent false negatives in low-grade, low-stage lesions
     b. Sixty percent of high-grade lesions have positive voided cytologies
     c. Retrograde brush biopsy, ureteroscopic biopsy extremely accurate

H. Treatment
  1. *Transitional Cell Carcinoma of the Renal Pelvis.* Recognition of the multifocal potential of urothelial neoplasms resulted in the adoption of nephroureterectomy with excision of a cuff of bladder as the standard surgical approach to upper tract urothelial neoplasms. Less extensive surgical procedures have been reserved for patients with solitary kidneys, bilateral tumors, or compromised renal function. Correlation of survival with stage and grade of tumor rather than with treatment employed has prompted the occasional consideration of more conservative therapy. The incidence of

tumor recurrence in the ureteral stump after nephrectomy alone has been reported to be as high as 20 to 30%.

2. *Transitional Cell Carcinoma of the Ureter.* Although nephroureterectomy with excision of a cuff of bladder is the standard procedure of choice for this malignancy, more conservative therapy in specific situations is gaining popularity. The more proximal the location of the primary tumor, the more distal recurrence is likely. The risk of a tumor developing proximal to a distal ureteral malignancy is considerably lower. Patients with low-grade, noninvasive distal ureteral tumors may be successfully managed with partial ureterectomy and reimplantation. The use of routine ureteroscopy for postoperative tumor surveillance may make this choice of therapy more common in the future.

III. CARCINOMA OF THE BLADDER

A. General Considerations

Bladder cancer is the second most common urologic malignancy. The volume of literature on the subject is enormous. Investigators and clinicians alike have been intrigued by the variability of the natural history of the disease. Although over 70% of bladder cancer cases occur in superficial form, a relatively small proportion of these patients have been observed to progress to life-threatening muscle-invasive disease. In contrast, the majority of patients with muscle-invasive disease have reached this advanced stage upon initial clinical presentation and do not have a long history of clinically diagnosed superficial disease. Although treatment approaches differ and more conservative treatment modalities seem to be gaining favor in certain circumstances in many medical centers, there is general agreement on the need for radical treatment methods to combat advanced stages of the disease.

B. Incidence

1. 40,000 new cases estimated in United States in 1985
2. 10,800 estimated deaths in United States in 1985

C. **Etiology**

A variety of occupational and environmental exposures have been associated with an increased risk factor for the development of bladder cancer.

1. *Industrial Carcinogens.* The initial four case reports linking bladder cancer to industrial carcinogens appeared in 1895. The chemicals responsible are aromatic amines, and they may be absorbed through the skin, gastrointestinal tract, and respiratory mucosa. Occupations at risk include chemical dye stuff manufacture, rubber manufacture, gas works producing coal gas, metallurgy, sewage work, and textile printing. The original studies postulated a 10- to 50-fold increased risk of dying from bladder cancer for dye stuff workers. The latency period for industrial exposure risk may vary from 18 to 45 years.

2. *Cigarette Smoking.* A two- to threefold increased relative risk for developing bladder cancer has been postulated in cigarette smokers (one-half to two or more packs per day). The mechanism is probably increased carcinogen excretion (? tryptophane metabolites, ? 2-naphthylamine) in the urine.

3. *Artificial Sweeteners.* Saccharin in very high doses has been shown to cause cancer in rodents. However, relative risk studies in humans have shown no change in risk in nondiabetics or diabetics who use generally increased amounts of artificial sweeteners. It is currently impossible to impute any carcinogenic risk in humans to artificial sweeteners.

4. *Coffee.* If there is an association between coffee drinking and occurrence of bladder cancer, it is a very weak one. Epidemiologic studies suggesting an association are biased by the strong correlation of cigarette smoking with coffee drinking.

5. *Pelvic Irradiation.* Pelvic irradiation has been associated with a two- to fourfold increased incidence of bladder carcinoma. It is not certain, however, if the incidence of bladder cancer in patients who have already developed a gynecologic malignancy is the same as that of a control population.

6. *Schistosomiasis*. In Egypt, where 70% of bladder cancers have squamous cell pathology, the prevalence of schistosomiasis is 45%. The disease characteristically damages the whole bladder wall and the urine is commonly infected. Whether the parasitic infestation itself or the frequently accompanying chronic infection is responsible for the high incidence of squamous cell carcinoma is unknown.

7. *Cyclophosphamide*. There have been several reports of bladder cancers developing in patients who had been treated with cyclophosphamide 6 to 13 years earlier. As much as a ninefold increased risk has been suggested, although some feel this relationship remains unproven.

8. *Phenacetin*. The *N*-hydroxy metabolite of phenacetin is probably the active carcinogen responsible for the incidence of urothelial carcinomas in patients exposed to constant phenacetin intake. Induction time is about 20 years and required intake is usually 1 g daily. Upper tract tumors are most common.

9. *Chronic Irritation and Infection*. Patients with indwelling urinary tract catheters over many years are subject to chronic bacterial infection, stone formation, foreign body reactions, and a 16- to 20-fold higher risk of squamous cell carcinoma of the urinary tract. Patients with pyocystitis in a defunctionalized bladder are also at risk.

10. *Bladder Exstrophy*. This condition has been associated with an increased risk of bladder cancer, primarily adenocarcinoma. Whether this is secondary to irritation is unknown.

11. *Tryptophan Metabolites*. An increased rate of excretion of tryptophan metabolites in patients with bladder cancer has been described. The significance of this finding is unknown.

D. Epidemiology

1. *Age*. Bladder cancer is extremely rare in the first two decades of life, and the incidence begins to rise sharply after the fifth decade of life, reaching a peak be-

tween 50 and 70 years of age. The overall incidence in populations over 40 years of age is 20 per 100,000.

2. *Race.* Bladder cancer occurs twice as frequently in white males as in black males and 44% more often in white females than in black females. The incidence is lower for Japanese than for Caucasians.

3. *Sex.* The male-to-female ratio in most Western countries is approximately 3:1.

4. *Demography.* Age-adjusted mortality is highest in South Africa, Great Britain, North America, and Western Europe. Lowest figures are from Japan, Ireland, Sweden, and Finland.

5. *Association with Other Urothelial Tumors.* Carcinoma in situ in one or both ureters in cystectomy specimens occurs in about 8 to 20% of cases. Carcinoma in situ of the urethra is found 10 to 15% of the time. There is a substantial incidence of carcinoma of the bladder in patients who have had a neoplasm of the renal collecting system or ureter. Periodic cystoscopy is necessary in these patients. Between 30 and 40% of patients with renal pelvic tumors either have had or will develop another urothelial tumor. Seven to sixteen percent of patients with bladder tumors have a history of a previous urothelial tumor elsewhere. The development of bladder cancer subsequent to a diagnosis of ureteral carcinoma has been reported in 15 to 35% of patients.

Thus, one must consider the urothelial lining of the urinary tract as almost one organ system in terms of its propensity for neoplasia.

E. **Symptoms**

1. *Hematuria.* Either gross or microscopic hematuria is present in 85% of cases. The amount of hematuria is not necessarily proportional to the severity of the tumor. The fact that hematuria is intermittent does not mean investigation is not warranted. There are a number of seemingly reliable reports in the literature that show that older patients with asymptomatic microhematuria have as much as an 11% chance of a neoplasm in the urinary tract, 90% of which are transitional cell tumors. The hematuria is usually not

accompanied by other symptoms and is referred to as painless. *"Hematuria means cancer until proven otherwise!"* is perhaps the most important urologic aphorism for medical students to remember.

2. *Vesical Irritability.* Increased frequency of urination, dysuria, urgency, and pain related to urination may herald bladder carcinoma, particularly diffuse, flat, carcinoma in situ.

3. *Bladder Filling Defect on Urography.* One must remember, however, that a normal bladder on the cystographic phase of a urogram or on cystography does not mean that a bladder lesion is absent.

4. *Symptoms of Metastatic Disease.* Bladder cancer can present with symptoms of metastatic disease (as can any cancer).

5. *Serendipitous Finding at Cystoscopy.* Bladder carcinoma may be discovered at the time of cystoscopy for a totally different reason, i.e., bladder outlet obstruction secondary to presumed benign prostatic hypertrophy.

F. Diagnosis

1. Cystourethroscopy

a. Transurethral resection. Diagnosis is generally made either by excisional or incisional biopsy. At the time of cystoscopy, if a lesion is discovered, it is generally resected at that time using a standard technique of transurethral resection. An effort is made to resect into bladder muscle, as the criteria of muscle invasion is critical in staging and in making further treatment decisions. Alternatively, lesions may be biopsied with one of a variety of "cold punch" or "cold cup" biopsy forceps.

b. Random biopsy. Because spatial multicentricity of malignant or premalignant change(s) has an influence on prognosis and treatment, and because transitional cell cancer is considered a "field disease," multiple random biopsies of apparently "normal" urothelium are commonly taken at the time of resection of an initial tumor. Findings of dysplasia or carcinoma in situ may harbor a more ominous prognosis than the pathology of the visible tumor suggests.

2. *Urinary Cytology.* Urinary cytology, especially of bladder washings, may provide useful information in screening groups at increased risk for bladder carcinoma. A positive cytology mandates a complete urologic evaluation to discover the source of the malignant appearing cells. Recently, computerized systems have been utilized to discriminate between normal and cancerous cells based on DNA content of individual cell nuclei (flow cytometry). The value of microscopic urinary cytology depends on the expertise of the cytopathologist. Well-differentiated lesions may be missed. Poor "track records" for other types of lesions should prompt review of collection, preparation, and interpretation techniques.

G. Pathology

Transitional cell carcinoma accounts for about 90% of bladder cancers, squamous cell for 7 to 9%, and adenocarcinoma for 1 to 2%.

1. *Epithelial Dysplasia.* Epithelial dysplasia is a term used to describe a "preneoplastic" lesion composed of a proliferation of cells with characteristic but non-neoplastic histologic and cytologic features that are associated in space or time with the development of carcinoma of the same histologic type. It is usually graded in severity as mild, moderate, or severe; mild is difficult to distinguish from reactive urothelium and severe may be difficult to distinguish from carcinoma in situ. The presence of dysplastic cells at the margin of superficial tumors has been associated with progression to cancer in 10 to 15% of cases.

2. *Carcinoma in Situ.* Urothelial carcinoma in situ carries more threatening implications than in nonurothelial malignancies. When present in association with cystoscopically evident bladder carcinoma, the recurrence rate has been reported to be over 80%, with 73% of patients developing infiltrating cancers. On the other hand, more recent studies have indicated a more benign, nonprogressive form of carcinoma in situ. It would appear that certain forms lack the capability to

infiltrate and probably pose little immediate threat for progression, while some carcinoma in situ may have the capability to infiltrate the submucosal connective tissue and underlying muscle and carry a significant threat. Carcinoma in situ may present with irritative symptoms and must be ruled out before classifying a patient as having ''urethral syndrome.'' A significant number of men initially diagnosed as having interstitial cystitis have been found to have carcinoma in situ.

3. *Superficial Transitional Cell Carcinoma.* Superficial tumors are generally papillary and confined to the mucosa, although some extend into the lamina propria. Any muscle invasion indicates a higher stage and poorer prognosis. When discussing the natural history of superficial bladder cancer one must be cognizant of two properties: the tendency for tumors to be multifocal in time and place, and the tendency for tumor recurrences to undergo progression in grade and stage. An easy way to remember the statistics for counseling patients is that about two-thirds of superficial bladder tumors will recur and, of those that do, one-third will increase in grade or stage. Superficial bladder cancer is a heterogeneous group of tumors. Many patients will follow a benign course and others will progress and die of metastatic disease if aggressive therapy is not undertaken in time. Grade is as important as stage in determining prognosis.

4. *Muscle-Invasive Transitional Cell Carcinoma.* Muscle invasion carries an ominous prognosis, with the patient surviving the disease only about 50% of the time. Twenty-five to thirty-five percent of patients presenting with the disease already have muscle invasion. Cases without clinically evident distant metastases can be considered for curative therapy. At least 50% of these patients fail with distant metastatic disease within 2 years of radical therapy. Solid tumors tend to be associated with a worse prognosis than papillary tumors and with a greater depth of penetration.

5. *Squamous Cell Carcinoma.* Etiologically this is probably related to chronic inflammation.

6. *Adenocarcinoma.* Adenocarcinoma of the bladder generally originates at the bladder base near the tri-

gone or, when urachal in origin, at the dome. It is not considered to be a field disease of the urothelium as transitional cell carcinoma is. It accounts for less than 1% of muscle-invasive tumors.

7. *Sarcomas of the Bladder.* Embryonal rhabdomyosarcomas or botryoid tumors may arise in the urinary bladder, vagina, prostate, or spermatic cord of infants and young children. Sarcomas of the bladder are rare in adults.

8. *Degrees of Histologic Abnormality.* Well-differentiated tumors are classified as grade 1, intermediate tumors as grade 2, and poorly differentiated pleomorphic tumors as grade 3. Favorability of prognosis is inversely related to tumor grade.

9. *Blood Group Isoantigens.* Blood group isoantigens are normally expressed on the membranes of normal transitional epithelial cells. Deletion of blood group antigens from the surface of bladder tumor cells may portend a poor prognosis, whereas retention of blood group antigens is considered a favorable sign. Although helpful, major therapeutic decisions are not as yet being made on the basis of these tests.

H. **Routes of Dissemination**

1. *Local Spread.* The great majority of grade 3 tumors and as many as 50% of grade 2 tumors are invasive into muscle when first diagnosed. Direct spread can occur through the wall of the bladder into the perivesical fat and beyond. Extensive local spread and fixation may occur, creating intractable symptoms.

2. *Lymph Node Metastases.* The lymphatic spread is to the regional pelvic lymph nodes (obturator, hypogastric, and iliac). The paraaortic nodes can also be involved as the next echelon.

3. *Distant Metastases.* Lymph nodes, liver, lungs, and bone are the most common sites of metastatic disease. The relative incidence of bony metastasis is decidedly less than that of prostatic carcinoma.

I. **Staging**

1. Systems
   a. Victor Marshall's modification of Jewett and Strong system

        (1) Stage 0: Tumor confined to mucosa (includes carcinoma in situ)

        (2) Stage A: No tumor penetration beneath lamina propria

        (3) Stage B1: Tumor invasion into superficial muscle

        (4) Stage B2: Tumor invasion into deep muscle

        (5) Stage C: Tumor penetration into perivesical fat or connective tissue

        (6) Stage D1: Metastatic involvement of pelvic lymph nodes. Some include invasion of contiguous viscera.

        (7) Stage D2: Juxtaregional lymph node involvement, distant metastasis

    b. TNM system. This system classifies tumors by the anatomic extent of the disease, and two classifications are described for each site: (1) the pretreatment clinical classification (TNM) and (2) the postsurgical pathological classification (pTNM):

        (1) T0: No evidence of primary tumor

        (2) TIS: Preinvasive carcinoma (carcinoma in situ)

        (3) Ta: Papillary noninvasive carcinoma

        (4) T1: Invasion not beyond lamina propria

        (5) T2: Superficial muscle invasion

        (6) T3: Deep muscle invasion or through bladder wall

        (7) T4: Tumor fixed or involving neighboring structures

        (8) N0: No nodal involvement

        (9) N1: Single positive homolateral lymph node

        (10) N2: Contralateral, bilateral, or multiple regional nodal involvement

        (11) N3: Fixed regional lymph nodes

        (12) N4: Juxtaregional lymph nodes

        (13) M0: No distant metastases

        (14) M1: Distant metastases

2. Staging Procedures

    a. Cystourethroscopy with excisional biopsy. This study will disclose the depth of invasion of the lesion insofar as the bladder wall is concerned. This resection of the bladder tumor should be adequate and should always include underlying muscle, preferably sent as a separate specimen. In addition, a random biopsy of ostensibly normal areas of bladder mucosa is valuable in assessing prognosis, as the association of carcinoma in situ with a known bladder tumor is ominous. This procedure may be curative for many tumors.

b. Bimanual examination under anesthesia. This is generally carried out at the time of endoscopy and transurethral resection. Pelvic fixation generally denotes disease that is locally invasive through the bladder wall.

c. Random bladder biopsy

d. Excretory urography. This will disclose ureteral obstruction or deviation potentially secondary to locally invasive bladder cancer or lymph node involvement. Upper tract visualization (either urography or retrograde studies) is necessary to rule out concomitant tumors of the ureters or renal collecting systems, which occur with increased incidence in patients with bladder cancer.

e. Chest x-ray or tomography

f. Routine chemical studies to disclose azotemia or liver dysfunction

g. Bone scan. Bone x-rays are taken of areas positive on nuclear scan. Equivocal findings should be biopsied in a patient in whom a radical exenterative procedure is contemplated.

h. Computed tomography of the abdomen and pelvis. It is possible to assess the liver and detect gross lymphadenopathy in the pelvis through CT scanning. Enlarged nodes can be aspirated with a skinny needle to confirm metastatic disease. There are an appreciable number of false-negative lymph node evaluations, however. CT scanning has not proven to be terribly reliable in judging the extent of perivesical involvement, especially after a transurethral resection with resultant edema in the area or if appreciable fibrosis has occurred after a resection in a given area.

i. Lymphography. The increasing popularity of CT

may render lymphography obsolete in this setting. The study is time consuming and expensive. Although it can produce excellent visualization of the external, common iliac and paraaortic lymph nodes, the lymphatic drainage of the bladder is first to the perivesical and then to the obturator and internal iliac groups of nodes. There is a considerable variation in the reported accuracy of lymphography.

j. Fine-needle lymph node aspiration

k. Magnetic resonance imaging. As experience with this new modality grows, it will likely be found useful in staging and following patients with bladder cancer. It is unknown at this time whether information generated is the same as or complementary to CT scanning.

l. Pelvic lymphadenectomy. This is the ultimate staging procedure insofar as the status of lymphatic spread is concerned. This is generally done along with radical cystectomy and urinary diversion. It should be noted that there is a substantial incidence of understaging (positive pelvic lymph nodes), even with the most sophisticated staging evaluation.

J. Treatment

1. Superficial Bladder Cancer

a. Transurethral resection. This is the standard initial method of management. One must completely remove the tumor or tumors, assess the need for further therapy, and plan the follow-up. Patients with superficial disease are followed in our institution with cystoscopy every 3 months until negative for 12 consecutive months; they then undergo cystoscopic evaluation every 6 months to look for recurrence. Some decrease this follow-up frequency after 5 years have elapsed since the last tumor. There is a tendency in some centers to routinely use intravesical chemotherapy sometime after resection in order to try to decrease tumor recurrence, perhaps from preventing implantation of tumor cells.

b. Laser irradiation. The neodymium–yttrium aluminium garnet laser is gaining in popularity as a method of treating superficial tumors. The advantages in using a laser for the treatment are purported to be greater control of the depth of tissue damage than can be had with electrocautery, early sealing of lymphatics, which may prevent tumor spread, and the vaporization of the tumor, which may prevent tumor cell implantation. There may be less chance of bleeding and a shorter hospital stay. The major disadvantage is that tissue for pathologic evaluation is not obtained. If one obtains tissue by standard transurethral resection or biopsy with fulgeration, and then proceeds to use the laser on the remainder of the tumor, it is debatable whether a laser advantage remains. Several studies are in progress to determine the place of the laser in treatment of bladder cancer.

c. Interstitial irradiation. Although generally not used in the United States for superficial disease, radium implants for solitary superficial disease have been used in the Netherlands with spectacular results, in terms of diminished progression and recurrence rates.

d. Intravesical chemotherapy. Because more than half of patients with superficial disease will experience recurrence of their tumors if only endoscopic resection is performed, intravesical chemotherapy programs have evolved in an attempt to reduce the number of tumor recurrences, increase the duration between recurrences, and possibly eradicate disease when carcinoma is so widespread in the bladder that it is not amenable to transurethral resection alone. It is also used to try to abort the seemingly progressive course of rapidly recurrent superficial disease, and may be tried as a definitive treatment of carcinoma in situ. Intravesical therapy allows for a high regional drug concentration at the bladder surface with comparatively minimal systemic toxicity.

e. Thiotepa. This has been used as both definitive therapy for lesions that still remain after endoscopic resection, and for prophylactic therapy to attempt to decrease the number of subsequent recurrences. Between 30 and 60 mg (1 mg/cc) are administered according to various schedules, such as weekly for 6 weeks and then monthly. Complete plus partial response rates between 47 and 72% have been achieved. Myelosupression and thrombocytopenia may occur. Thiotepa is considered as first-line intravesical therapy, but many consider it relatively ineffective for carcinoma in situ.

f. Mitomycin C. This is another highly efficacious intravesical agent, and response rates of up to 78% have been reported in treatment of superficial disease. This agent is extremely expensive, and it is usually reserved for disease resistant to Thiotepa, and for carcinoma in situ. Myelosuppression has not been reported, but local irritation and skin toxicity are not uncommon.

g. Adriamycin. This drug has been used successfully for both prophylactic and definitive treatment. It is relatively well tolerated and exhibits no systemic absorption or myelosuppression.

h. Bacillus Calmette–Guerin (BCG). Intravesical BCG may prove to be the most effective intracavitary therapy as a prophylactic adjunct to transurethral resection in preventing new tumors and reducing the rate of recurrences, and as a therapeutically active agent for persistent tumor and potentially more ominous unifocal or multifocal carcinoma in situ. The mechanism may be immunologic and/or the result of local inflammation provoked by BCG within bladder epithelium.

2. Muscle-Invasive Transitional Cell Cancer

a. Cystectomy with or without preoperative radiation therapy. Fifteen to thirty percent of patients with muscle-invasive bladder cancers have been documented to progress from initially superficial disease. The patient with muscle invasion has at best a 50% chance of surviving the disease regardless of the treatment modality. Although local control can often be achieved, the challenge is to find effective chemotherapeutic regimens to treat microscopic metastatic deposits present but not recognized during staging.

Radical cystectomy is indicated when other less conservative modalities are not applicable or when there is recurrent disease following definitive radiation therapy or more conservative surgery. In the male the procedure entails en bloc removal of bladder, prostate, seminal vesicles, and proximal urethra. If tumor extends into the prostatic urethra a total urethrectomy will usually be carried out. In the absence of a total urethrectomy, patients should be followed with routine urethroscopy and cytology of urethral washings to diagnose possible urethral recurrence. In the female the urethra is included with the specimen, which comprises the bladder, anterior vaginal wall, uterus, cervix, fallopian tubes, and ovaries. A pelvic lymphadenectomy is included in both sexes.

Urinary diversion is an integral part of the cystectomy operation and is usually performed as a part of a one-stage procedure. Most of the complications and morbidity of radical cystectomy can ultimately be traced to the urinary diversion. Discussion of diversion is beyond the scope of this chapter other than to note that the main methods include an ileal conduit, colon conduit, ureterosigmoid diversion, and cutaneous ureterostomy. A continent, catheterizable urinary reservoir constructed from bowel may prove to be an alternative method of diversion, but currently the ileal conduit is the most common form of diversion in patients with bladder carcinoma. Postoperative mortality rates for cystectomy and diversion vary from 2 to 10%, with early and late complication rates in the 20 to 45% range.

An ongoing debate in urology concerns the efficacy and necessity of preoperative radiation regimens in patients undergoing radical cystectomy and diversion. A lack of contemporary randomized trials prevents firm conclusions being drawn on its value.

b. Partial cystectomy. This modality may be indicated in patients with a solitary lesion with well-defined margins and no other mucosal changes present. A low likelihood of vesical recurrence is important to the success of the procedure, thus making patients with no past history of a transitional cell tumor the best candidates, along with patients with localized adenocarcinomas (tumors not classically considered indicative of a field change in the urothelium). The location of the tumor should allow for a wide surgical margin without requiring either ureteral reimplantation, partial prostatectomy, or resection of the bladder neck. Preoperative radiotherapy is thought to reduce the likelihood of wound implantation.

c. Radiation therapy
   (1) Definitive external beam therapy (Chap. 15)
   (2) Interstitial radiation: Interstitial radiotherapy has been used primarily in only a few centers overseas. Irridium needles are placed at surgery directly into the tumor exposed through the open bladder. They are removed percutaneously several days later when the calculated radiation dosage is optimal. Generally, perioperative radiation is given as well. Patient selection is similar to that for partial cystectomy.
   (3) Salvage cystectomy: The therapeutic approach of giving definitive radiation therapy for invasive bladder cancer, evaluating tumor response endoscopically, and reserving cystectomy and diversion for patients with inadequate response or local recurrence is popular in England and followed by some urologists in the United States. Salvage cystectomy can be

a hazardous procedure because of radiation-induced fibrosis and radiation vasculitis. Ureters and bowel may not heal well and mortality and morbidity are significantly higher than in primary cystectomy. Transverse colon rather than irradiated ileum seems to fare better as a conduit in these patients. Some centers report results and 5-year survivals comparable to primary cystectomy and diversion, in older populations.

   d. Combination chemotherapy, radical surgery protocols. New protocols designed to take advantage of active chemotherapeutic agents combine preoperative chemotherapy and radical surgery. Some large, invasive T3–T4 lesions have been downstaged, making more curative extirpative procedures possible.

3. Metastatic Disease (Chaps. 13, 15)

4. Palliation of Extensive Local Disease—Intractable Hemorrhage
   a. Transurethral resection and fulgeration
   b. Transurethral laser irradiation of tumor
   c. Intravesical formalin
      (1) One- to four-percent solution instilled under low pressure 10 to 15 minutes under anesthesia
      (2) Ureteral reflux relative contraindication
      (3) Possibility of bladder contraction, especially with repetitive treatments
   d. Hypogastric artery embolization
   e. Urinary diversion
   f. Palliative cystectomy plus urinary diversion

K. Overall 5-Year Survivals (Compiled Series)

Stage	Percent Survival
0/A	60–83
B1	41–70
B2/C	17–53
D1	0–35
D2	0–5

IV. ADENOCARCINOMA OF THE PROSTATE

A. General Considerations

Prostatic carcinoma is rather unique among cancers in that a given patient with localized disease may be managed by radical surgery in one center, radical external beam radiation therapy in another, implantation into the prostate of radioactive iodine seeds in a third, hormonal treatment in a fourth, and, under certain circumstances, by watchful waiting. At this point in time, there is tremendous disagreement about proper management and little in the way of controlled studies to provide a definite answer. Moreover, the problem is compounded by the fact that, although many patients experience substantial morbidity from the disease, far more men with prostate cancer never know they have it, and die from other causes. The underlying cause of this uncertainty is that the great majority of patients that can be cured are precisely those who will live the longest without treatment.

B. Incidence

Adenocarcinoma of the prostate is the second most common carcinoma in males in the United States and the third leading cause of male death from neoplastic disease. It is estimated that 86,000 new cases of prostate cancer will be diagnosed in the United States in 1986, and that it will account for over 25,000 deaths. It will account for 19% of cancers diagnosed in males in 1986 and 10% of cancer deaths in males. Its reported incidence is second only to lung cancer in the male population. Its true incidence is unknown, but is certainly higher than that reported. Thirty percent of all men over the age of 50 were reported in one carefully done autopsy study to have at least microscopic foci of prostate carcinoma. The incidence of unsuspected carcinoma of the prostate found at transurethral resection for voiding dysfunction rises from 10% in the sixth decade to 37% in the ninth decade.

C. Etiology

1. *General.* The etiology is still unknown. Cancer occurs primarily in the peripheral as opposed to the periurethral prostatic glands. The bulk of the peripheral

prostate is posterior, and so it is often stated that it occurs primarily in the posterior portion of the prostate. It is found almost exclusively in man; rarely is it observed in the dog prostate.

2. *Endocrine Factors.* Carcinoma is usually found in active or hyperactive glandular epithelium. The growth and function of the normal prostate is dependent upon testosterone and dihydrotestosterone. Experimental studies have demonstrated that chronic administration of combined testosterone and estrogen induces a prostate cancer in Noble rats. Along with the observations that most prostate cancers exhibit some degree of androgen dependence and that eunuchs apparently do not develop prostate cancer, this suggests a possible hormonal etiology. It may be that hormonal factors sustain a permissive environment in which neoplastic transformation may be induced by as yet unknown mechanisms.

3. *Genetic Predisposition.* There are data to suggest a higher incidence of prostate cancer among blood relatives of prostate cancer patients. Although racial, national, and regional differences in the occurrence of the disease are well documented, the relative importance of genetic predisposition as opposed to environmental factors is unknown. The latter may play a greater role, as populations migrating from low- to high-incidence areas gradually tend to assume the risk of the new geographic location.

4. *Infectious Agents.* There is a question as to whether increased sexual activity predisposes to the development of prostatic carcinoma because of the association of an increased incidence risk factor with an increased number of sexual partners, an increased incidence of venereal disease, an increased frequency of intercourse, and an earlier age of intercourse. An increased incidence of carcinoma of the uterine cervix among the wives of prostate cancer patients has been reported. Several specific viral infectious agents have been investigated, but no direct causal relationship with prostatic cancer has been established. There are no defini-

tive data that benign prostatic hyperplasia, prostatitis, or gonnococcal infections increase the risk of development of prostate cancer. There is no decrease in the incidence of prostatic carcinoma or the mortality from this disease in priests.

5. *Industrial Exposure.* Exposure to chemicals and/or diet has been implicated by the increased incidence of prostatic cancer in those migrating from low-risk to high-risk areas. Cadmium exposure has been reported to be a risk factor, presumably through its properties as a zinc antagonist. Zinc is concentrated in the prostate and thought by some to be necessary for normal function. More recent studies have failed to confirm an association.

D. Epidemiology

1. *Age.* Stamey has pointed out that, based on autopsy studies and epidemiologic data, the ratio of those who have histologic evidence of prostate cancer to those who actually die from it each year approaches 1300:1. Although autopsy sections from men dying in their ninth decade reveal prostatic carcinoma in as many as 70% of cases, the incidence of clinically diagnosed disease ranges only from 0.02% of men aged 50 to 0.8% of men aged 80. The median age for all stages clinically diagnosed is 70.5 years. These figures give a clear indication of the disparity between incidence rates and mortality rates, a clear expression of the unusually wide range of biologic activity of carcinoma of the prostate. Some patients suffer rapid progression of their disease with early death, whereas others show a much slower progression, and some even appear to live a normal life-span with normal quality of life in spite of a histologic diagnosis of prostatic cancer.

2. *Race.* In most developed countries, prostate cancer is the second most common cancer (after lung) occurring among males and the third leading cause of cancer death in males over 50 (after lung and colorectal). The mortality rate ranges from below 2 per 100,000 (Japan, Egypt, El Salvador) to more than 18 per 100,000

(Norway, Switzerland, Barbados, Sweden). The mortality in the United States is 15.5 per 100,000 for the white population and 28.7 for the black population. Oriental, American Indian, and Hispanic groups tend, in general, to have a low incidence. The importance of environmental influence is demonstrated by statistics that show a sixfold greater incidence of clinically manifest prostatic carcinoma in American blacks compared to Nigerian blacks, but a similar incidence in autopsy findings of occult carcinoma in the two groups.

E. **Signs and Symptoms**
   1. Prostatic Nodule or Induration Discovered on Routine Exam (50% Malignant)
   2. Bladder Outlet Obstruction (Less Common Than with Benign Hypertrophy)
   3. Bone Pain or Bone Lesions Found on X-Ray (Metastatic Disease)
   4. Ureteral Obstruction (Metastatic or Locally Advanced Disease)
   5. Hematuria (Less Common Than with Benign Hypertrophy)
   6. *Incidental Finding After Prostatectomy for "Benign Disease."* Unsuspected carcinoma ("occult carcinoma") is found in at least 10% of specimens examined histologically following removal or resection for voiding dysfunction secondary to apparent benign prostatic hypertrophy.

F. **Diagnosis**
   1. Incidental Finding at Transurethral or Open Prostatectomy
   2. *Core-Needle Biopsy in Suspected Cases.* Prostatic biopsy can generally be done under local anesthesia as an outpatient procedure. Transperineal or transrectal biopsies using a core type of needle are currently the most common means of establishing the diagnosis. Although transrectal biopsy may be slightly more accurate for very small lesions, the complication rates of urinary infection, sepsis, and significant bleeding are

higher. Implantation of tumor cells along the biopsy tract is extremely rare and reportable.

3. *Fine-Needle Aspiration Biopsy*. This method has been popular in Scandinavia and is gaining supporters in the United States. An excellent cytologist is essential. Complications are minimal, as an extremely fine needle is used to obtain an aspirate that is fixed and stained on a slide for cytologic evaluation.

G. Grading

Several different grading systems have been devised in an effort to accurately predict the biologic potential of a given prostate cancer in an individual patient. There is a general correlation between tumor grade and tumor volume. Most small tumors are well differentiated and most poorly differentiated tumors are large. The Gleason system is based on the degree of glandular differentiation and the growth pattern in relation to prostatic stroma. Five different patterns are described. A grade five pattern would portend the poorest prognosis. The Gleason ''score'' takes into account the variability of tumor grades in a malignant gland. The two most common patterns are added together, yielding a score of up to nine. This score has been directly correlated with the incidence of lymphatic involvement. The Mostofi system looks at cellular anaplasia as well as the glandular differentiation and growth pattern. There are three grades, with grade three being the most anaplastic and predictive of the poorest prognosis.

H. Routes of Dissemination

1. *Local Invasion*. Direct tumor extension into the periprostatic area rarely involves the rectum because of the presence of a natural barrier known as Denonvilliers' fascia. Between 10 and 35% of patients may suffer ureteral obstruction, usually from local extension, during the course of their disease.

2. *Lymphatic*. The primary field of lymphatic drainage includes the hypogastric nodes, nodes surrounding the obturator nerve, and the external iliac, presacral, and

presciatic nodes. Common iliac and paraaortic node
involvement may occur secondarily.

3. *Hemotogenous.* Skeletal metastases are usually osteoblastic, most commonly involve the pelvis, sacrum,
and other axial bones, and occur in about 85% of
patients dying of prostate cancer. Visceral metastatic
sites include lung, liver, and adrenal gland. Rarely is a
visceral site the only site of metastasis.

I. Staging

1. *Whitmore–Jewett System.* This is the most commonly
used staging system in the United States. It must be
remembered that there is a difference between clinical
and pathologic stage, especially when comparing and
contrasting the results of different treatment regimens.
The clinical stage assigned to the disease is the stage
assigned after the diagnosis has been made and noninvasive staging procedures carried out. Pathologic stage
is in fact the stage assigned after extensive metastatic
evaluation, including surgical examination of the pelvic lymph nodes, and, perhaps, radical prostatectomy
as well.

a. Stage A. This includes tumors that are not suspected on digital rectal examination but are detected on pathologic examination of prostatectomy
specimens—tissue removed for what apparently
was symptomatic clinically benign disease. Stage
A1 is further designated as focal, well-differentiated disease. In our institution this refers to tumors
that account for no more than three foci in a transurethral specimen. Definitions of this stage vary
from institution to institution. The tumors must be
well differentiated, but some include such tumors
comprising as much as 5% of a specimen. A1 is
designated a separate and special category because
the prognosis, with no treatment, is accepted as
identical to the general population. Stage A2 refers
to more diffuse or less differentiated but still unsuspected disease. About 10% of patients undergoing prostatectomy are found to have clinical stage

A disease, and this group comprises about 10% of patients with prostate cancer.

b. Stage B. Palpable carcinoma confined to the prostate on digital rectal examination is considered to be stage B. B1 tumors are less than 1.5 cm and confined to one lobe whereas B2 tumors are larger and have a poorer prognosis.

c. Stage C. Carcinoma locally extended to extracapsular structures but confined to the pelvis is classified as stage C. About 30% of tumors are pathologic stage C. Acid phosphatase may or may not be elevated.

d. Stage D. This comprises prostatic carcinoma with demonstrable lymphatic or hematogenous metastasis. Pelvic lymph node involvement alone is designated D1 disease, while more widespread disease is in the D2 category.

2. *TNM System*. In the tumor, node, and metastasis system the following equivalents roughly apply:

- T0 = A1
- T1 = B
- T2 = small C (invades capsule without penetration)
- T3 = large C
- T4 = massive C (fixed to periprostatic tissue or invading viscera)

Nodal involvement is characterized by the N score (0 to 4) and visceral metastasis by the M score. The system places more emphasis on tumor volume than does the Whitmore–Jewett system.

3. Staging Procedures

a. Physical examination. Approximately 30% of patients present with locally advanced disease and 40% present with metastatic disease. The staging procedures are directed at trying to assess whether the disease is inside the prostatic capsule, through the capsule but not metastatic, or metastatic. A careful digital examination of the prostate is obviously essential. A discrete, hard nodule and a difference in consistency in one area of the gland are the most frequent signs of early prostate carcinoma. As the disease progresses, there is a loss of the median sulcus, and further growth usually takes place in an upward and outward direction around the seminal vesicals and the bladder base. Fixation to the pelvic walls may also occur. The remainder of the pertinent physical examination involves examination of the lymph node bearing areas, including the supraclavicular area.

b. Laboratory tests

   (1) Complete blood count

   (2) Serum blood urea nitrogen and creatinine

   (3) Serum alkaline phosphatase

      (a) more often elevated than acid phosphatase

      (b) nonspecific

   (4) Serum acid phosphatase: This is a group of enzymes that hydrolyze ester of orthophosphoric acid in an acid milieu. The test is extremely important in staging and in following response to treatment. The value is generally determined by one of a variety of enzymatic methods. Newer and much more sensitive radioimmunoassays (RIA) are available.

      Nonprostatic causes of an elevated enzymatic acid phosphatase may include myeloma, osteogenic sarcoma, Gaucher's Disease, bony metastases from nonprostatic causes, osteoporosis, hyperparathyroidism, and hyperthyroidism. Prostatic infarction may be responsible for elevated levels, and they may exist simply with benign prostatic hypertrophy. In general, however, only prostatic carcinoma is associated with consistently marked (greater than twice normal) elevations of enzymatically measured acid phosphatase.

      Enzymatic acid phosphatase is elevated in 30% of untreated stage C patients and 70 to 80% of untreated stage D patients. The effect of digital examination on determinations is open to question. A conservative approach is to obtain prostatic acid phosphatase values before digital examination or 24 hours afterward.

An elevated level of enzymatic acid phosphatase generally indicates metastatic disease or significant extracapsular disease and is therefore a very valuable tool in planning therapy. Studies suggest that even in the presence of a negative lymph node dissection, an elevated serum acid phosphatase in a patient with documented prostatic cancer has significant prognostic import and indicates a strong likelihood of future metastatic disease, thus contraindicating radical curative treatment. The RIA acid phosphatase, on the other hand, is positive in many cases of localized disease and is therefore not useful for differentiating intracapsular from extracapsular disease, or for judging prognosis.

It has been conclusively shown that serum acid phosphatase is not a good screening test for prostatic cancer. The enzymatic test does not detect early disease. The RIA suffers from a high incidence of false-positive tests relative to the incidence of prostatic cancer in the population. Thus it is useful neither for screening nor staging, but may be informative in following patients undergoing therapy for the disease.

c. Chest x-ray. Lymphangitic spread is reported to be more common than "cannonball" pulmonary metastases, but this is based on only one study. Solitary pulmonary lesions are uncommon as the only evidence of metastatic disease.

d. Intravenous urogram. During this study the bones commonly involved with metastatic disease (lumbosacral spine and pelvis) are well seen. Delayed renal function may be indicative of obstruction. Ureteral deviation or dilatation suggests nodal disease or transcapsular extension.

e. Pedal lymphangiography. Lymph node metastases may distort the internal architecture of the lymph nodes and appear as filling defects within the involved nodes or prevent their visualization entirely. False-positive and false-negative lymphangiograms do occur; their incidence is dependent upon the interest and expertise of the lymphangiographer, and therefore may vary greatly from institution to institution. In our institution, at least at one point in time, the total incidence of false-positives and false-negatives exceeded 50% in patients with carcinoma of the prostate. Some feel that lymphangiography does not routinely visualize the obturator and major internal iliac (hypogastric) nodes.

f. Computer tomography (CT). The CT scan cannot accurately distinguish intranodal pathology, and unless the nodes are at least moderately enlarged they will appear as normal. Grossly enlarged pelvic lymph nodes strongly suggest metastatic disease. Ideally, locally invasive disease can be identified, but capsular penetration or seminal vesical involvement alone are difficult to assess, especially in patients who have undergone recent prostatectomy.

g. Percutaneous fine-needle aspiration biopsy. Transabdominal percutaneous fine-needle aspiration biopsy is relied upon to make the definitive diagnosis of lymph node involvement when positive findings are suggested on lymphangiography or CT. A negative aspiration in such a situation must be considered nondiagnostic, but a finding of class V cells indicates stage D disease and affects treatment decisions accordingly.

h. Skeletal survey. This has largely been replaced with the bone scan and specific spot films of positive areas. Bone lesions are most often osteoblastic but may be lytic or mixed. If blastic, they must be differentiated from Paget's disease, thyroid or breast metastases, fluorine intoxication, and other causes of dense bone deposition.

i. Bone scan. Before a lesion can be seen on a conventional radiograph, it must have replaced bone mass by 30 to 50% and be 10 to 15 mm in diameter. Nuclear scans with technetium-labeled phosphate, which concentrates in areas of active bone turnover, are considerably more sensitive. Approximately 25% of patients with bony metastases will have a normal acid phosphatase and be without symptoms of bone pain. Twenty-five percent of patients with prostate cancer judged to be free of disease by routine bone survey will have positive bone scans. When the bone scan is positive but other imaging modalities fail to demonstrate metastatic disease or uncover another cause, and the enzymatic acid phosphatase is negative, bone biopsy may be required.

j. Transrectal ultrasonography. This new modality may improve the accuracy of detecting extracapsular extension of tumor and aid in determining the amount of intracapsular disease. It may increase the accuracy of needle biopsy localization. It may also be useful in following patients after implant or external beam radiotherapy and after hormonal treatment or chemotherapy.

k. Bilateral pelvic lymphadenectomy. Bilateral pelvic lymphadenectomy is essential to achieve a high degree of staging accuracy if other staging studies are negative for metastatic disease. It is generally considered to be prognostic rather than therapeutic, and should only be employed when the results are likely to change therapeutic management. Positive nodes will be found in approximately 20 to 40% of patients thought to have stage A2 disease on the basis of the diagnostic studies mentioned, in 15 to 30% of patients with clinical stage B disease, and in 40 to 60% of patients with clinical stage C disease.

A limited dissection confined to the area between the external iliac vein and the obturator nerve, including the hypogastric vessels, will maximize information and minimize morbidity, including the delayed edema sometimes noted after full-course radiation therapy. In some patients, however, lymphadenectomy alone for staging may carry a greater risk than benefit. The patient with a poorly differentiated clinical stage C tumor has such a high likelihood of lymphatic spread that it may often be possible to confirm using thin-needle aspiration biopsy of an imaged abnormal lymph node, which would obviate the necessity for surgery. Lymphadenectomy is indicated in the group of patients who are candidates for curative treatment based on their life expectancy and who have negative clinical staging evaluations.

J. Treatment

1. *General Comments.* The great problem in discussing the treatment of prostatic carcinoma is that the natural history in an individual patient is extremely difficult to predict. Many patients live in apparent symbiosis with their tumor and the tumor does not appear to cause an appreciable decrease in their life-span. On the other hand, prostatic adenocarcinoma can be a rapidly progressive and extremely malignant disease in some individuals. To complicate the situation still further, prostate cancer occurs at an age when the disease competes heavily with other conditions for patient demise. Therefore, when making any management decisions in patients with prostate cancer, the patient's age and state of health must be considered along with other issues such as family history of longevity. Localized prostate cancer will begin to exert a negative biologic effect on patient survival during the first 5 years and this effect will increase further as time passes. With the actuarial life expectancy of the American male estimated to be 77 years, localized prostate cancer should be considered to represent a biologically significant illness in the "average" man below the age of 72. To see a difference in actual survival or quality of life with curative treatment, between 5 and 15 years may be necessary. Thus, one can reasonably consider the risks of radical curative treatment to be worthwhile

in patients with a 5- to 10-year or greater life expectancy.

Philosophies of management for individual stages vary greatly from institution to institution. A patient who solicits multiple consultations regarding his own management may well wind up having to choose between the same number of opinions as consultants. Regardless of one's preference, all reasonable modalities should be discussed and their more common potential side effects thoroughly described, as the factors that affect quality of life may be perceived differently by different patients. Treatment results also vary widely, and it is of critical importance, when comparing these, to make sure that similar populations are being discussed. This may not be the case, even within a particular pathologic stage. The ranges of survival by stage are shown below. Especially in carcinoma of the prostate, one must remember that these must be compared to the expected percent survival of the age group under consideration.

Stage	Survival		
	5 Years	10 Years	15 Years
A	54–80%	39–71%	18–35%
B	54–88%	38–73%	15–40%
C	15–72%	5–60%	0–29%
D	6–32%	3–10%	?

2. *Stage A1 Disease.* Philosophies of management vary, even in this good prognostic stage. Some clinicians simply follow these patients and initiate therapy only if symptoms develop or rapid progression occurs. Others are more aggressive and restage with four-quadrant transurethral biopsy and needle biopsy 8 to 12 weeks after the diagnosis of A1 disease. If these are negative for residual tumor, careful follow-up alone is instituted. If any residual disease is found, the stage is reclassified and treated as A2.

3. *Stage A2 Disease.* Stage A2 disease can be treated with either external beam radiation therapy or radical prostatectomy. The rim of prostatic tissue left follow-

ing the initial surgery is usually inadequate for interstitial implantation of iodine-125 (I-125) seeds. Some older series employed only hormonal treatment after detection of occult disease, with respectable survival rates.

4. *Stage B Disease*. Stage B disease can be treated with interstitial radiation, external beam radiation, or radical prostatectomy. Commonly anticipated potential side effects of these are listed below. Radical prostatectomy has been associated with the most favorable survival rates for this stage. B1 disease has a more favorable prognosis than B2, as about 50% of patients with clinical B2 disease will be pathologically stage C (versus 5 to 10% of clinical B1 patients). The operation involves total removal of the prostate, including the capsule and seminal vesicles, leaving a cuff of bladder neck to anastomose to the urethra just distal to the veru montanum. It may be done either with a retropubic or perineal approach. The former has become more popular, as it allows simultaneous sampling of the pelvic lymph nodes. The incidence of postoperative erectile impotence has recently been lowered substantially, from almost 95% to less than half that with the aid of a new nerve sparing retropubic technique developed by Patrick Walsh at Johns Hopkins.

Potential complications of curative therapies for Stage B carcinoma of the prostate are listed below, with relative risks in parentheses:

Complication	Radical Prostatectomy	External Beam Radiation	Interstitial I-125 Radiation
Urinary incontinence	Occasional (+)	Rare (0)	Rare (0)
Bladder neck contracture/ urethral stricture	Occasional (0–+)	Occasional (0–+)	Rare (0)
Impotence	Frequent (++–+++)	Frequent (++)	Unusual (+)
Cystitis (permanent)	Rare (0)	Occasional (0–+)	Rare (0)
Proctitis (permanent)	Rare (0)	Occasional (0–+)	Occasional (0–+)

5. *Stage C Disease.* Although there are some proponents of radical prostatectomy with or without hormonal therapy for stage C disease, most urologists favor external beam irradiation: at some institutions, this is combined with interstitial irradiation. Because of the high incidence of pelvic node involvement in clinical stage C patients, approximately 40 to 60% of them may avoid external beam radiotherapy if they undergo staging pelvic lymphadenectomy.

6. *Stage D Disease.* Systemic palliation of patients with symptomatic stage D tumors is primarily with an endocrine modality. When the tumor becomes refractory to endocrine manipulation, cytotoxic chemotherapeutic regimens may be tried. Focal palliation (radiation therapy for bone lesions, transurethral outlet reduction) may be extremely useful as well.

   a. Methods of hormonal manipulation. Normal prostatic epithelial cells are dependent on androgen to carry out their metabolic processes. Approximately 90% of testosterone, the major circulating androgen, is produced by the testes. If androgen is removed from the environment, prostatic cells are unable to produce certain proteins and subsequently atrophy. Most prostatic cancers are composed of a heterogeneous population of cells that differ in their requirements for androgen. Thus, tumors composed predominantly of androgen-dependent cells respond better to androgen withdrawal therapy than tumors that are not. Eventually, even in predominantly androgen-dependent tumors, the nondependent cell population will grow and the tumor will "escape" from endocrine control.

   Orchiectomy is perhaps the safest form of androgen ablation. There are no untoward side effects other than the very minimal risks associated with the procedure. Erectile dysfunction and loss of libido are commonly associated with all forms of androgen ablation.

   Diethylstilbestrol, an estrogen, can be given to feed back on pituitary luteinizing hormone (LH) and decrease testicular testosterone production. A dose of 1 mg/day will suppress serum testosterone to castrate levels in 50% of patients. A dose of 1 mg every 8 hours will suppress androgens to castrate levels in nearly all patients. Side effects include gynecomastia (which can be prevented with a short course of radiation therapy to the breasts) and sodium retention and subsequent fluid retention. Thromboembolic cardiovascular complications have been associated with estrogen therapy and seem to be dose dependent. It is not unreasonable to start a patient on 1 mg/day of diethylstilbesterol and follow the clinical response and serum testosterone level in symptomatic patients.

A newer treatment now being heavily promoted in pharmaceutical advertisements is the use of gonadotropin-releasing hormone analogues. After causing an initial flair in testosterone production, continued use of the drug decreases follicle-stimulating hormone (FSH) and LH, and decreases testosterone production to castrate levels. Although it avoids the gynecomastia and cardiovascular side effects associated with estrogens, the drug must be injected subcutaneously on a daily basis (a depot preparation is under study) and is extremely expensive.

Other means of endocrine control include progestational agents (megestrol acetate and hydroxyprogesterone) and antiandrogens such as cyproterone acetate and the still investigational drug flutamide.

b. Timing of endocrine therapy. It has never been proven statistically that overall survival is affected by earlier institution of hormonal treatment in asymptomatic patients. Some feel that early treatment prolongs the symptom-free interval and preserves quality of life longer than delayed treatment does. Sexually active asymptomatic patients obviously benefit by delay of therapy until symptoms of metastatic disease begin, as only a few patients will retain sexual potency after endocrine therapy.

Treatment should be begun promptly in symptomatic patients.

c. Secondary therapy for relapse. Results of secondary endocrine therapy for patients who relapse after responding to initial endocrine treatment have been poor. This is because the androgen-dependent cells have been suppressed, and the androgen-independent population will rarely respond to further minor decreases in circulating androgens. Some secondary treatments include high-dose intravenous diethylstilbestrol diphosphate, aminoglutethimide to effect a "medical adrenalectomy" (must give steroid replacement), and hypophysectomy, which has been associated with some subjective responses but no increase in survival.

Patients refractory to hormonal treatment can be treated symptomatically with outlet-reducing surgery for obstruction, radiation therapy for painful bone metastases, and chemotherapy protocols if their physical condition permits.

d. Prognosis. Between 70 and 80% of stage D2 patients will respond to hormonal treatment with an improvement in some parameter(s), though clinical significance must be considered. Survival is poor, as most of these patients will exhibit a relapse within 2 to 3 years. In patients developing soft-tissue metastases, 50% do not survive past 15 months. In patients developing bony metastases, 50% are dead in 11 months. In patients who develop new metastases where there are some already present, or who develop an increase in size of existing ones, or who experience a return of their serum acid phosphatase to elevated levels after one remission, 50% are dead in 6 months. These figures are reasonably accurate regardless of treatment.

K. Concluding Remarks

As can be deduced from the multitude of methods used to treat prostate cancer, the entire area is very controversial. Four pertinent questions attributed to Wilet Whitmore should be asked about each patient with stage A to C disease, as they tend to highlight the problems: (1) Is cure necessary? (2) Is cure possible? (3) If cure is possible, is it necessary? (4) If cure is necessary, is it possible?

V. URETHRAL CANCER

A. Carcinoma of the Female Urethra

1. *Anatomy.* The female urethra measures 2.5 to 4 cm in length and is lined with transitional epithelium in the proximal portion and stratified squamous epithelium in the distal portion. The boundaries between these types are not discrete or constant, and areas of multilayered columnar epithelium may also be present. The wall of the urethra also contains glands and smooth muscle bundles. The lymphatics of the proximal segment drain primarily to the internal and external iliac nodes. The distal segment drains primarily to the inguinal and subinguinal lymph nodes.

2. *Epidemiology.* Carcinoma of the urethra is a relatively rare tumor. It is more common in older women, with most cases occurring in patients over 50 years of age. It is reportedly more common in Caucasians. Caruncle and urethral stricture are felt by some to have a higher incidence of association with urethral cancer than would be expected by random association.

3. *Pathology.* Squamous cell carcinoma is the most frequent primary type, accounting for 60 to 70% of cases. Adenocarcinoma also occurs as a primary lesion and accounts for almost 20% of cases. Urethral carcinoma may constitute a direct continuation of a bladder cancer or may represent a portion of a multifocal malignant urothelial process, in which case the histology is usually transitional cell.

4. *Presentation.* Urethral bleeding or spotting is the most common symptom. Other symptoms may include urinary frequency, dysuria, and obstruction. The possibility of malignancy should at least be considered with any urethral mass or stricture.

5. *Diagnosis.* Physical examination, urinalysis and urine cytology, endoscopy, and biopsy usually are sufficient to make the diagnosis. Differential diagnosis includes caruncle, urethral prolapse, leukoplakia, stricture, fistulas, erosion, and, rarely, nephrogenic adenoma. Spread is initially by local infiltration, then by lymphatic invasion. Visceral metastases generally occur late. The staging evaluation is similar to that described in the section on bladder cancer. Several staging systems have been described. One system commonly used is as follows: stage 0—carcinoma in situ; stage A—tumor limited to submucosa; stage B—periurethral muscle invasion; stage C—tumor invading vagina, bladder, labia, or clitoris; and stage D—regional or distant metastases.

6. *Management.* Distal-third carcinomas can be managed by wide surgical excision, interstitial irradiation, external beam irradiation, or a combination of two of the three. Proximal and/or extensive urethral tumors carry a very poor prognosis and have a high local recurrence rate. Anterior exenteration is generally indicated. External beam radiation may be used as a pre- or postoperative adjuvant or as primary treatment.

7. *Carcinoma and Urethral Diverticula.* Less than 50 cases of carcinoma arising in female urethral diverticula have been reported, and, given the relatively high incidence of diverticula in the population, the association with carcinoma must be considered rare. Ten percent of documented cases were associated with calculi in the sac. About half of reported cases are adenocarcinomas, with transitional cell and squamous cell tumors making up the pathology of the majority of the remainder. A high index of suspicion is important if the diagnosis is not to be missed. Blood per urethra and elevation of the bladder base are suggestive of tumor and mandate a careful physical examination. Contrast studies, ultrasound, and CT may be useful if the index of suspicion is high; a filling defect found within a diverticulum demands exploration.

B. Carcinoma of the Male Urethra

1. *Anatomy.* The male urethra measures about 20 cm in length and is divided into prostatic, bulbomembranous, and penile segments. The prostatic segment is lined by transitional epithelium, and the distal segment is lined by pseudostratified columnar epithelium, except for the external meatus, which is covered by stratified squamous epithelium. Lymphatics of the prostatic and posterior urethra are drained by the internal and external iliac nodes. The anterior and penile segments are drained primarily by the inguinal lymph nodes.

2. *Epidemiology.* The incidence of urethral carcinoma in males is only about one-third of that in females. Chronic inflammation may have an etiologic role, as most patients have a history of urethritis or urethral stricture. Patients are generally over 50 years of age.

3. *Pathology.* Up to two-thirds of these neoplasms originate in the bulbar or bulbomembranous portions. The majority of the remainder arise from the anterior urethra, and most of these are located at the meatus of the fossa navicularis. Squamous cell carcinoma accounts for the majority of lesions, followed by transitional tumors. Urethral adenocarcinoma and primary melanoma are rare types, adenocarcinoma occurring almost exclusively in the bulbomembranous urethra.

4. *Presentation.* Carcinoma of the urethra is initially a locally invasive and destructive lesion. Clinically detectable distant metastases are rare at presentation, and death is often a result of local complications. Symptoms may include urinary obstruction, a bloody urethral discharge, a palpable perineal mass, urethral stricture, abscess or fistula, perineal pain, and inguinal adenopathy.

5. *Diagnosis.* Endoscopic biopsy under anesthesia is the mainstay of diagnosis. Urinary or urethral washing cytology may be useful. Retrograde urethrography, intravenous urography, and CT are helpful in assessing the extent of disease. The staging evaluation is similar to that of bladder carcinoma. It is important to

rule out the presence of simultaneous bladder carcinoma. A common staging system is as follows: stage 0—in situ; stage A—confined to the submucosa; stage B—direct extension into tissue beyond the corpus spongiosum; and stage D—metastasis.

The differential diagnosis includes benign stricture disease, periurethral abscess, and inflammatory phlegmon.

6. *Management.* Management is dependent upon the location of the tumor. The 10 to 15% of tumors that are transitional are predominantly in the prostatic urethra, and as such are sometimes difficult to distinguish from primary transitional cell bladder carcinomas. Infiltration of the prostatic stroma portends a poor prognosis. Transurethral resection can be effective therapy for low-grade superficial lesions. More aggressive and extensive disease mandates an en bloc removal of the urethra, prostate, seminal vesicles, and bladder, sometimes with a resection of the inferior rim of the pubis. Preoperative radiation therapy may have a place, although there is little established data to refer to.

Localized anterior urethral carcinoma can be managed with total or distal urethrectomy (where applicable). This may allow preservation of erectile function. In most cases, partial or total penectomy is required. Inguinal lymphadenectomy is indicated in the presence of malignant adenopathy. Bulbomembranous tumor generally requires radical exenterative surgery.

VI. PENILE AND SCROTAL CANCER

A. Penile Carcinoma

1. *General Considerations.* The incidence of penile carcinoma in Britain and the United States is about 1 per 100,000 males per year. The incidence in underdeveloped countries or in areas in which early circumcision is not practiced is much higher, and it accounts for up to 10 to 20% of all malignancies in some African tribes. It is unknown among Jewish people, who practice ritual circumcision shortly after birth. If cir-

cumcision is delayed until puberty, penile carcinoma is slightly more common. The rarity of the disease in the United States—it accounts for less than 2% of all cancer deaths in men—and the lack of controlled prospective studies of various treatment methods has led to the development of a considerable literature on the proper management of this tumor, especially in its early stage.

2. Potentially Premalignant Lesions
   a. Condylomata acuminata. Penile warts are due to infection with a filterable papova virus and are transmissible through sexual contact as well as being autoinoculable. They may involve the glans, prepuce, or shaft of the penis, and 5% of patients will have urethral involvement. A small number of patients with penile warts will subsequently develop penile carcinoma. Local treatments have included podophyllin, 5-fluorouracil cream, diathermy, and laser photoirradiation.
   b. Buschke–Loewenstein tumor. Also known as "giant condyloma accuminata" and "verrucous carcinoma," this growth has an entirely benign histologic appearance. It does not metastasize, but grows into a large necrotic exophytic lesion that can ultimately destroy much of the penis. The etiology may be viral. This tumor destroys adjacent tissue, unlike condyloma acuminata, which may grow to a large size but always remain superficial. Treatment is by wide local excision.
   c. Erythroplasia of Queyrat and Bowen's disease. These conditions are histologically carcinoma in situ of the skin of the glans penis. The former presents as a localized, velvety red lesion on the glans or prepuce. The latter can develop on the skin anywhere and is associated with internal carcinomas. Circumcision and biopsy will confirm the diagnosis. Topical 5-fluorouracil and radiation have both been used to treat these lesions effectively.
   d. Leukoplakia. This term describes a white cut-

aneous plaque that may be hypertrophic or atrophic. It may coexist with or precede the development of squamous cell carcinoma. It is usually secondary to chronic irritation. Circumcision, surgical excision, and irradiation have all been used in treatment. Close follow-up to detect malignant degeneration is essential.

3. Invasive Carcinoma

   a. Etiology. The development of penile carcinoma has long been associated with poor hygiene and exposure to still undefined irritants or carcinogens in the smegma of uncircumcised patients. The neonatal circumcision ritual in Jews as opposed to the ritual circumcision of Moslems between the ages of 3 and 14 may account for the increased incidence of the tumor in the latter group. A case can be made that personal hygiene is more important than circumcision in the prevention of penile carcinoma. In all countries, it is usually found in men of the lowest economic level, generally with sordid living conditions and habits.

   b. Natural history. Carcinoma of the penis usually begins with a small lesion on the glans or prepuce, or, rarely, on the shaft. Lesions may be exophytic and accompanied by considerable secondary infection. The penis, corpora, and urethra may be destroyed, and only biopsy may differentiate the tumor from a huge Buschke–Loewenstein condylomata. Ulcerative tumors are more common, and grow inwardly, destroying the glans and the prepuce and invading the corpora cavernosa and urethra. Microscopically, the exophytic tumors are usually well-differentiated squamous cell lesions, whereas ulcerative tumors are often less-differentiated squamous cell malignancies or of the spindle cell variety.

    Ulcerative lesions tend to metastasize earlier. The regional inguinal and iliac nodes are the earliest sites of dissemination. The lymphatic anatomy of the penis is extremely important. The lymphatics of the prepuce end in the upper inner group of superficial inguinal lymphatics. The lymphatics of the glans divide to follow the femoral canal and end in the superficial inguinal nodes, the node of Cloquet, and the retrofemoral nodes, or follow the inguinal canal and end in the external retrofemoral lymph nodes. Both left and right nodes have a rich subcutaneous communication with each other.

Distant metastases may involve the abdominal lymph nodes, liver, and lungs. Death is usually secondary to involvement of the regional nodes, eventually resulting in skin necrosis, chronic infection and inanition, sepsis, or hemorrhage secondary to erosion into the femoral vessels.

c. Clinical features. Carcinoma of the penis generally begins as a painless nodule, wartlike growth, ulceration, or vesicle. Phimosis is present in up to 50% of patients. The lesion may be ignored by the patient until it reaches a considerable size, and, in fact, medical attention is not sought by many patients for up to 1 year. Local growth at diagnosis can be massive. Inguinal lymph nodes are palpably enlarged in approximately one-half of patients, but in many patients adenopathy is secondary to chronic infection associated with the carcinoma rather than metastatic disease.

d. Diagnosis and staging. Diagnosis depends on pathologic examination of biopsied tissue. Size, location, fixation, and involvement of the corporal bodies is noted. Careful bilateral palpation of the inguinal areas is of extreme importance.

The following is a commonly used staging system:

• Stage 1: tumor limited to the glans or prepuce.
• Stage 2: induration indicating invasion of the shaft of the penis proximal to the glans, yet limited enough to allow partial amputation of the penis.

- Stage 3: primary tumor too large to allow for any operative procedure short of total penectomy.
- Stage 4: fixed inguinal nodes with biopsy-proven metastases, distant metastases, or primary tumor encroachment into the perineum or anterior abdominal wall.

Staging evaluation should include a CT scan or lymphangiogram to assess the regional nodes with thin-needle aspiration biopsy of suspicious adenopathy. Routine superficial femoral node biopsy (''sentinel node'') has been advocated by some. Distant metastatic disease can be evaluated with the usual modalities for lung, liver, and bone.

e. Treatment
   (1) Primary lesion. Lesions confined to the glans or prepuce can be treated by partial amputation, with a 2-cm margin proximal to the tumor to guard against local recurrence. Local wedge excision is associated with recurrence rates approaching 50%. If the lesion is so proximal that partial penectomy with a 2-cm margin would leave a stump inadequate for sexual function or upright voiding, a total penectomy can be done. Partial penectomy in the absence of inguinal metastases can produce a 5-year survival of up to 80%. Extensive local spread of tumor may mandate radical surgical procedures such as hemipelvectomy or hemicorporectomy if cure is to be attempted.

   Modern radiotherapeutic techniques can be curative in selected patients, and have the advantage of preserving the penis (Chap. 15). Recently the Nd–YAG laser has been reported to control certain primary lesions.
   (2) Inguinal lymph nodes. The presence of inguinal metastases is a more important prognostic factor than tumor grade or gross appearance. Between 25 and 50% of patients present with palpable inguinal nodes, of whom

between 33 and 66% are tumor free on histologic examination. For that reason, some
urologists advocate a 4- to 6-week course of
antibiotics after penectomy in patients with inguinal adenopathy in an effort to separate out
patients with adenopathy on the basis of
chronic infection often associated with penile
carcinoma. Between 20 and 25% of nodes not
clinically palpable contain metastases. If the
lymph nodes are involved on one side, the
contralateral nodes are involved in 50% of
cases. If the inguinal nodes are positive, the
iliac nodes are involved in 30% of cases.

Such a considerable controversy exists regarding the management of the regional lymph
nodes after treatment of the primary site (as-
suming no known distant metastases exist) that
more than a brief mention is beyond the scope
of this section. Initial management of the patient with palpably negative groins ranges
from close observation alone to "sentinel
node" (at the junction of the greater saphenous and femoral vein) biopsy to unilateral or
bilateral groin dissection. For those who are
followed and who subsequently develop abnormal inguinal lymph nodes, a groin dissection (in the absence of other demonstrable disease) is generally recommended. For the
patient with an initially abnormal groin examination, most would advocate antibiotic therapy first, followed by groin dissection, for
those in whom abnormal findings persist. The
extent of the groin dissection also varies from
institution to institution and may or may not
include the pelvic lymph nodes. All agree on a
grim prognosis implied by pelvic nodal
extension.

    (3) Chemotherapy (Chap. 13)

  f. Prognosis. The 5-year survival rate of patients

without palpable adenopathy is 65 to 80%. Patients with positive lymph nodes have 5-year survival rates of 20 to 50%, with the poorest survivals recorded in patients with iliac as opposed to solely inguinal metastases. Up to 90% of patients with negative inguinal nodes on node dissection survive 5 years.

B. Carcinoma of the Scrotum

Carcinoma of the scrotum used to be common among chimney sweeps. It was one of the first environmentally related cancers described—the association noted by Percival Pott in the 18th century. Mule spinners also suffered from scrotal carcinoma, as their clothes became saturated with lubricating oil from the spinning jenny. Squamous cell carcinoma arose from exposure to the hydrocarbons in soot, tars, and petroleum products. These tumors are now rare. Lesions present as ulcerated or exophytic growths. Wide local excision with or without ipsilateral ilioinguinal lymphadenectomy is the treatment of choice. Nonoccupational tumors of the scrotum include reticulum cell sarcoma, rhabdomyosarcoma, leiomyosarcoma, liposarcoma, and melanoma.

VII. TESTICULAR TUMORS

A. Classification

Primitive totipotential germ cells are thought to undergo malignant transformation. These cells are recognized as embryonal carcinoma. Differentiation can proceed along germ cell lines to seminoma or along pathways to embryonic tissues—either extraembryonic, such as choriocarcinoma and yolk sac tumors, or intraembryonic. If the embryonal cells become committed to intraembryonic development, somatic germ cell layers form as a teratoma with either mature or immature elements. The combination of teratoma and embryonal cell elements in one tumor is then easily understood as evidence of a transformation state.

1. Schema of primary testicular neoplasms
    a. Germinal neoplasms
        (1) Seminoma
            (a) classic
            (b) anaplastic
            (c) spermatocytic
        (2) Embryonal carcinoma
        (3) Teratoma (with or without malignant transformation)
            (a) mature
            (b) immature
        (4) Choriocarcinoma
        (5) Yolk sac tumor
    b. Nongerminal neoplasms
        (1) Specialized gonadal stromal tumors
            (a) Leydig cell tumor
            (b) other gonadal stromal tumor
        (2) Gonadoblastoma
        (3) Miscellaneous neoplasms
            (a) carcinoid
            (b) adrenal rest
            (c) mesenchymal neoplasms

B. Adult Germ Cell Tumors

Testicular cancer has become the most curable solid tumor in man, largely owing to the development of effective combination chemotherapy programs during the last 20 years.

1. *Epidemiology.* Five thousand new cases of testicular cancer and 1000 deaths from the disease are reported annually in the United States. The probability of a white American male developing the disease in his lifetime is approximately 1 in 500; the incidence in blacks is about one-fourth that of whites. The Scandinavian countries have the highest annual rate of testicular cancer. The highest incidence is in young adults, making these tumors the most common solid malignancies of men between 20 and 34 years of age. Other incidence peaks occur in men over 60 years and males under 10 years of age. Seminoma is the most

common histologic type, with a peak incidence in the late 30s. Spermatocytic seminoma tends to occur in men over 50. Embryonal and teratocarcinoma tend to occur between the ages of 25 and 35. Choriocarcinoma makes up 1 to 2% of germ cell tumors, and occurs in young adults. Yolk sac tumors are the predominant lesions of infancy and childhood.

Two to three percent of tumors are bilateral, either synchronously or asynchronously, and 90 to 95% of primary testicular tumors are germinal tumors. Seminoma makes up 40%, embryonal 20 to 25%, teratocarcinoma 25 to 30%, teratoma 5 to 10%, and pure choriocarcinoma 1%. Often there are combined cell types within one tumor.

2. *Etiology*. The observation that testicular maldescent and tumor formation are related was made 135 years ago. Of patients with testicular tumors, 7 to 12% have a prior history of cryptorchidism. The risk of tumorigenesis in a man with a history of maldescent has been thought to be 48 times that of men with normally descended testes, although more recent studies suggest an incidence of only 3 to 14 times the normal expected incidence. In 5 to 15% of patients with a history of cryptorchidism and testicular tumor, the malignancy occurs in the contralateral, normally descended gonad.

3. *Natural History*. Intratubular carcinoma in situ grows beyond the basement membrane to eventually replace some or all of the testicular parenchyma. Epididymal and cord involvement is hindered by the tunica albuginea. Lymphatic or hematogenous spread may occur first. Half of patients with nonseminomatous tumors present with disseminated disease. Tumors confined to the testis spread to the retroperitoneal nodes, although pelvic and inguinal adenopathy is noted when there is cord or epididymal involvement. Lung, bone, and liver are sites of hematogenous spread.

Complete spontaneous regressions are rare. All germinal tumors in adults, including teratoma, should be regarded as malignant. Lymphatic metastases are com-

mon to all of these tumors, although pure choriocarcinoma almost always shows hematogenous dissemination as well. Right testis drainage is to the
interaortocaval region at the level of L2. Left testicular
drainage is primarily to the paraaortic nodes at the
same level. Most blood-borne spread occurs following
lymphatic involvement, a fact critical in prognosis and
treatment. The growth rate of nonseminomatous tumors tends to be rapid, with doubling times less than
30 days. Seminomas may follow a more indolent
course.

4. *Clinical Manifestations and Diagnosis.* Testicular cancer is relatively rare and affects an age group generally
not attuned to the possibility of cancer. As such, a 4-
to 6-month delay in diagnosis is unfortunately not uncommon. The most common symptoms are testicular
enlargement or mass. Testicular pain, though not classically described, may be present in almost 50% of
cases. Patients may present with constitutional symptoms or cough, abdominal mass, back pain, or adenopathy, all from metastatic disease.

Physical examination is the key in establishing a
diagnosis. A mass that cannot be clearly identified as
separate from the testis should be explored. Testicular
ultrasound is helpful in equivocal cases. Between 5
and 25% of patients with testicular cancer are mis-
takenly treated for epididymitis before the true diagnosis is made. If physical examination or ultrasound
suggests that a mass is intratesticular, an exploration
of the testis through an inguinal incision is needed. A
transscrotal biopsy of the testis puts inguinal nodes at
risk for metastases, markedly increases the potential
for implantation in the scrotal skin, and may make
chemotherapy, hemiscrotectomy, and/or inguinal
node dissection advisable in cases where these
modalities might not otherwise be indicated. There is
some controversy as to the advisability of orchiectomy
versus biopsy-frozen section followed by orchiectomy
in patients with scrotal masses. Inguinal orchiectomy
is performed except in cases where the benign nature

of the lesion is unequivocal. The most common benign mass in the testicle is an epidermoid cyst.

5. Staging
    a. Representative staging system—nonseminomatous tumors. Stage 1: disease limited to testis. Stage 2A: pathologically positive retroperitoneal lymph nodes at lymphadenectomy, but five or less involved and not grossly positive. Stage 2B: grossly positive retroperitoneal lymph nodes and/or greater than five positive nodes. Stage 2C: palpable abdominal mass. Stage 3: supradiaphragmatic or visceral involvement.

    There is a wide variance among institutions in terms of staging systems.

    b. Representative staging system (wide variance)—seminoma. Stage 1: disease limited to testis. Stage 2A: positive retroperitoneal nodes on lymphangiogram or abdominal CT scan. Stage 2B: palpable abdominal mass. Stage 3: supradiaphragmatic adenopathy, mediastinal and/or cervical. Stage 4: visceral metastases—pulmonary, osseous, hepatic, and/or CNS.

    c. Imaging studies
        (1) Chest radiography
        (2) Intravenous urography
        (3) Pedal lymphangiography. This technique was introduced in 1955 and is valuable in visualizing nodal architecture. Although testicular lymphangiography would better serve to visualize the nodal drainage area, it is not practical. Lymphangiography can identify metastatic nodes in 70 to 85% of cases and is widely used by radiotherapists for treatment planning in seminoma. The false-positive rate may be as low as 5%.
        (4) CT of retroperitoneum. This study is extremely helpful in evaluating the retroperitoneum. Approximately 75% of cases with metastases will be detected, with a false-positive rate of 15 to 20%. It can obviate the

need for an intravenous urogram, as the information desired from the latter study can be obtained.

(5) CT of chest. Whole lung tomography or chest CT can identify a small number of patients with chest metastases whose standard chest film is normal.

d. Tumor markers

(1) Human chorionic gonadotropin (hCG). This glycoprotein usually circulates at concentrations less than 1 ng/ml among normal individuals. Both hCG and its pituitary counterpart, LH, bind to the same specific plasma membrane receptors and essentially induce the same biochemical effects. Young boys with hCG-secreting tumors may present with signs of precocious puberty because hCG stimulates Leydig cells to increase testosterone synthesis and secretion. Men who present with hCG-secreting testicular cancers frequently have no signs or symptoms of excess circulating hCG. Some men will present with gynecomastia not because of hCG secretion but because of concomitant estradiol synthesis by their tumor.

Men presenting with seminomas may have abnormally high circulating levels of hCG approximately 5 to 20% of the time, depending on assay sensitivity. Synctiotrophoblasts within the seminoma are responsible for hCG secretion. Virtually all men with pure choriocarcinomas will have abnormally high circulating levels of hCG. Men presenting with embryonal cell carcinoma will have elevated hCG prior to treatment approximately two-thirds of the time. As with α-fetoprotein, it is imperative that hCG levels be determined prior to orchiectomy so that concentrations may be monitored postoperatively to help ascertain whether residual disease persists. Persistent elevation following treatment suggests residual tumor, whereas normalization of previously elevated markers at a rate consistent with their serum half-life is compatible with (but not necessarily indicative of) eradication of tumor. One can appreciate that it is helpful to be dealing with a tumor that is marker positive. Postorchiectomy determinations may provide a very important clue as to tumor eradication and subsequent recurrence. A marker-negative tumor is much more difficult to manage. The plasma half-life for hCG is 24 to 30 hours.

(2) α-fetoprotein (AFP). AFP was the first oncofetoprotein to be used as a tumor marker and was thought to be uniquely present among patients with tumors. More sensitive assays revealed low levels circulating in normal individuals. AFP is not secreted by seminomas. Consequently, if a patient is thought to have a pure seminoma but AFP levels are elevated in the face of no known underlying liver dysfunction, then occult nonseminomatous disease is considered present and therapy adjusted accordingly. Approximately 85% of men with nonseminomatous germ cell testicular tumors have elevated levels of either hCG or AFP or both. The plasma half-life for AFP is about 7 days.

6. Treatment

   a. Seminoma. The radiosensitivity of seminoma favors relatively modest amounts of megavoltage irradiation as the treatment of choice in patients with stage 1 and 2A disease (Chap. 15). Five-year survival rates for stage 1 approach 95%, and corresponding rates for stage 2A are about 87%.

     Platinum-based chemotherapy regimens are currently favored as initial treatment for advanced seminomas. Following inguinal orchiectomy, the role of surgery in treatment of pure seminoma is limited.

   b. Nonseminoma (chemotherapy discussed in
      Chap. 13)
      (1) Stage 1 and 2A disease. If staging procedures
          are negative for tumor, the patient is consid-
          ered to have clinical stage 1 disease. Contro-
          versy exists over the role of elective retro-
          peritoneal lymph node dissection versus
          observation alone in this setting. Of clinical
          stage 1 patients, 15 to 25% will have patholog-
          ic involvement of the retroperitoneal lymph
          nodes at surgery (stage 2A) and would there-
          fore be expected to clinically relapse after or-
          chiectomy alone. Of those found to have
          positive nodes at surgery, 50 to 70% will be
          cured by the node dissection alone. Less than
          1% of recurrences will occur in the retro-
          peritoneum after node dissection. Relapses are
          usually discovered on chest x-ray or by eleva-
          tion of serum markers, and early chemother-
          apy should provide almost a 100% cure rate.
              Advantages of retroperitoneal node dissec-
          tion include (a) accuracy of staging, (b)
          proven efficacy in terms of survival, (c) a fa-
          vorable relapse ''model'' in that chemothera-
          peutic rescue is higher when relapse involves
          the chest alone rather than chest and retro-
          peritoneum, and (d) excellent patient com-
          pliance to rigorous follow-up. Disadvantages
          include (a) it is not therapeutic for the 75% of
          patients with negative nodes on pathologic ex-
          amination, (b) newer combination chemother-
          apy regimens may give a rescue rate as high as
          that after recurrence post node dissection, (c)
          significant incidence of inability to ejaculate
          after node dissection despite operative modifi-
          cations to preserve sympathetic plexus, and
          (d) 8% of patients with negative node dissec-
          tions will still relapse with chest recurrence
          and require chemotherapy anyway.
              The management of clinical stage 1 disease

is an area of current urologic controversy, and trials are in progress throughout the world to answer the questions as to the best mode of therapy. The ultimate aim of such studies is to try and define two groups of patients: those with a high risk of tumor dissemination, in whom postorchiectomy therapy is certainly justifiable, and those with a low risk of metastases, in whom an observation alone policy postorchiectomy seems reasonable.

(2) Stage 2B, 2C, and 3 disease. Initial cytoreductive chemotherapy in patients with advanced nonseminomatous testicular tumors is now the treatment of choice. Patients with clinical staging suggesting 2B disease fall into a "gray" zone. In some centers they may be treated with chemotherapy as initial therapy, whereas in others retroperitoneal node dissection may be considered.

(3) Postchemotherapy surgery. Patients who initially present with unresectable stage 2 disease or with stage 3 disease should receive chemotherapy and undergo restaging at the completion of therapy. Patients who have normalization of their tumor markers with chemotherapy but have persistent, potentially resectable disease radiographically, are termed "resectable partial remission cases." Surgical removal of residual disease then is undertaken 4 to 6 weeks after the last course of chemotherapy. About one-third of resected specimens will show only fibrous or necrotic material, one-third will have some elements of persistent viable carcinoma, and one-third will show teratoma. Patients with viable carcinoma are given further chemotherapy. Presence of teratoma is associated with increased risk for relapse. As it does not appear to be eradicated by chemotherapy, a meticulous dissection is recommended and can be therapeutic. Those

patients who do not become marker negative after current standard chemotherapy courses are candidates for other chemotherapeutic–surgical protocols.

C. Other Testis Neoplasms
    1. Leydig Cell Tumors
        a. Make up 1 to 3% of testis tumors
        b. Are malignant in 10% of cases
            (1) Histologic criteria for differentiation unreliable
            (2) Diagnosis of malignancy by presence of metastases
            (3) Never malignant in prepubertal (25%) cases
    2. Sertoli Cell Tumors
        a. Less than 1% of testis tumors
        b. Malignancy diagnosed by presence of metastases
        c. Are malignant in 10% of cases

BIBLIOGRAPHY

Prostate Cancer

Catalona WJ: Prostate Cancer. Orlando, FL: Grune & Stratton, 1984.

Catalona WJ, Scott WW: Carcinoma of the prostate. In Walsh PC, Gittes RF, et al (eds): Campbell's Urology. Philadelphia: W.B. Saunders, 1986, pp 1463–1534.

Chisholm GD: Carcinoma of the prostate. In Whitfield HN, Hendry WF (eds): Textbook of Genitourinary Surgery. New York: Churchill Livingston, 1985, pp 1001–1018.

Labrie F, Dupont A, Belanger A: Complete androgen blockade for the treatment of prostate cancer. In DeVita VT, Jr, Hellman S, Rosenberg SA (eds): Important Advances in Oncology. Philadelphia: J.B. Lippincott, 1985.

Olsen S: Tumors of the Kidney and Urinary Tract. Philadelphia: W.B. Saunders, 1984.

Olsson CA (ed): Prostate cancer: Current concepts and controversies. Part I. Semin Urol 1(3), 1983.

Olsson CA (ed): Prostate cancer: Current concepts and controversies. Part II. Semin Urol 1(4), 1983.

Paulson DF (ed): Prostatic carcinoma. World J Urol 1(1), 1983.

Stamey TA: Cancer of the prostate. Monogr Urol 3(3), 1982.

Bladder Cancer

Droller MJ: Transitional cell cancer: Upper tracts and bladder. In Walsh PC, Gittes RF, et al (eds): Campbell's Urology. Philadelphia: W.B. Saunders, 1986, pp 1343–1462.

Kaufman JJ (ed): Current Urologic Therapy. Philadelphia: W.B. Saunders, 1986, pp 288–312.

Smith PH, Prout GR (eds): Bladder Cancer. Butterworths International Medical Reviews. Boston: Butterworths, 1984.

Whitmore WF: Urothelial tumors. Semin Urol 1(1), 1983.

Zingg EJ, Wallace DMA (eds): Bladder Cancer. New York: Springer-Verlag, 1985.

Renal Cell Carcinoma

deKernion JB: Renal tumors. In Walsh PC, Gittes RF, et al (eds): Campbell's Urology. Philadelphia: W.B. Saunders, 1986, pp 1294–1392.

del Regato JA, Spjut HJ, Cox JD: Cancer of the genitourinary tract. In Cancer: Diagnosis, Treatment, and Prognosis. St. Louis: C.V. Mosby, 1985, pp 637–659.

Harris DT, Maguire HC: Renal cell carcinoma. Semin Oncol 10(4), 1983.

Lieskovsky G, Pritchett R, Skinner DG: Surgical management of renal cell carcinoma. Monogr Urol 5(4), 1984.

Pontes JE: Metastatic renal cell carcinoma. In Kaufman JJ (ed): Current Urologic Therapy. Philadelphia: W.B. Saunders, 1986, pp 92–94.

Smith RB: Bilateral renal cell carcinoma and renal cell carcinoma in the solitary kidney. In Kaufman JJ (ed): Current Urologic Therapy. Philadelphia: W.B. Saunders, 1986, pp 94–96.

Woodhouse CRJ, Hendry WF, Bloom HJG: Renal carcinoma. In Whitfield HN, Hendry (eds): Textbook of Genitourinary Surgery. New York: Churchill Livingstone, 1985, pp 945–961.

Urothelial Tumors of the Renal Pelvis and Ureter

Droller MJ: Transitional cell cancer: Upper tracts and bladder. In Walsh PC, Gittes RF, et al (eds): Campbell's Urology. Philadelphia: W.B. Saunders, 1986, pp 1343–1462.

Grabstald H: Renal pelvic tumors. In Kaufman JJ (ed): Current Urologic Therapy. Philadelphia: W.B. Saunders, 1986, pp 103–105.

Hendry WF, Bloom HJG: Urothelial neoplasia. In Whitfield HN, Hendry WF (eds): Textbook of Genitourinary Surgery. New York: Churchill Livingstone, 1985, pp 971–1000.

McCarron JP, Mills E, Vaughn ED: Tumors of the renal pelvis and ureter: Current concepts and management. Semin Urol 1:75–81, 1983.

Olsen S: The renal pelvis and ureter. In Olsen S (ed): Tumors of the Kidney and Urinary Tract. Philadelphia: W.B. Saunders, 1984, pp 136–148.

Carcinoma of the Penis and Scrotum

Catalona WC: Role of lymphadenectomy in carcinoma of the penis. Urol Clin North Am 7:785–792, 1980.

del Regato JA, Spjut HJ, Cox JD: Male genital organs/penis. In del Regato JA, Spjut HJ, Cox JD (eds): Cancer. St. Louis: C.V. Mosby, 1985, pp 721–729.

Fraley EE, Zhang G, Sazama R, Lange P: Cancer of the penis: Prognosis and treatment plans. Cancer 55:1618–1624, 1985.

Grabstald H: Controversies concerning lymph node dissection for cancer of the penis. Urol Clin North Am 7:793–799, 1980.

Hendry WF: Tumours of penis and scrotum. In Whitfield HN, Hendry WF (eds): Textbook of Genitourinary Surgery. New York: Churchill Livingstone, 1985, pp 1034–1039.

Kaufman JJ: Carcinoma of the penis and erythroplasia of Queyrat. In Kaufman JJ (ed): Current Urologic Therapy. Philadelphia: W.B. Saunders, 1986, pp 410–412.

Schellhammer PF, Grabstald H: Tumors of the penis. In Walsh PC, Gittes RF, et al (eds): Campbell's Urology. Philadelphia: W.B. Saunders, 1986, pp 1583–1606.

Carcinoma of the Urethra

Hanno PM, Wein AJ: Female urethral diverticulum. Am Urol Assoc Update Ser, lesson 3, volume 5, 1986.

Hopkins SC, Grabstald H: Benign and malignant tumors of the male and female urethra. In Walsh PC, Gittes RF, et al (eds): Campbell's Urology. Philadelphia: W.B. Saunders, 1986, 1441–1462.

Melicow MM, Roberts TW: Pathology and natural history of urethral tumors in males. Review of 142 cases. Urology 11:83, 1978.

Olsen S: Tumors of the female and male urethra. In Olsen S (ed): Tumors of the Kidney and Urinary Tract. Philadelphia: W.B. Saunders, 1984, chap 10.

Skinner DS: Urethral carcinomas, including cowper's gland carcinoma. In Kaufmann JJ (ed): Current Urologic Therapy. Philadelphia: W.B. Saunders, 1986, pp 384–385.

Roberts TW, Melicow MM: Pathology and natural history of urethral tumors in females. Review of 65 cases. Urology 10:583, 1977.

Carcinoma of the Testis

Donohue JP, Rowland RG: The role of surgery in advanced testicular cancer. Cancer 54:2716–2721, 1984.

Einhorn LH, Donohue JP, et al: Cancer of the testes. In DeVita VT, Hellman S, Rosenberg S (eds): Cancer: Principles and Practice of Oncology. Philadelphia: J.B. Lippincott, 1985, pp 979–1012.

Morse MJ, Whitmore WF: Neoplasms of the testis. In Walsh PC, Gittes RF, et al (eds): Campbell's Urology. Philadelphia: W.B. Saunders, 1986, pp 2933–2954.

Roth BJ, Loehrer PJ: Testicular cancer: New directions in therapy. Curr Concepts Oncol, Spring 1985, pp 7–16.

Skinner DG (ed): Testicular carcinoma. Semin Urol 2:189–277, 1984.

15

Radiation Therapy

Philip Littman
Robert E. Krisch
James M. Galvin

I. HISTORY

A. In 1895 Roentgen described x-rays that emanated from a vacuum tube developed by Crookes several years previously.

B. At about the same time Henri Bacqueral noticed similar rays emanating from a natural material that was later isolated as radium by Madam Curie.

C. Two physicists were responsible for the use of x-rays in medicine.
1. Bacqueral noticed that radioactive material left in his waistcoat pocket caused skin inflammation.
2. Madam Curie lent radium to M. Danlos to be used at the St. Louis Hospital in Paris.

D. The first reported use of x-rays in the treatment of cancer was by Pratt in 1896.

E. By 1904 textbooks appeared on the use of radiation therapy for the treatment of cancer.

II. PHYSICS

A. Radiation Therapy
Radiation used for therapy falls into two categories: electromagnetic waves or particles. Both x-rays and gamma-rays are electromagnetic waves and are sometimes re-

353

ferred to as photons. Particles used for therapy can be charged (electrons, protons, heavy nuclei) or uncharged (neutrons). Gamma-rays are characterized by the radioactive nucleus from which they are emitted, whereas x-rays and charged particles are described by their energy. For x-rays, the energy of the electrons that produce (see below) the beam is stated. Typically, the range of electron energies (and therefore the photon energies) is from 50,000 to 40 million electron volts (eV). An electron volt is the energy gained by an electron when it is accelerated across a potential difference of 1 v (cathode to anode).

B. Electromagnetic Radiation

1. Gamma-rays are produced by certain unstable nuclei called radioactive isotopes, e.g., cobalt-60, radium-226, cesium-137, gold-198, iodine-125, and iridium-197.

   a. Each radioisotope emits photons at a discrete set of energies.

   b. The activity of any radioisotope decreases exponentially with time. This emission of radiation is expressed by the half-life of the material—the time it takes for one-half of the atoms in a sample to decay. Because radioactive isotopes decay, they are only clinically useful for the specific period of time determined by their half-life (Table 1).

TABLE 1. HALF-LIFE AND PHOTON ENERGIES OF COMMONLY USED RADIONUCLIDES

	Half-Life	Photon Energies MeV
Cesium-137	30.0 years	0.662
Gold-198	2.698 days	0.41–1.09
Iodine-125	60.25 days	0.035
Radium-226	1604 years	0.0247–2.44
Iridium-192	115.0 days	0.043–1.45
Cobalt-60	5.26 years	1.17–1.33

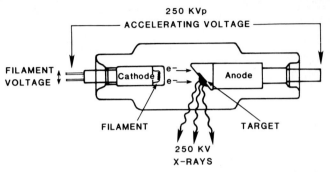

Figure 1. Production of x-rays from an x-ray tube. Electrons are emitted from the cathode and bombard the target at the anode.

    2. Electromagnetic radiation can also be produced electrically.
       a. The simplest means of production involves accelerating electrons across a potential difference, as is done in a basic diagnostic x-ray tube (Fig. 1). The x-rays are produced when the accelerated electrons bombard a high-atomic-number metal target such as tantalem or gold. As the electrons pass by the nuclei of the target atoms they are slowed and deflected by the coulomb field and x-rays are produced. These x-rays are called Bremsstrahlung radiation. A spectrum of x-ray energies results from Bremsstrahlung production because some interactions are weak while others are strong. The maximum photon energy cannot exceed that of the bombarding electrons (Fig. 2).
       b. Higher-energy electrons (and therefore x-rays) are available with linear accelerators and betatrons.
    3. Important characteristics of electromagnetic radiation.
       a. The greater the energy of the electromagnetic radiation, the greater is its ability to penetrate tissue.
       b. As the energy increases, the dose at the entrance surface of the irradiated material decreases and a

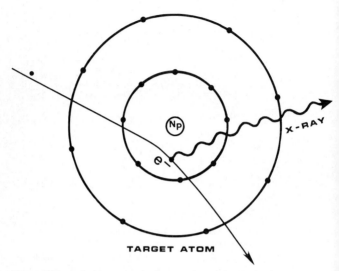

Figure 2. Bremsstrahlung occurs when an electron bombards a target atom of high atomic number and a photon is emitted.

> dose maximum is reached at several millimeters to centimeters below the surface. This initial build-up of dose is called skin sparing.
>
> c. Sparing of the surface tissues and increased penetration make high-energy electromagnetic radiation particularly useful in the management of deep-seated cancers.

C. Particulate Radiation

1. Electrons are the most commonly used particulate radiation and are extracted from linear accelerators or betatrons by allowing them to pass through a thin vacuum window without using the metal target that produces Bremsstrahlung radiation. As is the case with gamma radiation, electrons (called beta particles) can also be obtained from radioactive nuclei.

   a. Electrons, in contrast to photons, do not penetrate deeply into tissue. They dissipate their energy up

to a fixed depth, which depends on their initial energy, and then stop.
   b. They do not spare the skin surface to the degree seen with high-energy electromagnetic radiation.
   c. Electrons are particularly useful for treating malignancies that are near the surface, while sparing underlying structures.
2. Though the other kinds of particulate radiation are not commonly used, both neutron beams and proton beams are actively being studied to determine their possible advantages.

III. RADIOBIOLOGY

A. Ionization

The major effect of irradiation on tissue is ionization. Since water is the most common substance in tissue, the ionization primarily occurs in water.
1. The irradiation of water causes multiple interactions, resulting in the formation of free radicals.
2. These free radicals are very reactive substances and interact readily with cellular molecules.
3. The most important molecule damaged by free radicals is DNA. DNA damage is believed to account for essentially all cell killing by ionizing radiation.
4. Ionizing radiation has little effect on proteins at clinical doses.
5. Although ionizing radiation can kill cells immediately, usually cells are able to divide several times before division ceases (Fig. 3).

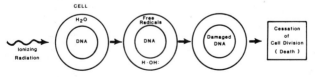

Figure 3. Ionizing radiation causes indirect damage to DNA as a result of the migration of free radicals formed in cellular water. This DNA damage results in cessation of cell division.

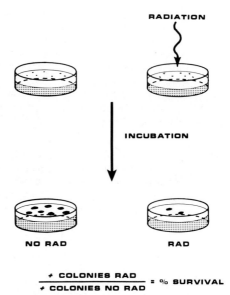

Figure 4. When cell cultures are irradiated with several hundred rads of ionizing radiation most cells will be unable to form colonies.

B. Response of Cells in Vitro
It was not until 1955 that Puck described the effects of ionizing radiation on cells in culture.
1. Surviving colonies that developed from individual cells that had been irradiated were counted and cell survival curves were generated (Figs. 4 and 5).
2. Cells from normal tissue or malignant tissue have similar survival curves and no obvious difference in radiosensitivity. This has been demonstrated in cell culture experiments.

C. Tumor Cell Sensitivity
It is not clearly understood why radiation can destroy tumors while damaging normal tissues to a lesser extent, since the sensitivity of tumor cells and normal tissue cells

does not seem to differ very much. Tumor cells tend to proliferate somewhat more rapidly than normal cells and their proliferation tends to be disorderly or asynchronous. It is thought that this disorganization of tumor cell proliferation is probably primarily responsible for their greater sensitivity to radiation. Multiple dose (fractionated) or continuous (interstitial) irradiation is much more effective in destroying tumor while preserving normal tissue than is a single dose of irradiation.

D. Tumor Resistance
Tumor resistance, an all too frequent clinical problem, may be due to a combination of several factors.
1. The presence of hypoxia in tumors which may have areas of poor blood supply could be a factor in tumor resistance. Cell culture studies have demonstrated that hypoxia can make tumor cells more resistant to radiation.

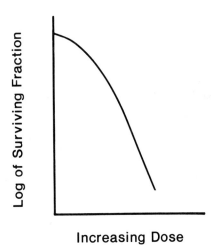

Figure 5. The reduction of colony formation in cell culture experiments is proportional to the dose of radiation. A typical cell survival curve shows an initial shoulder followed by a slope.

2. Some tumor cells may be in a resting state, which could make them more radioresistant.

3. Tumors of large size may be incurable because a very large amount of radiation would be needed to reduce the cell population to a level where complete eradication could occur. This amount of irradiation would exceed normal tissue tolerance.

E. Successful Radiotherapy

Tumor control with radiotherapy depends on the ability to eradicate tumor tissue while sparing normal tissue. This is called a favorable therapeutic ratio.

IV. RADIOTHERAPY EQUIPMENT

A. External Beam (Teletherapy)

1. As stated above, electromagnetic radiation is produced by accelerating electrons across a potential difference and having them strike an appropriate target material. A simple x-ray tube is shown in Figure 1. This approach can be used to obtain photon energies up to about 300,000 eV.

2. Superficial x-ray equipment accelerates the electrons to an energy which falls in the range of 50,000 to 100,000 eV. Therefore, the resulting Bremsstrahlung spectrum will have a maximum energy lying in this range. Those photon beams are commonly used in the treatment of skin cancer.

3. Orthovoltage units accelerate the electrons to an energy that falls in the range of about 150,000 to 300,000 eV. X-rays produced at these energies were for many years used to treat deep-seated cancer.

4. Starting in the mid-1950s, orthovoltage equipment was gradually replaced by van de Graaff generators or treatment units using the gamma radiation from the radioisotope Co-60. These were the first supervoltage units and marked the beginning of the modern radiotherapy era.

   a. These units exhibited the skin sparing discussed above. Skin, due to its relatively high sensitivity to radiation had previously often been the limiting tissue when deep structures were treated.

b. Linear accelerators producing energies from approximately 4 million to 35 million electron volts are now commonly used. Above about 6 million electron volts, it is easy to extract the electron beam for direct use.

c. Both Co-60 units and linear accelerators can be mounted so that they can rotate around a fixed point (isocenter) in space. This allows for precision treatment from different directions without moving

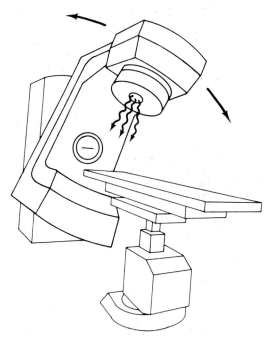

Figure 6. A modern isocentric radiation therapy unit and treatment couch. The patient can be put into proper position and the machine can treat from multiple positions, all focusing on the tumor.

the patient (Fig. 6). Also, this simple method for increasing the number of fields further spreads the skin dose. Betatrons, another device for producing high-energy electrons and photons, are not easily mounted using this isocentric mounting due to their larger size.

B. Interstitial and Intracavitary Techniques (Brachytherapy)

1. Radiation can also be delivered by the use of radioactive elements placed in tissues or in body cavities.

   a. These materials can be in the form of needles, wires, seeds, or tubes. The most commonly used materials are I-125, Ir-192, Cs-197, and Au-198. These sources are favored because they are somewhat safer than the older, commonly used radium, which has a higher energy and can give off radioactive gas if a tube is accidentally fractured. Different sources are particularly useful for specific areas of the body.

   b. Au-198, I-125, and Ir-192, most commonly used in urologic practice, are useful only for a relatively short period of time and must be ordered for each patient.

   c. Ir-197 must be removed from the body at completion of treatment.

   d. Au-198 and I-125 both remain permanently in place as an inactive (decayed) element.

V. BASIC APPROACH TO RADIOTHERAPY TREATMENT

A. Tumor Localization

1. In order to achieve the maximum therapeutic benefit for a particular patient, a thorough knowledge of the location of the tumor is necessary. A proper workup, frequently including computed tomography, is essential. If the patient is treated, careful determination of the extent of the tumor is needed and surgical clips

defining the edge of the tumor are helpful. These should be used sparingly so as not to cause artifact in future computed tomography studies.

2. Once a decision has been made to treat a patient and the tumor volume has been defined, the patient undergoes a procedure called treatment planning, which includes simulation. A simulator unit has the same geometry and movements as a therapy machine, and it produces diagnostic quality x-ray films rather than the poorer quality port films taken with the therapy unit (Fig. 7). The tumor can be outlined by localizing lines on x-ray film. In a complex treatment of deep tumors,

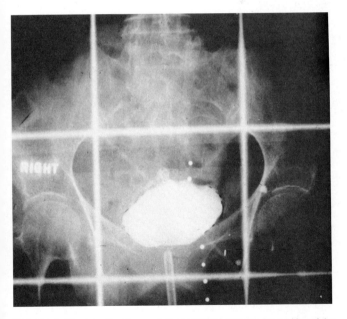

Figure 7. A. Simulator films from anterior and lateral showing the position of the bladder.

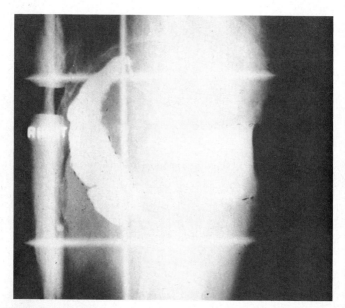

Figure 7. B. Simulator films from anterior and lateral showing the position of the rectum.

simulation and CT scans of the patient are used to help localize the tumor and determine the direction of treatment beam (Fig. 8).

B. Tumor Dose

1. Computers are helpful in calculating dose distributions and determining directions for the radiation beams. Careful attention to simulation and the other aspects of treatment planning will deliver the desired dose to the tumor while minimizing the dose to surrounding normal tissues (Fig. 9).

2. Before treatment actually begins, a dose schedule must be prescribed. Shortly after the introduction of x-rays for therapy, it was appreciated that treatment was

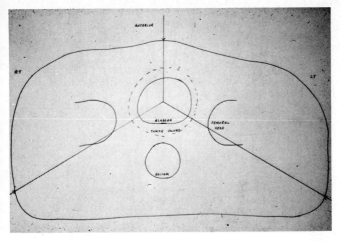

Figure 8. Cross section of a patient with the important structures located by the help of simulation films and CT scans.

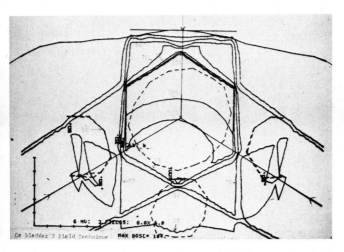

Figure 9. Computer-derived dose distribution around a bladder tumor treated with one anterior and two posterior oblique radiation fields.

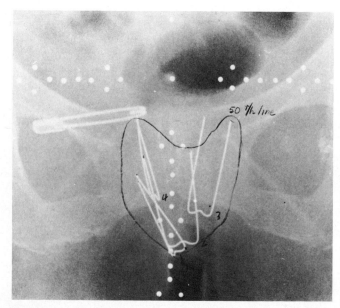

Figure 10. Ir-192 implant of the urethra. These sources are removable and treatment is determined by the length of time they are in place.

much better tolerated by normal tissues if it was given in multiple doses, usually two to five times per week. Most treatment is now delivered on a 5-day schedule.
3. The total dose is determined by the type of tumor, the sensitivity of the surrounding tissues, and the treatment goal, e.g., radiotherapy combined with surgery, tumor eradication with radiotherapy alone, tumor reduction by radiotherapy for palliation.

C. **Interstitial Therapy (Brachytherapy or Implant Therapy)**
1. Some tumors lend themselves to treatment with radiation from interstitial implants. This allows for a higher dose for the tissue where the radioactive material has

been inserted, while the surrounding normal tissue receives a very small dose. This dose differential cannot always be achieved with external beams.

2. For a particular radioisotope, the dose delivered by interstitial therapy is determined by a combination of the activity of the sources inserted and the length of time they are left in place. The dose for I-125 or Au-198 is determined only by the amount of material inserted since these sources are not removed. The dose delivered by Ir-192, which is removed after a specific amount of time, is determined by the number of sources inserted and the time they are left in place (Figs. 10 and 11).

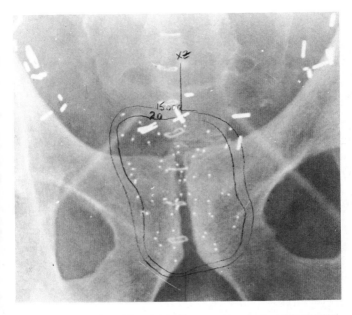

Figure 11. I-125 implant of the prostate. These are permanent sources and total dose to the tumor is determined by the number of sources inserted and their locations.

VI. PROSTATE CANCER

A. Tumor Response

Except for pathologically staged A1 tumors, which appear to do well without any form of treatment, stage A2, B, C, and some stage D tumors can be treated with curative radiation therapy. However, radical prostatectomy is considered by some urologists to be the best treatment for stage A2 and B.

B. Treatment Modalities

Radiation therapists generally feel that radiation therapy is as effective as any other treatment in the curative management of nonmetastatic carcinoma of the prostate. There is no good randomized study that compares radiation to surgery.

1. External Beam Therapy
   a. External beam radiation must be given with a supervoltage x-ray therapy unit. A dose of 6500 to 7000 rads is delivered to the prostate gland in approximately 6 to 7 weeks.
   b. Many radiotherapists use pelvic radiation, 4500 to 5000 rads, to treat the lymph-node draining areas; however, there are no good data for prostate to support that practice (Fig. 12).
2. Interstitial Therapy
   a. Radiation therapy can be delivered by inserting (implanting) radioactive seeds, usually I-125, suprapubically into the prostate (Fig. 11). The I-125 seeds deliver a radiation dose of about 15,000 to 20,000 rads over a period of 1 year to the prostate only. A total of 50% of this dose is delivered within the first 60 days. These seeds are never removed. At the time of operation a limited lymph node dissection, which is considered to be diagnostic only, can be done.
   b. Au-198 has also been used in conjunction with some amount of external beam therapy.
   c. Ir-192, inserted through the perineum, has had some limited use.

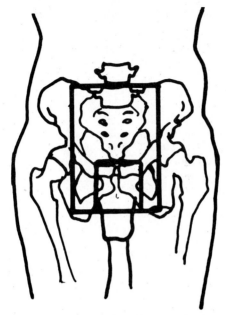

Figure 12. Outline of the smaller x-ray field used to treat the prostate gland alone and the large pelvic x-ray field used to treat lymph node draining areas.

3. I-125 and External Beam Radiation

These are the two standard radiotherapeutic approaches in the management of localized prostate carcinoma, and each has specific advantages and disadvantages.

a. I-125 seed insertion can be done as part of a lymph node dissection, which allows for determination of the presence of positive nodes. Although there is no good treatment for the presence of positive nodes, the status of the nodes has great prognostic importance. With iodine seed implants, treatment of prostate cancer can be done during surgery with no further treatment necessary. The procedure is of low risk, and seems to have a lower incidence of impotence when compared to external beam radiation. Most patients develop irratative bladder symptoms, which can last as long as 6 months. Proctitis is occasionally seen.

b. External beam radiation can be delivered without any surgical procedure; however, the true status of pelvic nodes cannot be determined. The incidence of proctitis and cystitis are similar to the incidence when I-125 is used. The risk of impotence may be higher than with I-125.

4. Palliative Care

a. Patients with metastatic bone disease can usually be effectively palliated with radiation therapy. Irradiation can decrease pain and produce healing of lytic lesions. If fracture occurs, the bones can be pinned and radiation can be given postoperatively. Doses of 2000 to 3000 rads delivered over 1 to 2 weeks are quite effective in decreasing pain and some bone healing occurs in most patients. In general, radiation therapy for bone metastases can be repeated once but not more than that since further radiation could lead to severe soft tissue fibrosis. The use of radiation therapy must be carefully considered in a patient with metastatic carcinoma of the prostate since these patients may live a number of years. Furthermore, treatment of multiple areas of the body can lead to profound bone marrow depression. As a general rule patients with metastatic carcinoma of the prostate should be treated for pain that is not relieved by moderate pain medication.

b. Frequently, patients with metastatic carcinoma of the prostate respond very well to estrogen therapy. However, in many patients estrogens are associated with swelling and tenderness of the breasts (painful gynecomastia). Three doses of 500 rads each using superficial radiation therapy delivered to each nipple can be very effective in preventing this side effect. Breast irradiation should always be given before estrogen treatment since it is ineffective if given after symptoms occur.

c. Occasionally, patients have severe bleeding from the prostate gland, obstruction requiring frequent transurethral resections (TURs), or rectal obstruction. In these cases, it might be beneficial to give a short course of radiotherapy to the prostate gland, delivering 3000 to 3600 rads over 2 to 3 weeks. Patients with metastatic prostate carcinoma rarely need local radiation to the prostate. Urinary obstruction is usually treated with TUR alone.

d. Patients with metastatic carcinoma of the prostate can present with extradural metastases resulting in compression of the spinal cord. This is a radiotherapeutic emergency and patients should have radiation immediately after the location of the block is determined by a myelogram. Initial daily doses should be high, approximately 400 rads and then reduced after several treatments to deliver a total of about 3000 rads. High doses of steroids initially are usually recommended as part of the management.

VII. BLADDER CANCER

A. Superficial Tumors

Although superficial bladder tumors and in situ cancer have been treated by various forms of radiation therapy, urologists generally manage these lesions by using intravesical chemotherapy or local resection.

B. Invasive Tumors

Invasive bladder cancers have been treated by radiotherapy using doses of 6000 to 7000 rads over 6 to 7 weeks. Interstitial radiation therapy of the bladder has been used in Europe. The general recommendation for treatment of invasive bladder cancer is surgery. However, for very elderly or inoperable patients, external irradiation should be given and will be curative for some patients.

C. **Pre- and Postoperative Radiotherapy**

1. There has been considerable interest in the use of radiation therapy precystectomy. Many centers recommend 1600 to 4500 rads given over 1 to 5 weeks. The value of preoperative radiation therapy has not been proven. Many urologists, however, feel more comfortable doing a cystectomy after a dose of preoperative radiation therapy has been delivered, particularly if the lesions are high grade and high stage.

2. If preoperative radiotherapy has not been given and, if margins of resection are found to be positive, lymph node metastases are found in the pelvis, or tumor extends into the perivesical fat, postoperative radiation therapy is generally recommended. This may improve local control but it is very uncertain if there would be any effect on survival.

3. Radiotherapy for palliation in bladder cancer can be of some benefit. Patients who have advanced bladder cancer with metastases often get relief of bone pain with doses of 3000 rad over 2 weeks. In contrast to prostate cancer, bone metastasis in carcinoma of the bladder is usually associated with very short survival. Occasionally patients with unresectable carcinoma of the bladder have severe bleeding. This sometimes can be controlled with a dose of 3000 rads delivered over 2 weeks.

VIII. TESTIS

A. **Seminoma**

1. The only testicular tumor for which radiation is regularly used is seminoma.

2. Over 90% of patients with stages I and II seminomas can be cured by resection of the testis and postoperative radiation therapy to draining lymph nodes.

3. Doses in the range of 2500 to 3500 rads over approximately 3 to 4 weeks are used and have few side effects.

4. In stage I seminoma, patients receive radiation therapy to the ipsilateral iliac and paraaortic lymph nodes up to the level of the diaphragm (Fig. 13).

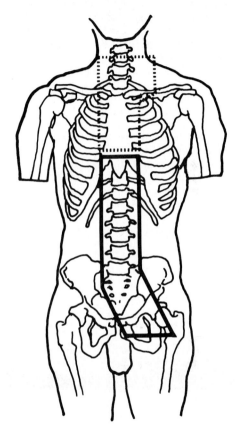

Figure 13. An outline of the x-ray field used to treat a stage I seminoma. The dotted x-ray field can be used to treat the mediastinum and left supraclavicular areas for patients with stage II disease.

5. In stage II seminoma, there is considerable controversy over whether mediastinal and supraclavicular area radiation should be given in addition to infradiaphragmatic treatment. Since there is excellent salvage chemotherapy some oncologists would prefer that su-

pradiaphragmatic radiation therapy not be given so that if patients recur they can receive chemotherapy without the problems of bone marrow suppression secondary to previous extensive radiation therapy. However, others claim that radiation therapy to the supradiaphragmatic areas in stage II seminoma gives such a good survival rate that the chances of failing and needing chemotherapy are very small. No randomized trials have been done to answer this question and the treatment for stage II seminoma varies from institution to institution.

6. Very bulky stage II and stage III seminoma is generally managed by chemotherapy. Radiation therapy may be used for areas of disease that do not respond completely to chemotherapy.

7. The recommended surgical management of seminoma is radical orchiectomy, removing the testis through an inguinal incision. There are, however, patients who have had a testis removed through the scrotum. This is inadvisable because scrotal lymphatics could be seeded with tumor, which can then lead to local recurrence or metastasis to inguinal nodes. Furthermore, in some patients the tumor has grown through the capsule of the testis and contaminated the scrotum. In either case it has been recommended that radiation therapy be delivered to the scrotum. This, however, is somewhat difficult to do without radiating the other testis and a hemiscrotectomy is the preferred management.

B. Nonseminomatous Testicular Cancer
Nonseminomatous testicular cancer is primarily managed by chemotherapy.

IX. PENILE AND URETHRAL CANCER

A. Penile Cancer
Tumors of the penis can be effectively treated with radiation therapy. Superficial tumors can be managed using superficial radiation therapy. Interstitial treatment and external beam to the entire penis has also been used with

success for more extensive lesions. No general treatment recommendation can be made regarding carcinoma of the penis since it is a rare disease. Most often the treatment is surgical resection of the primary with inguinal lymph node dissection.

B. **Urethra**
1. Carcinoma of the urethra in the male is usually managed surgically. These lesions tend to do very poorly.
2. In the female, urethral lesions that are not large can be managed very effectively with interstitial radiation therapy. The area tolerates this form of treatment fairly well. Since the surgical management would require removal of the bladder, radiation therapy is a good initial treatment reserving radical surgery for failures. If the urethral tumor is very large and involves the bladder, then radical surgery should be performed.

X. URETERAL CANCER
Ureteral carcinoma is very rare. There is some evidence that postoperative radiation therapy may be of benefit when the tumor extends beyond the wall of the ureter, there are positive margins, or there is tumor spillage.

XI. RENAL CANCER
Preoperative radiation therapy has not been shown to be of benefit.

For patients with positive margins, tumor spill, or positive nodes, postoperative radiation therapy has been given to some patients. Doses of 4500 rads are recommended. It is difficult to give more than that amount because of the large volume of tissue that requires treatment. The value of this treatment is uncertain.

Unfortunately palliation in renal cell carcinoma is difficult to achieve since these tumors tend to be quite radioresistant. The usual dose of 3000 rads over 2 weeks for bone metastases from other tumors may not be helpful for renal cell carcinoma metastases, and higher doses are sometimes necessary. Patients with local problems such as bleeding or pain from renal carcinomas that are unresectable are best managed with embolization.

XII. PEDIATRIC UROLOGIC CANCER

Although pediatric cancer is fortunately a rare disease, it is the second highest cause of death in children under age 15. Great strides have been made in the management of childhood cancer. One of the main reasons for this success is the availability of effective chemotherapy. Furthermore, most of these tumors have been carefully studied in randomized trials and the best forms of management have been established.

A. Renal Tumors

1. Wilms' tumor is one of the most common types of pediatric malignancy. Overall survival exceeds 80%. Wilms' tumor is occasionally seen in adults where the patients do not do as well as those in the pediatric age group. Postoperative radiation therapy to the renal bed is delivered for all patients with positive margins, residual disease, spillage of tumor, or positive nodes but is not necessary when the tumor has been completely resected (Fig. 14). Doses of 1000 to 2000 rads are given except for patients with a specific histologic appearance that is considered "poor." This represents a small group of Wilms' tumor patients. Patients with "poor" histology should receive 3500 to 4000 rads postoperatively to their renal bed. Patients with gross spillage of tumor into the abdominal cavity receive 1000 to 2000 rads to the entire abdomen and patients with metastatic lung disease receive 1200 rads to both lungs. All Wilms' tumor patients receive concurrent chemotherapy.

2. Renal cell carcinoma is rare in childhood and is usually managed like Wilms' tumor. Some of these tumors respond like Wilms' tumors although others respond like adult renal cancer and do very poorly.

B. Bladder, Prostate, and Testis Tumors

1. Tumors of bladder and prostate in children are usually rhabdomyosarcomas. Because of the great reluctance to perform radical surgery in small children, radiation

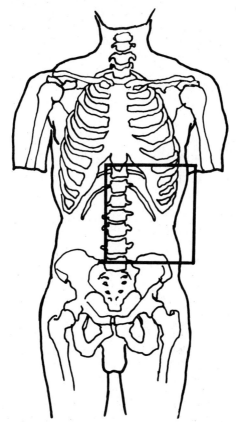

Figure 14. Outline of radiation field used to deliver postoperative treatment for a patient with Wilms' tumor. A significant number of vertebral bodies, several ribs, and sometimes part of the pelvis may be included in this field.

therapy (4000 to 5000 rads) and chemotherapy are used for primary treatment, reserving surgery for salvage. Organ preservation can sometimes be achieved.

2. Testis tumors are rare in childhood and the management is similar to that of adults. A very young child

with seminoma may, however, be managed with chemotherapy rather than radiation therapy. Paratesticular
rhabomyosarcomas are managed with surgery and chemotherapy. Radiation therapy is only used for treating
nonresectable lymph node disease, which is very
infrequent.

XIII. COMPLICATIONS OF RADIOTHERAPY

A. Acute Effects

1. Since supervoltage radiation therapy spares the skin,
    skin reactions are seldom seen except in skin folds
    where sparing is reduced. Hair loss is common even
    with very modest doses of radiation. Loss of hair in the
    pubic area secondary to radiation may be of concern to
    patients; however, the hair usually grows back.

2. Nausea is the most commonly asked about side effect
    of radiation therapy and is frequently seen during the
    first few days of treatment even if the gastrointestinal
    tract is not in the treatment field. Even when the gas-
    trointestinal tract is in the field, however, nausea
    rarely lasts more than a few days, but may occasion-
    ally last longer and require medication. Diarrhea is
    usually seen 2 to 3 weeks after the start of radiation
    and can sometimes be managed just with restriction of
    vegetables, fruits, and milk products. Antidiarrheal
    medication is frequently needed in patients who re-
    ceive pelvic irradiation greater than 4000 rads.

3. Proctitis and exacerbation of hemorrhoids may also
    occur during prostate irradiation. Sterile cystitis is usu-
    ally seen after 3 to 4 weeks of pelvic radiation. This
    can   be   managed   symptomatically   with   anti-
    cholinergics, and resolves several weeks after the
    completion of radiation therapy.

4. After several weeks of radiation therapy, patients com-
    plain of fatigue. The cause of this is unknown, and it
    resolves a few weeks after completion of treatment.

5. A reduction in blood counts can be significant if large
    volumes of bone marrow are treated and/or the patient
    has received or is receiving chemotherapy. Weekly

counts should be carefully monitored, particularly when the pelvis is in the treatment field.

6. In general, acute effects of radiation therapy are transient, fairly well tolerated, and can in most cases be treated symptomatically.

B. Late Effects

1. Late effects of radiation therapy are strongly dose dependent, tissue dependent, and can be very severe. The degree of late effects cannot be predicted by the degree of acute effects. Furthermore, patients react differently to radiation therapy, with some reacting much more severely than expected. Since the goal of radiation therapy is to cure cancer, some degree of late effects must be accepted and a certain occurence of severe late effect is unavoidable.

2. Late gastrointestinal effects following high doses of radiation can include fibrosis, obstruction, and fistula formation. These complications can require surgical intervention and can be fatal. Surgery of heavily irradiated bowel must be done very cautiously since it is often technically difficult secondary to adhesions. In addition, previously irradiated tissue may not heal as well as unirradiated tissue.

3. The kidney is very sensitive to radiation and doses above 1500 to 1800 rads can lead to radiation nephritis, which may result in renal failure. Radiation therapy to a single kidney can occasionally lead to hypertension.

4. The ureter is felt to be resistant to radiation therapy. However, stenosis is seen occasionally after high-dose radiation therapy for carcinoma of the cervix.

5. Bladder late effects can be seen after high doses of pelvic radiation. These problems consist of chronic nonbacterial cystitis, hemorrhagic cystitis, radiation ulcers, and loss of bladder capacity. Sometimes cystectomy is needed. Complications in the bladder are most commonly seen after radiation therapy for carcinoma of the cervix and after definitive radiation therapy for bladder cancer.

6. Late effects due to radiation of the prostate are gener-

ally not related to the prostate but rather are due to damage of the bladder and/or rectum. Chronic cystitis secondary to definitive radiation therapy of the prostate is rare. However, rectal problems are occasionally seen. One of the most significant side effects secondary to irradiation of the prostate is impotence. It may be as high as 50% with external beam and 20% with interstitial therapy. The cause of this is thought to be secondary to radiation effect on small blood vessels. Radiation therapy to the prostate does not seem to affect orgasm or ejaculation.

7. Sperm production is extremely sensitive to radiation and very low doses can drop sperm counts profoundly, and in some cases permanently. Even when the testes are not in the radiated field, the dose to the testis from scattered radiation may be sufficient to cause significant drops in sperm count. This is frequently seen in patients who are treated for Hodgkin's disease. There is no evidence that the offspring of patients who have been previously exposed to therapy with ionizing radiation have an increase in either birth defects or cancer. Testosterone production is relatively resistant to radiation therapy. However, loss of Leydig cells is seen in leukemic children who get repeated courses of irradiation to the testes for leukemic infiltration.

8. The ovary is moderately sensitive to irradiation. Any ovulating female patient who requires a dose of radiation therapy to the pelvis exceeding 2400 rads is very likely to be sterilized by radiation therapy.

9. Growth is a major consideration in children who receive radiation therapy, as bone and soft tissue growth can be profoundly affected. Wilms' tumor has been a particular problem because of the large fields necessary to cover the entire renal bed. Even with reduced doses now given to Wilms' tumor patients, a mild degree of scoliosis may be seen.

10. The induction of neoplasia due to therapeutic radiation is well known. These second malignant neoplasms are seen 5 to 30 years posttreatment. This is a

particular problem in treating children or young adults. Certain chemotherapeutic agents are also carcinogenic and when given in conjunction with radiation therapy can increase the risk of second malignant neoplasms. In general the risk of a second malignant neoplasm is small and not a particular issue in the adult population.

XIV. FUTURE DEVELOPMENTS IN RADIOTHERAPY

A. **Like surgery, radiation therapy can only deal with local tumor.** A cause of failure for most urologic malignancies is metastatic disease. Further progress must be made in dealing with that problem. Except for testicular tumors, chemotherapy has not been particularly helpful in urologic cancer. More effective use of radiation therapy for local tumor control in urologic malignancy is needed to achieve organ preservation. Drugs for increasing radiosensitivity of tumors or decreasing the radiosensitivity of normal tissues are being studied.

B. **The use of different forms of radiation,** which may be more useful in dealing with gross tumor, such as neutrons and protons, are under active investigation.

C. **The use of radiation therapy given intraoperatively** either through direct application of external beam radiotherapy through the surgical wound or the insertion of radioactive materials into the tumor is being explored in many centers.

XV. CONCLUSION

A. **Radiation therapy** plays an important role in the management of urologic cancer.

B. **Although it can destroy malignant tissue** it can cause significant side effects.

C. **Radiation therapy for urologic malignancy** is used best when urologists and radiotherapists work closely together.

BIBLIOGRAPHY
Coia L, Moylan DJ: Therapeutic Radiology. Baltimore: Williams & Wilkins, 1984.
Fletcher GH: Textbook of Radiotherapy. Philadelphia: Lea & Febiger, 1978.
Galvin JM: The physics of radiation therapy equipment. Semin Oncol 8:18–37, 1981.
Hall EJ: Radiobiology for the Radiologist. Philadelphia: Harper & Row, 1978.
Johns HE, Cunningham JR: The Physics of Radiology. Springfield, IL: Charles C Thomas, 1983.

16

Voiding Function and Dysfunction

Alan J. Wein
Philip M. Hanno

I. INTRODUCTION

For the purposes of description and teaching, micturition is best divided into two relatively discrete phases, one of bladder filling and urine storage, and one of bladder emptying. Particular aspects of anatomy, physiology, and pharmacology may relate more to one phase than to another. We first summarize relevant facts regarding the anatomy, neuroanatomy, pharmacology, and physiology of the lower urinary tract. We then attempt to answer, on the basis of the science so presented, certain important functional questions related to the filling/storage phase and to the emptying phase of micturition. Certain "rules" will be formulated that must be satisfied for the lower urinary tract to function normally. By extrapolation, these rules can be used as a basis for a very simple functional classification of voiding dysfunction, which can be easily extended to include urodynamic evaluation and treatment. Voiding dysfunction is considered from the standpoint of the neurologic evaluation and from the standpoint of diagnosis and treatment. Lastly, common problems are briefly discussed.

II. VOIDING FUNCTION

A. Relevant Anatomy and Terminology

The designation lower urinary tract includes the bladder, the urethra, and the periurethral striated muscle. Anatomically and embryologically the bladder has traditionally been divided into detrusor and trigone regions. The terms bladder body and bladder base refer to a functional rather than anatomic division of bladder smooth muscle, which is based on distinct differences in neuromorphology and neuropharmacology between the smooth muscle lying circumferentially above (body) and below (base) the level of the ureterovesical junction. Bladder smooth muscle bundles are, to a greater or lesser extent, loosely organized in the area of the bladder base into an outer longitudinal, middle circular, and inner longitudinal layer. There is a great deal of disagreement regarding the continuity of some longitudinal smooth muscle from the bladder into the urethra. The entire urethral length of the female and the proximal portion (down to the urogenital diaphragm) in the male contains smooth muscle that is capable of affecting urethral resistance. The "smooth sphincter" refers to the smooth muscle of the bladder neck and proximal urethra. This is not an anatomic sphincter, but a physiologic one. Normally, resistance increases in the smooth sphincter during bladder filling and urine storage and decreases in this area during a bladder-emptying contraction.

The classical view of the "external sphincter" is that of a striated muscle within the leaves of the urogenital diaphragm that, on contraction, is capable of stopping the urinary stream. This concept has been expanded to include an intramural and extramural portion. The extramural portion corresponds roughly to the classical external urethral sphincter and the urogenital diaphragm. The intramural portion denotes skeletal muscle intimately associated with the urethra in both sexes above the urogenital diaphragm, continuous from that level for a variable distance to the bladder neck, and forming an integral part of the outer muscle layer of the urethra. In the male, though some striated muscle is seen in the prostatic capsule and parenchyma, this is primarily located between the verumontanum and the urogenital diaphragm. Activity increases in the striated sphincter during the filling/storage phase of micturition and virtually disappears during normal emptying.

B. Receptor Function and Innervation of the Lower Urinary Tract

The physiology and pharmacology of the lower urinary tract cannot be separated from that of the autonomic nervous system. There are many differences between the autonomic nervous system and the somatic nervous system, but the easiest for clinicians to understand and remember is that the autonomic nervous system includes all efferent pathways having ganglionic synapses outside of the central nervous system (CNS). There are no somatic nerve synapses outside of the CNS. The terms sympathetic and parasympathetic refer simply to anatomic divisions of the autonomic nervous system. The sympathetic division consists of those fibers that originate in the thoracic and lumbar regions of the spinal cord, whereas the parasympathetic division refers to those fibers that originate in the cranial and sacral spinal nerves. The classical view of the peripheral autonomic nervous system involves a two-neuron system: preganglionic neurons emanating from the central nervous system and making synaptic contact with cells within ganglia, from which postganglionic neurons emerge to innervate peripheral organs (Fig. 1). This relatively simple concept, however, though still useful for the purposes of discussion, has undergone much contemporary expansion and modification. Most innervation of the lower urinary tract actually emanates from peripheral ganglia that are at a short distance from, adjacent to, or within the organs they innervate (the ''urogenital short neuron system''). Additionally, the efferent autonomic pathways do not necessarily conform to the classical two neuron model, as they are often interrupted by more than one synaptic relay. Furthermore, for many years the only autonomic neurotransmitters recognized were acetylcholine and norepinephrine. It has become obvious that other transmitters are involved in various components of the autonomic nervous system, and a once relatively simple concept of chemical neurotransmission has been expanded to include synaptic systems that involve modulator transmitter mechanisms, prejunctional inhibition or enhancement of transmitter release, postjunctional modula-

Neurohumoral Transmission

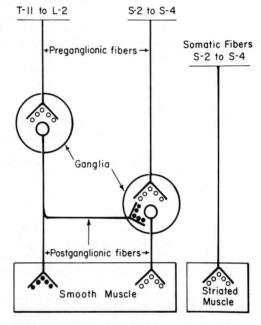

Sympathetic Fibers Parasympathetic Fibers
T-11 to L-2 S-2 to S-4

←Preganglionic fibers→

Somatic Fibers
S-2 to S-4

Ganglia

←Postganglionic fibers→

Smooth Muscle

Striated
Muscle

Nature of chemical transmitter

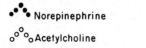

•••• Norepinephrine

○○○○ Acetylcholine

Figure 1. Classical neuroanatomic and neuropharmacologic description of the innervation of the smooth muscle of the bladder and urethra and the striated muscle of the external urethral sphincter. Note the termination of some postganglionic sympathetic (adrenergic) fibers on parasympathetic ganglion cells, providing the morphologic substrate for sympathetic inhibition of parasympathetic ganglion cell transmission.

tion of transmitter action, cotransmitter release, and the secondary involvement of locally synthesized hormones and other substances such as prostaglandins. All of these are subject to neuronal and hormonal regulation, desensitization, and hypersensitization. Finally, these relationships may be altered by changes that occur secondary to disease or destruction in the neural axis, obstruction of the lower urinary tract, aging, and hormonal status.

The classical model of smooth muscle contraction involves synaptic release of neurotransmitter in response to neural stimulation, with the transmitter agent subsequently combining with a recognition site, or receptor, on the postsynaptic smooth muscle cell membrane. The transmitter–receptor combination then initiates changes in the postsynaptic effector cell that ultimately result in what we consider the characteristic effect of that particular neurotransmitter on that particular smooth muscle. Clinicians are often confused because they assume that the terms sympathetic and parasympathetic imply particular neurotransmitters. These terms imply strictly anatomic origin within the autonomic nervous system. Other adjectives are used to describe the nature of the neurotransmitter involved.

The term cholinergic refers to those receptor sites where acetylcholine is the neurotransmitter. Peripheral cholinergic fibers include somatic motor fibers, all preganglionic autonomic fibers, and all postganglionic parasympathetic fibers. The cholinergic receptor sites on autonomic effector cells are termed muscarinic, while such sites on autonomic ganglia and on motor end plates of skeletal muscle are designated nicotinic. Atropine competitively inhibits muscarinic receptor sites.

The term adrenergic is applied to those receptor sites where a catecholamine is the neurotransmitter. Most postganglionic sympathetic fibers are adrenergic receptor sites, including those to the lower urinary tract smooth muscle, where the catecholamine responsible for neurotransmission is norepinephrine. Adrenergic receptor sites are further classified as alpha (α) or beta (β) on the basis of the differential effects elicited by a series of catecholamines and their antagonists. Classically, the term α-adrenergic effect designates vasoconstriction and/or contraction of smooth musculature in response to norepinephrine. These are inhibited by phentolamine, phenoxybenzamine, and prazosin. The term β-adrenergic effect implies smooth muscle relaxation in response to catecholamine stimulation and also includes cardiac stimulation, vasodilatation, and bronchodilatation. These effects are stimulated most potently by isoproterenol, much more so than by norepinephrine.

The pelvic and hypogastric nerves supply the bladder and urethra with efferent parasympathetic and sympathetic innervation, and both convey afferent sensory impulses from these organs to the spinal cord. The parasympathetic efferent supply is classically described as originating in the grey matter of sacral spinal cord segments S2 to S4. This preganglionic supply is ultimately conveyed by the pelvic nerve. Efferent sympathetic fibers to the bladder and urethra are thought to originate in spinal cord segments T11 to L2, and are carried within the hypogastric nerves. Bilaterally, at a variable distance from the bladder and urethra the hypogastric pelvic nerves meet and branch to form the pelvic plexus. Divergent branches of this pelvic plexus innervate the pelvic organs. Efferent innervation of the striated sphincter is classically thought to be somatic and to emanate from sacral spinal cord segments S2 to S4 via the pudendal nerve. Some feel that the striated sphincter is innervated by branches of the autonomic nervous system as well.

Cholinergic innervation is abundant to all areas of the bladder of animals and of man. Though most authorities agree on the existence of a cholinergic innervation at least of the proximal urethra in animals, there is considerable disagreement regarding the extent (and in some cases existence) of a similar innervation in man. It is generally agreed that abundant muscarinic cholinergic receptor sites exist throughout the bladder body and base of various animal species and of man. A sustained bladder contraction is produced by stimulation of the pelvic nerves, and it is generally agreed that reflex activation of this pelvic nerve excitatory tract is responsible for the emptying bladder contraction of normal micturition, and for the involuntary bladder contractions seen with various diseases of the neural axis and response to lower urinary tract obstruction. Whether acetylcholine is the sole neurotransmitter released during such stimulation is highly controversial. Atropine resistance refers to the only partial antagonism exhibited by atropine of the bladder response to pelvic nerve stimulation or of isolated bladder strips to electrical field stimulation. It is generally agreed that atropine resistance occurs in various experimental animal models, and the most logical explanation seems to be release of additional neurotransmitter(s) besides acetylcholine in response to nerve stimulation. Whether atropine resistance actually occurs in normal man is a matter of controversy. However, one should not ignore the possibility that different types of atropine resistance may exist in various types of bladder hyperactivity, regardless of the normal state of affairs.

Adrenergic innervation of the bladder and urethral smooth musculature has been extensively demonstrated in animals. These studies have shown that the smooth musculature of the bladder base and proximal urethra possesses a rich adrenergic innervation, while the bladder body has a sparse but definite adrenergic innervation. The density of innervation seems in all areas to be less than that of the cholinergic systems. Considerable disagreement exists, however, as to even the presence of postganglionic sympathetic innervation in the bladder and proximal urethra of man. There is general agreement that the smooth muscle of the human male bladder neck possesses a dense adrenergic innervation, but little consensus otherwise. Even those authorities who ascribe a significant influence of the sympathetic nervous system on the micturition cycle have difficulty demonstrating more than a sparse adrenergic innervation in other areas of the bladder and urethra. There is general agreement, however, that the smooth muscle of the bladder and proximal urethra in a variety of animals and in man contains both α- and β-adrenergic receptors. α-adrenergic responses predominate in the bladder base and proximal urethra, where-as β-adrenergic responses predominate in the bladder body. Additionally, there is general agreement that there is a significant inhibitory influence exerted on parasympathetic ganglionic transmission by postganglionic sympathetic fibers (Fig. 1). Those who advocate a major role for the sympathetic nervous system on the micturition cycle summarize the influences as follows. The sympathetic nervous system is felt to act primarily to facilitate the filling/storage phase of micturition, and does so by three mechanisms:

1. Increasing outlet resistance, by stimulation of the predominantly α-adrenergic receptors in the bladder base and proximal urethra.
2. Inhibiting bladder contractility via a blocking effect on parasympathetic ganglionic transmission.
3. Increasing accommodation by stimulation of the predominantly β-adrenergic receptors in the bladder body.

It should be noted, however, that many noted authorities are of the opinion that the sympathetic nervous system plays a very minor role in the micturition cycle.

Other peripheral neurotransmitters doubtless exist in the lower urinary tract, and this is the object of much contemporary investigation. Adenosine triphosphate (ATP) has been postulated as the "other" excitatory neurotransmitter in cases of atropine resistance. Vasoactive intestinal polypeptide (VIP) has been generally shown to have an inhibitory effect on bladder muscle contractility, and has been postulated to act as a modifier of bladder activity during filling.

C. Central Influences on Lower Urinary Tract Function
Micturition is basically a function of the peripheral autonomic nervous system. However, the ultimate control of lower urinary tract function obviously resides at higher neurologic levels. There is general consensus that the micturition "center" in the spinal cord is primarily localized to segments S2 to S4, with the major portion at S3. However, there is little question

that the brainstem, specifically the neurons of the pontine–mesencephalic gray matter, contains the nuclei that are the origin of the final common pathway to bladder motor neurons. Input to this area is derived from the cerebellum, basal ganglia, thalamus and hypothalamus, and cerebral cortex. Bladder contraction elicited by stimulation at or above this area seems to occur with a decrease in activity of the paraurethral striated musculature, as in normal micturition. The region of the cerebral hemispheres primarily concerned with bladder function consists of the superomedial portion of the frontal lobes and the genu of the corpus callosum. Transection experiments indicate that the net effect of these areas is inhibitory.

Strong evidence is accumulating that endogenous opioid peptides influence micturition by a tonic inhibitory effect on detrusor reflex pathways. These inhibitory effects could be mediated at several levels, including the peripheral bladder ganglia, the sacral spinal cord, and the brainstem micturition center. Different types of opioid receptors may be responsible, at different sites, for different types of effects on bladder contractility.

D. Important Functional Questions

1. *What Determines Bladder Response During Filling?* The normal bladder response to filling at a physiologic rate is an almost imperceptible change in intravesical pressure. There is little question that, during the initial stages of filling, this very high compliance is due primarily to purely passive properties of the bladder wall, summarized by the concepts of elasticity and viscoelasticity. At a certain level of bladder filling, a spinal sympathetic reflex is clearly evoked in animals, and there exists indirect evidence to support such a role in humans. The effects of this reflex are to facilitate the filling/storage phase of micturition and have been previously described. There is little question that a strong tonic inhibitory effect on bladder activity is contributed by endogenous opioids, at least at the level of the spinal cord and brainstem.

2. *What Determines Outlet Response During Filling?* There is a gradual increase in urethral pressure during bladder filling. Both smooth and striated sphincteric

elements contribute to this pressure by different reflex mechanisms through their respective efferent innervation. The passive properties of the urethral wall also doubtless contribute to the maintenance of continence. The tension that develops in the urethral wall is a product not only of the active characteristics of smooth and striated muscle, but of the passive characteristics of the elastic and collagenous tissue composition of the urethral wall as well. This tension must be exerted on a soft or plastic inner layer capable of being compressed to a closed configuration. Moreover, whatever the compressive forces, the lumen must be capable of being obliterated by a watertight seal (the mucosal seal mechanism).

3. *Why does voiding ensue with a normal bladder contraction?* During voluntarily initiated micturition, the bladder pressure becomes higher than the outlet pressure, certain adaptive changes occur in the shape of the bladder outlet, and urine passes into and through the proximal urethra. There is a reflex coordination between a voluntarily induced bladder contraction of adequate magnitude and active responses of the proximal urethra. Urethral pressure actually decreases prior to bladder contraction. The decrease in pelvic floor striated musculature electromyographic (EMG) activity prior to voluntary bladder contraction would strongly suggest that at least a portion of this decrease in urethral response is secondary to a reflex mechanism involving the striated sphincter. It is tempting to speculate that a similar reflex coordination of smooth sphincter activity exists, mediated through a decrease in efferent hypogastric nerve activity. Additionally, there may be an active mechanism that occurs to decrease urethral smooth muscle activity which involves stimulation of β-adrenergic receptors.

4. *Why does urinary leakage not occur with abdominal straining?* First of all, a coordinated bladder contraction does not occur in response to such stimuli, and this fact clearly points out the fact that increases in intravesical pressure are by no means equivalent to

emptying ability. For urine to flow through a normal bladder neck and into a normal proximal urethra, not only must an increase in intravesical pressure occur, but it must be a product of a coordinated bladder contraction, occurring through a neurally mediated reflex mechanism associated with characteristic changes in the bladder neck and proximal urethra area. A major factor in the prevention of urinary leakage during increases in intraabdominal pressure is the location of the bladder neck and proximal urethra (the ''sphincter unit''). Normally this is situated within the abdominal cavity to allow equal transmission of any increase in intraabdominal pressure to the bladder neck and proximal urethra. Ligamentous and fascial structures normally support the sphincter area and prevent its descent into a position where intraabdominal pressure increases are not transmitted at least equally. Alteration of these structures such that pathologic descent does occur with abdominal straining occurs secondary to many etiologic factors, predominantly in the female, and stress incontinence is the result. To correct this, it is necessary only to substitute a mechanism to prevent this descent and to restore the normal resting position of the sphincter unit. This is accomplished by any of the standard vesicourethral suspension procedures.

E. Summary and Extrapolation

What follows is a concise and simplified description of the normal processes involved in lower urinary tract function that seems consistent with existent data and opinions. The two functions of the lower urinary tract are the storage and active expulsion of urine. During bladder filling at physiologic rates, intravesical pressure initially rises slowly despite large increases in volume. This phenomenon is due primarily to the passive properties of the smooth muscle and connective tissue of the bladder wall. There is little neural efferent activity until a certain critical intravesical pressure is reached, following which there is a gradual reflex increase in somatic nerve activity that causes increased activity in the striated sphincter. In animals, and perhaps in humans as well, an additional spinal sympathetic reflex also results. The efferent limb of this reflex is through the hypogastric nerve, resulting in inhibition of bladder contractile activity through an effect on parasympathetic ganglionic transmission and also in an increase in outlet resistance because of active stimulation of the adrenergic receptors in the smooth sphincter. A decrease in bladder body contractility mediated through β-adrenergic receptors may also play a role. It is very probable that a tonic inhibitory influence exerted by endogenous opioids contributes to maintaining bladder stability during filling. Intraurethral pressure is normally greater than intravesical pressure, and this relationship is maintained during increases in intraabdominal pressure because of the anatomic localization of the sphincter unit and the positive pressure transmission ratio to this area with respect to intravesical contents.

Although many factors are involved in the micturition reflex, it is intravesical pressure producing the sensation of distention that is primarily responsible for the initiation of voluntarily induced emptying of the lower urinary tract. The origin of the parasympathetic neural outflow to the bladder is in the sacral spinal cord. However, the actual organizational center for the micturition reflex in an intact neural axis is in the brainstem. The final step in voluntarily induced micturition involves inhibition of the somatic neural efferent activity to the striated sphincter and an inhibition of all aspects of the spinal sympathetic reflex evoked during filling. Efferent parasympathetic pelvic nerve activity is ultimately what is responsible for a highly coordinated contraction of the bulk of the bladder smooth musculature. A decrease in outlet resistance occurs, with adaptive shaping or funneling of the relaxed bladder outlet. This involves reflex inhibition of striated and smooth sphincter tone, and may involve an active mechanism of smooth muscle relaxation in this area as well. Superimposed on these autonomic and somatic reflexes and modifying factors are complex peripheral and central inputs, both facilitory and inhibitory, which allow for the full conscious control of micturition.

Whatever disagreements exist, all ''experts'' would agree on certain points. The micturition cycle involves two relatively discrete processes: bladder filling and urine storage, and bladder emptying. Whatever the neuromorphologic, neurophysiologic, neuropharmacologic, and mechanical details involved, one can succinctly summarize these processes from a conceptual point of view. Bladder filling and urine storage requires

1. Accommodation of increasing volumes of urine at a low intravesical pressure and with appropriate sensation.
2. A closed bladder outlet at rest that remains so during increases in intraabdominal pressure.
3. Absence of involuntary bladder contractions.

Bladder emptying requires

1. A coordinated contraction of adequate magnitude of the bladder smooth musculature.
2. A concomitant lowering of resistance at the level of the smooth sphincter and the striated sphincter.
3. Absence of anatomic obstruction.

Any type of voiding dysfunction must result from an abnormality of one or more of the factors listed as involved in the two phases of the micturition cycle. This division, with its implied subdivisions under each category into causes related to the bladder and causes related to the outlet, provides a perfect rationale for the classification of all types of voiding dysfunction into disorders related to bladder filling or urine storage and disorders related to bladder emptying. There are indeed some types of voiding dysfunction that represent a combination of filling/storage and emptying disorders. Within this scheme, these combined disorders become readily understandable. Further, one may take all aspects of urodynamic and video urodynamic evaluation and classify the individual component studies as to exactly what they evaluate in terms of either bladder or outlet activity during filling/storage or emptying. Finally, one can then easily classify all known treatments for voiding dysfunction under the broad categories of whether they facilitate filling/storage or emptying, and whether they do so by an action primarily on the bladder or on the components of the bladder outlet.

III. VOIDING DYSFUNCTION

Abnormalities of the micturition cycle are responsible for a large number of patient visits to the urologist. The symptoms produced by these disorders can range from annoyance to complete disability. These abnormalities may occur on the basis of bladder outlet obstruction, neurogenic disease or neurologic injury, loss of the supporting structures of the lower urinary tract secondary to surgical and nonsurgical trauma, or as a consequence of aging, and on a strictly psychogenic basis.

A. The Neurourologic Evaluation (Table 1)

1. *History.* In general, clinicians commonly speak of obstructive as opposed to irritative symptoms. Obstructive symptoms are supposed to indicate abnormalities of emptying, whereas irritative symptoms are supposed to connote abnormalities of filling/storage. However, objective assessment often correlates poorly with subjective symptomatology. Hesitancy and straining are generally symptoms of emptying failure. Although urgency, frequency, and incontinence are generally symptoms of filling/storage failure, they can also be symptoms of emptying failure in a patient with a large residual urine and resultant decrease in functional bladder capacity.

2. *Physical and Neurologic Examination.* Especially relevant to the urologist is the evaluation of deep tendon reflexes that provide some indication of segmental spinal cord function as well as suprasegmental function.

TABLE 1. THE NEUROUROLOGIC EVALUATION

History	Intravenous urogram
Physical examination	Voiding cystourethrogram
Neurologic evaluation	Endoscopic examination
Renal function studies	Urodynamic studies
Urine bacteriologic studies	Videourodynamic studies

Particularly relevant is anal sphincter tone, considered representative of the perineal striated musculature. Normal anal sphincter tone and the ability to voluntarily contract this muscle indicates integrity of pelvic floor innervation, both sacral and suprasacral. Preservation of tone in the absence of voluntary contraction indicates a suprasacral lesion, whereas diminished tone implies a sacral or peripheral nerve abnormality. The bulbocavernosus reflex is elicited by squeezing the glans penis or clitoris and monitoring external anal sphincter or bulbocavernosus contraction. The spinal cord segments involved are primarily S2 to S4, and spinal cord injury above these segments will generally cause hyperactivity, while the bulbocavernosus reflex will be lost or decreased with sacral or peripheral nerve damage. Other deep tendon reflexes, as well as a sensory assessment, may be useful in localizing a particular neurologic lesion. Other specialized laboratory studies, more properly within the province of the neurologist, may be necessary.

3. *Urodynamic Evaluation (Table 2).* Urodynamics of the lower urinary tract consist simply of methods designed to generate quantitative data regarding what occurs in the bladder and in the bladder outlet during the filling/storage phase and during the emptying phase of micturition. The subject has become far more complicated than need be—90% of pertinent and relevant urodynamic information can be obtained by a logical clinician using relatively simple studies. It is important to remember that the clinical symptoms or problem must be reproduced during whatever testing sequence is utilized; otherwise the urodynamic testing is irrelevant and worthless.

   a. Flow—residual urine. Flowmetry and residual urine determination are simply methods of integrating the activity of the bladder and the outlet during the emptying phase of micturition. If the flow rates and the flow pattern are normal, it is unlikely that there is any significant abnormality of the emptying phase of micturition. Important factors to

TABLE 2. URODYNAMICS MADE EASY

	Bladder	Outlet
Filling/storage	P_{det}(FCMG)[a]	P_{ureth}[b] Fluoro[c]
Emptying	P_{det}(VCMG)[d]	P_{ureth}[b] Fluoro[c] EMG[e]
	---------------Flow[f]--------------	
	--------------- RU[g]---------------	

[a]Filling cystometrogram (recording of detrusor pressure during filling)
[b]Urethral Pressure(s)
[c]Fluoroscopy
[d]Voiding cystometry (recording of detrusor pressure during voluntary or involuntary emptying)
[e]EMG of periurethral striated muscle
[f]Flowmetry
[g]Residual Urine Determination

consider include the pattern of flow (normally a parabola), and the mean and peak flow rates (15 and 25 ml/sec, respectively, in younger individuals). Reproducibly low flow rates generally indicate either increased outlet resistance, decreased bladder contractility, or both. This situation is usually associated with a pattern abnormality consisting of low acceleration and a broad plateau. An intermittent phasic flow pattern generally indicates either abdominal straining or sphincter dyssynergia. A consistently increased residual urine volume generally indicates increased outlet resistance, decreased bladder contractility, or both. Minimal residual urine is seen with normal lower urinary tract functioning during emptying but may coexist with either significant incontinence or outlet obstruction.

   b. Cystometry. A cystometrogram provides activity about the activity of the bladder during the filling/storage phase of micturition. As normally applied, the term refers to "filling cystometry," as opposed to "voiding cystometry," which refers to the measurement of intravesical pressure during voluntary or involuntary micturition. Cystometry is done simply by recording bladder pressure through a urethral or suprapubic catheter. As such, it measures total bladder pressure; in order to determine intrinsic or subtracted bladder pressure, it is necessary to simultaneously record some measure of intraabdominal pressure, and subtract this from the total bladder pressure. Filling cystometry can be done with either carbon dioxide or saline. At the filling rates commonly used, both are distinctly unphysiologic, and thus filling cystometry, in either case, is truly a screening test. Bladder filling normally occurs with a very low pressure rise in spite of a large increase in volume. Bladder compliance (rate of change of volume divided by rate of change of pressure) is high, until bladder capacity is reached. Bladder hyperactivity during cystometry occurs either because of involuntary bladder contractions that cause phasic increases in intravesical pressure, or because of decreased compliance, which causes a steep slope of the filling limb without phasic contractions. Detrusor hyperreflexia is the term applied to involuntary contractions that occur in a patient with known neurologic disease. Detrusor instability is the term applied to involuntary bladder contractions that occur without known neurologic cause. Cholinergic supersensitivity (bethanechol supersensitivity test) can be determined during cystometry, and a positive result indicates a reactive detrusor, and one that may be (but is not necessarily) neurologically decentralized.

c. Electromyography. For the average urologist, electromyography permits evaluation only of the activity of the striated sphincter during the emptying phase of micturition. EMG activity in the periurethral striated musculature is virtually absent at rest, increases during filling, and becomes virtually absent just prior to the onset of an emptying bladder contraction. Dyssynergia refers to inappropriate sphincter activity during bladder contraction and may be localized to either striated or smooth sphincter. Striated sphincter dyssynergia does not refer to the increase in periurethral striated muscle EMG activity seen in response to an involuntary bladder contraction during filling in an individual whose sensation is normal. In this case, the appropriate response is attempted inhibition of the bladder contraction by pelvic floor striated musculature contraction, a circumstance that will produce a simultaneous increase in pelvic floor EMG activity and intravesical pressure. Striated sphincter dyssynergia refers to the occurrence of involuntary striated sphincter activity during a voluntary bladder contraction or an involuntary bladder contraction in an individual with absent or markedly impaired sensation. Neurologists use electromyography to study motor unit potentials of striated muscle in order to be able to differentiate myogenic from peripheral neurogenic disease.

d. Cystography and voiding cystourethrography. A cystogram in the erect position at rest and during straining may be useful in diagnosing a nonfunctional bladder neck and stress urinary incontinence. Voiding cystourethrography is useful to diagnose the site of obstruction in a patient already known to have urodynamic evidence of obstruction.

e. Combined studies. Intraabdominal pressure, intravesical pressure, and flow may be measured simultaneously with or without EMG recording. The purpose of such studies is to determine whether or not obstruction is present and to be able to assess bladder contractility more precisely. Fluoroscopy may be combined with these studies, and all parameters displayed on a screen within a system with audio overlay and video playback capability. This is the most complete (as well as most expensive and time consuming) method of collecting data referable to the micturition cycle and should therefore be reserved for problem cases.

f. Urethral pressure studies. The usual static infusion urethral pressure profile records the pressure generated in response to infusion of either gas or liquid through the side hole(s) of a small catheter being withdrawn from the bladder past the urogenital diaphragm. As such, it may be useful in evaluating urethral resistance under certain circumstances, but its utility is limited because it is carried out at rest, and not really during filling/storage or emptying. Urethral pressure determinations are more useful when recorded simultaneously with bladder pressure during filling and emptying. This may be done at one site in the proximal urethra or it may be done by pulling the catheter out through the urethra during bladder emptying, a so-called micturition pressure profile. This latter study, though somewhat complicated, is an excellent way of determining the site of an obstruction.

g. Urography—ultrasonography—isotope studies. Many urologists believe that the intravenous urogram is the optimal screening study of the upper tracts (kidneys and ureters) in patients with significant voiding dysfunction. Dilatation of the ureters or renal collecting system, or a decrease in function, represents significant complications of lower urinary tract dysfunction and is an absolute indication for intervention. Other complications, such as renal scarring and calculi, are also easily seen. Ultrasonography can give adequate information about hydronephrosis, the presence of larger calculi, and occasionally hydroureter. Isotope studies may be useful to evaluate renal blood flow and function and to establish the presence of renal or ureteral obstruction.

h. Endoscopic examination. This is valuable to exclude irritative, neoplastic, or preneoplastic changes in the bladder epithelium as a cause of voiding symptomatology. The presence or absence of trabeculation (which is compatible with obstruction, involuntary bladder contractions, or neurologic decentralization) can also be determined. Endoscopic examination may likewise be confirmatory of obstruction at a particular site, but it should be recognized that not everything that appears obstructive endoscopically is obstructive urodynamically (all large prostates are not obstructive), and lack of a visually appreciated obstruction does not exclude functional obstruction (striated or smooth sphincter dyssynergia) during bladder emptying.

B. Classification of Voiding Dysfunction

There are many classification systems for voiding dysfunction, and these are generally based on either neurologic, urodynamic, or functional considerations. As previously implied, our center primarily employs a functional type of classification, describing voiding dysfunction in terms of whether the deficit produced is primarily one of the filling/storage phase of micturition (failure to store) or of the emptying phase (failure to empty). Either type of deficit can be further divided on the basis of whether it exists primarily because of bladder-related reasons or because of reasons related to the outlet. Situations exist that represent a combination of storage and emptying failure, and some of these are discussed subsequently.

Jack Lapides of the University of Michigan contributed significantly to the classification and care of the patient with neurogenic voiding dysfunction by popularizing a modification of a scheme originally proposed in 1939. Explanations and descriptions of the components of this system are descriptive and combine typical cystometric data with clinical setting and symptomatology. This is still probably the most common classification system used to explain neurogenic bladder dysfunction to the medical student. Sensory neurogenic bladder results from any disease that selectively interrupts the sensory fibers between the bladder and spinal cord or the afferent tracts to the brain. The disease most frequently associated with this type of dysfunction is diabetes. The earliest change consists of only a delay in the first desire to void. As bladder sensation becomes further blunted, unless voiding is initiated out of habit or on a timed basis, varying degrees of bladder overdistention result, with resultant decompensation of the bladder smooth muscle and hypotonicity. Significant amounts of residual urine are found, and the cytometric curve exhibits a marked shift to the right, with a flat low-pressure curve and a marked increase in bladder capacity. Motor paralytic bladder implies a disease process that has selectively destroyed the parasympathetic motor innervation of the bladder. Extensive pelvic surgery or trauma and herpes zoster can produce this type of dysfunction, which can be partial or complete. The early symptoms may vary from painful urinary retention to a relative inability to initiate and maintain normal micturition. If chronic overdistention and smooth muscle decompensation occurs, the cystometrogram resembles that of a late-stage sensory neurogenic bladder. Uninhibited neurogenic bladder describes a clinical situation characterized symptomatically by frequency, urgency, and sometimes urge incontinence, and cystometrographically by normal sensation with involuntary bladder contractions at low filling volumes. Residual urine volume is characteristically small or absent unless anatomic outlet obstruction exists, implying that the striated sphincter relaxes appropriately during detrusor contraction. The patient can usually initiate micturition voluntarily, but often is unable to store enough urine to do so because of bladder hyperactivity. Cerebrovascular accident and demyelinating disease are recognized as the most common causes of this type of lesion. Reflex neurogenic bladder describes the state of affairs that exists after complete suprasacral interruption of the sensory and motor pathways to and from the sacral spinal cord. This most commonly occurs after traumatic spinal cord injury, following the resolution of spinal shock. The typical patient has no bladder sensation, is unable to initiate micturition voluntarily, and is incontinent because of low-volume detrusor hyperreflexia. Large volumes of residual urine with respect to bladder capacity generally result, implying dyssynergia during detrusor hyperreflexia.

C. **Treatment**

The functional classification for voiding disorders previously described can be expanded into a system that categorizes all forms of therapy for voiding dysfunction on the basis of whether they facilitate urine storage, by inhibiting bladder contractility or increasing outlet resistance, or facilitate bladder emptying, by increasing bladder contractility or decreasing outlet resistance (Tables 3 and 4). If therapy is unsuccessful, circumvention can be accomplished either by continuous or intermittent catheterization or by urinary diversion.

D. **Common Problems**

1. *Outlet Obstruction Secondary to Prostatic Enlargement.* This is probably the most common voiding dysfunction seen by the urologist. Classically, the patient complains of hesitancy and straining to void, with the urodynamic correlates of low flow and high intravesical pressure during attempted voiding. This situation represents a pure failure to empty. Approximately 50% of the time, the patient with significant prostatic obstruction develops detrusor hyperactivity secondarily, with resultant urgency, frequency, and, if the hyperactivity cannot be inhibited, urgency incontinence. Under such circumstances, the voiding dysfunction becomes a combined emptying and filling/storage problem. Treatment is relief of the obstruction, generally by a transurethral prostatectomy. Relief of the outlet obstruction will result in the eventual disappearance of detrusor hyperactivity, where present, in about 70% of cases.

2. *Urethral Incontinence.* Involuntary leakage of urine per urethra (as opposed to incontinence that occurs because of a decreased mental status or secondary to a

fistula) may be due to bladder- or outlet-related causes. Involuntary bladder contractions and decreased compliance during filling represent different types of detrusor hyperactivity, each of which can give rise to urinary incontinence. With normal sensation,

TABLE 3. THERAPY TO FACILITATE BLADDER EMPTYING

I. Increasing Intravesical Pressure
  A. External compression, Valsalva
  B. Promotion or initiation of reflex contractions
    1. Trigger zones or maneuvers
    2. Bladder training, tidal drainage
  C. Pharmacologic therapy
    1. Parasympathomimetic agents
    2. Prostaglandins
    3. Blockers of inhibition
      a. α-adrenergic antagonists
      b. Opioid antagonists
  D. Electrical stimulation
    1. Directly to the bladder
    2. To the spinal cord or nerve roots
II. Decreasing Outlet Resistance
  A. At a site of anatomic obstruction
    1. Prostatectomy
    2. Urethral stricture repair/dilatation
  B. At the level of the smooth sphincter
    1. Transurethral resection or incision of the bladder neck
    2. Y-V plasty of the bladder neck
    3. Pharmacologic therapy
      a. α-adrenergic antagonists
      b. β-adrenergic agonists
  C. At the level of the striated sphincter
    1. External sphincterotomy
    2. Urethral overdilatation
    3. Pudendal nerve interruption
    4. Pharmacologic therapy
      a. Skeletal muscle relaxants
        1. Benzodiazepines
        2. Baclofen
        3. Dantrolene
      b. α-adrenergic antagonists
    5. Psychotherapy, biofeedback
III. Circumventing Problem
  A. Intermittent catheterization
  B. Continuous catheterization
  C. Urinary diversion

TABLE 4. THERAPY TO FACILITATE URINE STORAGE

I. Inhibiting Bladder Contractility/Decreasing Sensory Input
   A. Timed bladder emptying
   B. Pharmacologic therapy
      1. Anticholinergic agents
      2. Musculotropic relaxants
      3. Polysynaptic inhibitors
      4. Calcium antagonists
      5. β-adrenergic agonists
      6. α-adrenergic antagonists
      7. Prostaglandin inhibitors
      8. Tricyclic antidepressants
      9. DMSO
    10. Bromocriptine
   C. Biofeedback, bladder retraining
   D. Bladder overdistention
   E. Electrical stimulation (reflex inhibition)
   F. Interruption of innervation
      1. Subarachnoid block
      2. Selective sacral rhizotomy
      3. Peripheral bladder denervation
   G. Cystoplasty (augmentation)
II. Increasing Outlet Resistance
   A. Physiotherapy
   B. Electrical stimualtion of the pelvic floor
   C. Pharmacologic therapy
      1. α-adrenergic agonists
      2. Tricyclic antidepressants
      3. β-adrenergic antagonists
   D. Nonsurgical mechanical compression
   E. Surgical mechanical compression
   F. Vesicourethral suspension (SUI)
III. Circumventing Problem
   A. Antidiuretic hormone-like agents
   B. External collecting device
   C. Intermittent catheterization
   D. Continuous catheterization
   E. Urinary diversion

these give rise to the symptom of urgency. If voluntary inhibition of these phenomena is possible, only urgency is present, but if inhibition is not possible, then urge incontinence results. Pharmacologic management is the first type of treatment attempted, generally with an anticholinergic agent (such as propantheline), an antispasmodic agent (such as oxybutinin or dicyclomine), or a tricyclic antidepressant (such as imipramine, which inhibits bladder contractility by a non-adrenergic-noncholinergic-related mechanism). The most common type of outlet-related incontinence is stress urinary incontinence in the female. Classical stress incontinence occurs because of an abnormal descent of the "sphincter unit" (see previous discussion) during increases in intraabdominal pressure, such that these pressure increases are no longer transmitted equally to the sphincter unit as they are to the bladder. Optimum treatment consists of any of the forms of vesicourethral suspension that stabilize the bladder neck such that abnormal descent no longer occurs. α-adrenergic agonists, such as phenylpropanolamine, are sometimes employed for mild to moderate cases: these act by increasing urethral resistance through stimulation of the primarily α-adrenergic receptors of the smooth muscle of the bladder neck and proximal urethra. A nonfunctional bladder outlet generally results in a more severe degree of incontinence, with gravitational incontinence that increases during abdominal straining. This type of incontinence may be seen in the female after pelvic trauma or repeated pelvic surgery or in response to peripheral nerve injury. In the male, it is seen in postprostatectomy incontinence. Pharmacologic treatment or simple vesicourethral suspension is generally unsuccessful in such cases, which require either reconstruction of the bladder outlet or external compression, achieved most commonly with a sling type procedure or by placement of an artificial sphincter.

3. *Neurogenic Bladder Dysfunction.* Cerebrovascular accident may initially result in urinary retention followed by detrusor hyperactivity of the type described under the uninhibited neurogenic bladder (see previous section). Multiple sclerosis may result in this type of voiding dysfunction or in involuntary bladder contractions with striated sphincter dyssynergia. Suprasacral

spinal cord injury initially results in a period of spinal shock, with no measurable reflex activity below the neurologic level of injury. After spinal shock passes, a reflex neurogenic bladder results (see previous section). This represents a combined filling/storage–emptying deficit. There is an abnormality of filling/storage because of involuntary bladder contractions that occur without sensation, and emptying dysfunction results because of simultaneous striated sphincter dyssynergia. Two avenues of treatment are possible. The first involves suppression of the detrusor hyperactivity, that is, attempted conversion of the deficit to purely one of emptying. This is then circumvented using intermittent catheterization. Alternatively, the emptying portion of the disorder can be corrected with striated sphincterotomy, or an attempt can be made to correct it with pharmacologic management. In the male, an external collecting device can be utilized to circumvent the resultant urinary incontinence (which occurs because of the still present involuntary bladder contractions), but, in the female, a suitable collecting device has not been developed. Significant injury to the sacral spinal cord or to the peripheral nerve roots initially results in loss of measurable bladder reflex activity and an inability to voluntarily initiate micturition. Later, a very complicated picture may develop, involving decreased compliance during filling, but without a true bladder contraction, an open bladder neck down to the level of the striated sphincter, and a resultant inability to either fill or store urine normally, or to empty. This is best treated with intermittent catheterization and pharmacologic management to inhibit bladder contractility and augment outlet resistance.

4. *The Decompensated Bladder*. This situation may occur after long-standing bladder outlet obstruction or as a chronic response to neurologic injury. Attempts to produce emptying pharmacologically with a cholinergic agonist and an α-adrenergic antagonist have been generally unsuccessful, and the best treatment is

intermittent catheterization. One should resist the temptation to surgically decrease bladder outlet resistance in the hopes of "tipping the balance" in favor of emptying. This approach is seldom effective unless it produces a form of stress incontinence.

5. *Postoperative Retention.* Urinary retention can occur postoperatively for a number of reasons. Nociceptive impulses can inhibit the initiation of reflex bladder contraction, perhaps through an opioid-mediated mechanism. Transient overdistention of the bladder can occur under anesthesia or under the influence of analgesic medication. Purely neurologic injury during abdominal and pelvic surgery can also occur. Generally, in the absence of neurologic injury, a patient's voiding status will return pretty much to what it was prior to the surgery and anesthesia. Therefore, the optimal treatment is intermittent catheterization. Return of bladder function may be facilitated by the use of an α-adrenergic antagonist. When effective, the mechanism is probably blockade of the inhibitory sympathetic influence on parasympathetic ganglionic transmission. A patient with prostatism previously on the borderline of significant voiding dysfunction may indeed have his previously tenuous ability to empty satisfactorily (but not normally) compromised. In these cases, prostatectomy is justified.

BIBLIOGRAPHY

Barrett DM, Wein, AJ: Controversies in Neuro-Urology. New York: Churchill Livingstone, 1984.

Hald, T, and Bradley WE: The Urinary Bladder. Baltimore: Williams & Wilkins, 1982.

McGuire EJ: Clinical evaluation and treatment of neurogenic vesical dysfunction. In Libertino JA (ed): International Perspectives in Urology. Baltimore: Williams & Wilkins, 1984, vol. II.

Mundy, AR, Stephenson TP, Wein AJ: Urodynamics: Principles, Practice and Application. New York: Churchill Livingstone, 1984.

Raz S: Female Urology. Philadelphia: W. B. Saunders, 1983.

Wein AJ, Levin RM, Barrett DM: Voiding function: Relevant anatomy, physiology, pharmacology. In Gillenwater J, Grayhack J et al. (eds): Textbook of Urology. Chicago: Year Book, to be published.

17

Male Sexual Dysfunction

Philip M. Hanno
Alan J. Wein

I. GENERAL CONSIDERATIONS

Although sexual function and dysfunction were not subjected to rigorous scientific study until relatively recently, sexual health has long been a concern of physicians. To Hippocrates is attributed the belief that "Preoccupation with business and lack of attractiveness can cause impotence." Aristotle discussed "engorgement" and recognized some of the physiologic aspects of ejaculation.

The apparent increase in impotence as a presenting complaint can be attributed to (1) changes in sexual attitudes and expectations, (2) alteration in traditional male–female roles, and (3) advances in diagnosis and treatment. The incidence of erectile dysfunction is about 5% in the 5th decade, increasing to 35% by the 7th decade, and almost doubling to 60% the following decade. These figures are indicative of a problem much more common than cancer or heart disease, and one that deserves serious consideration.

II. PHYSIOLOGY OF SEXUAL FUNCTION

A. Erection

Erection is a neurologically mediated event producing vascular changes that result in engorgement and rigidity of the penis. Anatomic changes include a slight increase in length preceding an increase in circumference, followed by elevation of the penis from the resting position. Increases in volume and size do not necessarily parallel changes in rigidity and hence the ability to penetrate the vagina.

Penile erection is initiated by an increase in blood inflow over outflow to the penile corporal spaces. At the point of full erection a new steady state is reached where inflow equals outflow. The tunica albuginea of the corpora limit tissue expansion and account for penile rigidity in the tumescent state. It is generally believed that increased arterial inflow rather than decreased venous outflow is the major erectile event. Potential arterial and venous mechanisms are by no means mutually exclusive, however.

The many theories of the vascular mechanisms of erection have usually described shunting of blood through some mechanism away from or around the cavernous spaces in the flaccid state and closure of these shunts with diversion of blood into the cavernous spaces during erection. The basic theory is that of Conti, which postulates muscular ''polsters'' that are located in the arteries, A-V shunts, and veins that control the amount and distribution of blood flow. The actual existence of these structures has been questioned in recent years, and it may be that structures identified on anatomic studies and thought to represent muscular and connective tissue shunts are in reality early manifestations of atherosclerosis, occurring at branch points of vessels.

Although the exact mechanism is yet to be worked out, certainly blood is shunted into the corpora during erection. This process is under neurologic control. Two types of stimuli have been defined in eliciting erection: psychogenic and reflexogenic. A reflex nature implies that little voluntary control exists; just as one cannot always will or demand an erection, erection cannot willfully be suppressed at times. Stimuli defined as psychogenic include those of an auditory, visual, olfactory, gustatory, tactile, or imaginative nature. Reflexogenic stimuli include those of an exteroceptive nature associated with genital manipulation and afferent impulses traveling along fibers of the pudendal nerve. Often the two types of stimuli act synergistically in producing erection.

Thus neurogenic stimuli may increase arterial inflow through a combination of (1) intrinsic vasodilatation of the pudendal and penile arteries and arterioles, (2) opening of new pathways allowing a greater total cross-sectional area of the arterial vascular tree for runoff, and (3) decreasing intrinsic tone of cavernous tissue in which the arterial vessels run, resulting in increased tissue perfusion and decreased resistence to flow. Venous mechanisms may also be involved.

Neurally mediated erections may be reflexogenic, originating in the sacral spinal cord and mediated through the pudendal nerve (afferent) and the nervi erigentes (efferent), or psychogenic, originating in the cerebral cortex, and mediated through the sympathetic thoracolumbar and parasympathetic sacral tracts. Neurotransmitters involved may include vasoactive intestinal polypeptide, adrenergic, or cholinergic substances.

The role of male hormones in regard to erectile physiology and sexual behavior is unclear. Erectile function in males castrated before puberty is felt to be quite rare. The effects of postpubertal castration range from complete loss of libido and erectile ability to totally normal activity. Generally there is an overall decrease in sexual activity and ability following medical or surgical castration. After puberty, testosterone may well have more of an influence on libido than on erectile ability. The two may be hard to differentiate in the clinical setting.

The cerebral cortex plays a major role, as yet poorly understood, relative to erection. The limbic system, noted to be the oldest part of the brain phylogenetically, appears to contain most of the centers from which stimulation can elicit erection. These centers have a close physical relationship to areas associated with emotional functions, such as fear and rage, as well as with areas for olfaction and vision. Especially unknown are the pathways and centers that may be involved in inhibition of erection. Such centers may relate to psychogenic impotence, and the importance of delineating these is obvious.

B. Emission

Emission refers to the deposition of the glandular secretions from the prostrate and seminal vesicals and the contents of the distal vasa into the posterior urethra. Although emission and ejaculation are two reflex phenomena that are usually closely related temporally, occurring at the culmination of a sexually exciting situation, each has the potential in certain situations to be independent of the other, as well as independent of penile erection.

The exact nature of the afferent stimuli preceding emission is not clear, but, as for erection, exteroceptive stimuli from the genitalia as well as cerebral stimuli are probably involved. Cerebral control is such that emission may be halted voluntarily up to the sensation of ''inevitability'' which is due to filling and distension of the posterior urethra. Efferent neural control emanates from the T10 to L2 sympathetic outflow. Sympathectomy and α-adrenergic blockade can eliminate emission. Closure of the bladder neck occurs concomitant with emission and is also under sympathetic control.

C. Ejaculation

Ejaculation is a complex phenomenon involving rhythmic contractions of the pelvic floor musculature and compression of the urethra, such that, under normal conditions, the semen is expelled in an antegrade direction through the urethra and out the penile meatus. The afferent stimuli seems to be the passage of semen from the posterior urethra into the bulbous urethra. Little voluntary control probably exists at this point. Although the control center for ejaculation appears to be located at the T12 to L2 level, the outflow at the time of ejaculation also involves the sacral somatic nervous system. A coordinated neural output controls both smooth and striated muscles. The bladder neck remains tightly closed and external sphincter rhythmic relaxation allows semen to enter the bulbous urethra, where it is expelled by bulbocavernosus and ischiocavernosus muscle contraction.

D. Orgasm

Orgasm is a central nervous system phenomenon that relates genital experiences to whole-body physiology and is the goal of normal male sexual function. It can be described as an intense and profoundly satisfying cerebral sensation that represents the explosive discharge of accumulated neuromuscular tensions. Following orgasm, detumescence takes place and a refractory period ensues where the male is unable to achieve full erection or repeat orgasm. Detumescence may be a sympathetic event secondary to vasoconstriction.

III. SEXUAL DYSFUNCTION

A. Definitions

1. *Premature Ejaculation.* Cannot control ejaculation to satisfy partner 50% of the time. Generally this is a functional problem, a type of learned behavior, and it responds well to several techniques of behavioral therapy described in Masters and Johnson's books and several self-help books now available (see bibliography).

2. *Ejaculatory Incompetence.* Cannot ejaculate during intercourse. This form of dysfunction can be considered the opposite of premature ejaculation. It is relatively rare and usually psychogenic in nature.

3. *Primary Impotence.* Never able to maintain erection to achieve successful coitus. This always demands a full diagnostic evaluation to rule out an organic etiology.

4. *Secondary Impotence.* Previously potent, but subsequent failure to achieve successful coitus in at least 25% of coital opportunities.

5. *Libido Quantification.* This is very difficult, as what is adequate for one person or one couple may be inadequate for another. The frequency of intercourse varies. If a patient feels his libido is low, one may either attempt to increase it or modify expectations.

B. Problems in Evaluation

Until about 5 years ago it was generally felt that 80 to 90% of impotence was psychogenic and only 10% had an organic basis. It is now thought that up to half of all cases of secondary erectile impotence may have an organic cause, and that many patients with primarily psychogenic impotence may have a contributing organic disorder. Thus, urologists have assumed an increasingly important role and perhaps the primary role in the evaluation and treatment of sexual dysfunction. The goal of the urologist is to prevent unproductive, expensive psychotherapy for organic impotence, and prevent unnecessary prosthetic surgery or other invasive treatment modalities if psychologic help is possible. If in doubt, a conservative approach is certainly indicated.

G. F. Lydston, one of the early pioneers in the treatment of male sexual dysfunction, commented on the problems of evaluation and treatment of these disorders in 1908. ''The objection to operative measures based on a diagnosis of psychic impotence is absurd. The patient wants relief, not a psychic diagnosis. Scientific reasoning and psychopathic diagnoses fall to the ground before the absolute of a flaccid penis in a physiological emergency.''

C. Psychologic Factors

Normal sexual functioning requires a certain degree of self-confidence, absence of anxiety, presence of arousing mental and/or physical stimulation, and the ability to focus attention on sexual activity. A wide variety of psychologically based problems can interfere with these prerequisites, and determination of such an underlying problem is critical to successful treatment. A careful history and an appropriate selection of diagnostic tests to rule out a primary or concomitant organic problem are essential.

D. End-Organ Factors

Congenital problems include the extrophy/epispadius complex, microphallus, fusiform megalourethra, and severe penile chordee.

Peyronie's disease is characterized by the development of a fibrous plaque involving the tunica albuginea surrounding the erectile tissue of the corpora. The earliest pathologic finding is a vasculitis in the loose areolar tissue beneath the tunica. The etiology is unknown, although it has been associated with a more generalized fibrotic tendency. Patients have an increased incidence of Dupuytren's contractures and often display fibrous degeneration of the external ear cartilage. Most cases involve men in the 4th or 5th decade. Symptoms include the presence of a plaque or induration within the penis, penile curvature during erection, and painful intercourse. The natural history is variable and some patients improve spontaneously. Medical treatment has included steroids (orally or by injection into the plaque), vitamin E, paraaminobenzoate, and local dimethyl sulfoxide. Surgical options, generally resorted to after a year or so of watchful waiting, include excision of the plaque with placement of a graft, excision of a diamond-shaped portion of tunica opposite the plaque to foreshorten but straighten the penis, or placement of a penile prosthesis.

Priapism is the pathologic prolongation of a penile erection most often associated with pain but not with sexual excitement or desire. It may be idiopathic or secondary to a variety of processes including sickle-cell disease, trauma, leukemia, and medications. Overall, priapism is associated with a 50% rate of impotence secondary to corporal scarring regardless of the modality of treatment.

Finally, prostatitis and seminal vesiculitis can cause pain on arousal or ejaculation, and constitute end-organ causes of sexual dysfunction.

E. Vascular Disease

Arteriosclerosis, aortic aneurysm, trauma (pelvic fracture), and decreased cardiac output can all decrease the amount of blood flow available for erectile function and result in impotence.

F. Neurologic Disease

Tumor, trauma, and any disease affecting the central nervous system, spinal cord, or peripheral nerves can interfere with sexual functioning. From 26 to 43% of patients with multiple sclerosis have erectile dysfunction. This is generally due to spinal cord involvement.

G. Surgical Procedures

Radical pelvic surgery, prostatic surgery, perineal surgery, and vascular surgery can cause erectile or emission and ejaculatory problems. The incidence of erectile problems after transurethral prostatectomy is about 6%.

H. Endocrine/Metabolic Disorders

Disorders in the hypothalamic–pituitary–gonadal axis commonly cause sexual dysfunction. Primary gonadal failure (hypergonadotropic hypogonadism) is the most

common endocrinologic cause of impotence. Both hypo-
thyroidism and hyperthyroidism may cause decreased potency. On initial screening a careful history, physical examination, and appropriate laboratory tests, including
serum gonadotropin, prolactin, and testosterone levels, as
well as genetic screening when indicated, are important to
avoid missing a treatable disorder. If the patient is capable
of collecting an ejaculate for semen analysis, and subsequent analysis reveals normal motility, morphology, and
sperm count, an endocrinologic defect is unlikely to be
present.

I. Diabetes

In diabetic men impotence is more common than either
retinopathy or nephropathy. Half of male diabetics (2 to
2.5 million men) complain of sexual dysfunction. Thirty
to fifty percent of all diabetic men aged 50 are impotent.
Impotence does not correlate with severity of disease or
adequacy of control. Libido is usually normal. When age
is accounted for, there appears to be a greater risk of
developing impotence with increasing duration of diabetes. A high association of vascular risk factors, a tendency toward atherosclerosis, and diabetic microangiopa-
thy all contribute to high impedance of blood flow in the
arterial bed of the penis. Peripheral neuropathy is not
uncommon in diabetics and up to 30% of impotent diabetics in the Boston University series were felt to have neurologic impotence. In addition to neuropathic and vascular
causes of impotence in diabetics, these patients are just as
prone as the general population to have psychologically
based sexual dysfunction, so that a full evaluation is in
order. Retrograde ejaculation and lack of emission have
also been associated with diabetic neuropathy.

J. Drug-Induced Effects

Any agent that pharmacologically alters the normal hormonal milieu, somatic and autonomic neurotransmission,
or vascular flow, may produce changes in sexual function.
These effects may be reflected in the state of the libido,
erectile ability, or ejaculatory capacity. Virtually every
antihypertensive drug currently in use has been associated

with impotence or ejaculatory dysfunction. The frequency varies dramatically between drugs, however. The diuretic class rarely demonstrates side effects of sexual dysfunction. The vasodilators such as hydralazine and minoxidil are relatively free of sexual side effects. The sympatholytic agents, which include methyldopa, clonidine, and reserpine, are the ones most often associated with sexual dysfunction. α-adrenergic blockers (phenoxybenzamine, phentolamine, and prazosin) adversely affect emission and ejaculation on a peripheral level. β-blockers (propranolol and metroprolol) are not infrequent offenders.

Psychotropic agents, anticholinergic drugs, and commonly abused substances, including alcohol, amphetamines, barbiturates, cocaine, marijuana, and narcotics, are all potentially detrimental to sexual function. It is incumbent upon the physician to review all of the drugs a patient with sexual dysfunction is taking, in order to prevent diagnostic or surgical procedures or unnecessary psychotherapy in cases where a change in medication alone might be all that is needed.

K. Other Factors

Uremia is associated with a series of metabolic derangements influencing reproductive and sexual functioning. Low circulating levels of testosterone, Leydig cell abnormalities, elevations in luteinizing hormone and follicle-stimulating hormone, an increase in prolactin levels, and secondary hyperparathyroidism may occur. Reduced erectile ability exists in 40 to 80% of dialysis patients, and up to half may be completely impotent.

Any severely debilitating condition may adversely affect sexual function.

IV. EVALUATION OF SEXUAL DYSFUNCTION

A. History

1. *Physiologic Changes.* A good history is often the most valuable part of the erectile dysfunction evaluation. One must have an understanding of the normal physiologic changes that occur. Sexual drive and perfor-

mance in the male probably peaks between the ages of 15 and 25. Following this, there is a progressive decrease in function. After the age of 50 there is generally a longer stimulation time required for erection, the preejaculation period is longer, ejaculation may be shorter with decreased volume and expulsion force, and the refractory period is increased.

2. *Psychologic Dysfunction.* Psychologic dysfunction often has an abrupt onset and a careful history will usually disclose the inciting factors. The patient will usually admit to erections in certain situations (masturbation, extramarital coitus, in the early morning, or when awakening from sleep). Performance anxiety, while often a secondary phenomenon in organic impotence, can be the primary problem in psychologic dysfunction.

3. *Organic Deterioration.* Characteristically there is a gradual deterioration noted with organic impotence. The following sequence of deterioration is typical: decreased hardness, decreased frequency, failure with fatigue, erection achieved and not maintained, success only in morning or after waking with erection from a dream, success only in very exciting circumstances, loss of nocturnal erections, loss of erection with masturbation, and complete loss of erectile function despite no loss of libido.

B. Physical Examination

Look for changes compatible with endocrine disease. Examine the penis and testes, prostate, and seminal vesicles. Conduct a thorough neurologic examination, including evaluation of anal sphincter tone and voluntary contraction, bulbocavernosus reflex, perineal and genital sensation. Vascular examination should include search for bruits, characterization of peripheral pulses, skin temperature, color, and hair distribution.

C. Laboratory Data, Hormonal Evaluation

The usual screening blood chemistries to look for diabetes and renal failure are helpful as well as a hormonal evaluation including testosterone, prolactin, and luteinizing hormone (LH). Hypogonadotropic hypogonadism is diagnosed by a low LH and low testosterone. Hypergonadotropic hypogonadism (primary testicular failure) is associated with a high LH and low testosterone. Hyperprolactinemia is usually associated with a low testosterone and a low LH. The sexual dysfunction is not alleviated by testosterone supplementation alone, and the hyperprolactinemia must be corrected. Prolactin reduces end-organ responsiveness to LH and reduces conversion of testosterone to dihydrotestosterone. Prolactin secretion is inhibited by dopamine. Thus, drugs that affect prolactin and dopamine may affect sexual function. Bromocriptine, a dopamine agonist, may correct impotence related to elevated prolactin levels associated with pituitary adenomas.

One may suspect a hormonal etiology for sexual dysfunction when the libido is low or the testes are small. Impotence may not be absolute in this group, and successful intercourse may occur occasionally.

D. Assessment of Penile Blood Flow

    1. *Doppler Studies.* The most simple and most common erectile function test to detect impaired hemodynamic blood flow parameters is the use of Doppler ultrasound techniques to record systolic occlusion pressure in the cavernosal arteries of the penis. A pediatric blood pressure cuff is placed around the base of the penis and is inflated above brachial systolic pressure. A Doppler ultrasound probe is used to detect the return of pulsation in the right and left cavernosal arteries as the cuff is slowly deflated. If the penile systolic pressure is less than 60% of the brachial systolic pressure, this is considered compatible with arterial vasculogenic impotence.

    2. *Cavernosography.* European researchers have demonstrated that infusion of saline at high flow rates into the corpora cavernosa will result in a penile erection. Intravenous catheters are used to cannulate both corporal bodies, which are then infused with warmed, heparinized saline at the flow rate necessary to achieve an erection. Contrast is then infused into the penis, and

if the dorsal vein is visualized and the flow rate required to maintain erection is high, the patient is considered to have venous insufficiency syndrome of the corporal bodies and may be a candidate for ligation of the dorsal vein of the penis. The dorsal vein should not be able to be visualized during erection in normal individuals.

3. *Angiography.* Internal pudendal arteriography is the most sensitive procedure for precise evaluation of the anatomy of the entire hypogastric-cavernous arterial bed. Arteriography is an expensive, invasive procedure associated with significant risks and should be used only in individuals willing to consider penile revascularization procedures.

E. **Assessment of Autonomic Pathways**

When the index of suspicion for a neurologic basis for sexual dysfunction is high, helpful corroboratory data can be obtained from neurologic testing. Cystometrography and bethanechol supersensitivity testing evaluate the pelvic parasympathetic nerves at the vesical parasympathetic plexus. At present there is no reliable test of the corporal parasympathetic plexus, and only inference as to its integrity can be made from testing of the more proximal vesical pathway.

Perineal electromyography and sacral reflex latency testing can evaluate the somatic pudendal nerve. The pudendal nerves (S2 to S4) supply sensation from the penile skin and provide motor innervation to the bulbocavernosus, ischiocavernosus, and external urethral sphincter muscles. The sensory aspect is important in erection and the motor aspect in ejaculation.

Examination of the suprasacral afferent pathways is possible through testing of the genitocerebral evoked response. The penis is stimulated and evoked potentials at various sites within the central nervous system are measured.

F. **Nocturnal Penile Tumescence**

Nocturnal penile tumescence (NPT) was first described in infants in 1940 and in adults by Ohlmeyer in 1944. NPT usually occurs in conjunction with rapid eye movement (REM) sleep. Nocturnal erections are not affected by recent sexual gratification nor is the dream content necessarily erotic in nature. Normally there are three to five erectile episodes per night, lasting 10 to 25 minutes each, and associated with expansion in penile circumference of 15 to 30 mm. Although there is some question as to the ultimate significance of NPT and the possibility that NPT may possibly be affected by psychologic influences, it is generally believed that the occurrence of normal NPT in an individual with erectile dysfunction logically suggests a psychogenic origin for the problem, as the basic physiologic mechanisms for erection would appear to be intact. A similar inference can be drawn from the ability of a patient to get good erections with masturbation or with partners other than the spouse.

It has been conclusively demonstrated that "morning erections" are not secondary to a full bladder but merely represent the last NPT episode of sleep. NPT is best monitored for one to three nights at home or in a formal sleep laboratory with the aid of loop strain gauges that are placed around the penis and connected to a transducer and monitor that can give a recording of tumescence at the base and tip throughout the night. It is important to note that tumescence and not rigidity is generally measured, and the advantage of formal sleep laboratory testing is that a technician can evaluate penile rigidity and awaken the patient to obtain his own interpretation of the suitability of the erection for vaginal penetration.

G. Visual Sexual Stimulation

Visual sexual stimulation is a technique of evaluating erectile function during erotic stimulation, and, as such, is an eminently logical diagnostic procedure. It was pioneered in Scandinavia. There is little in the literature at present. It would seem that a positive test would have diagnostic importance while a negative test might have minimal significance. Generally, patients are shown a variety of explicit sexual videotapes and erectile responses monitored over closed circuit television or with the aid of NPT equipment.

H. Psychologic Testing

The Beck Depression Inventory can be a valuable aid in making a diagnosis of clinically significant depression, a common cause of decreased libido and erectile dysfunction. The questionnaire can be administered in 15 minutes and is a useful screening aid. The Minnesota Multiphasic Personality Inventory is perhaps the best known of many psychologic examinations that the patient can self-administer. Abnormal results serve as a "red flag" and suggest the need for further psychologic evaluation. Patients with depression, grave marital difficulties, or abnormal personality inventories should probably be referred for psychiatric evaluation in addition to undergoing a complete urologic evaluation.

V. NONSURGICAL TREATMENT

A. Time

Many psychologically based sexual problems will disappear with simple reassurance by the physician and time. Few men have not experienced an episode of erectile failure at some point.

B. Psychotherapy/Sexual Counseling (Various Grades)

Psychotherapy can run the gamut from reassurance, education, and modified sexual therapy by the urologist to formal marriage counseling and sexual therapy by psychologists and trained specialists to the psychiatric treatment of depression and even psychoanalysis. Generally, performance anxiety is targeted and various desensitization techniques are employed. Sensate focus and noncoital techniques are taught so that the sexual experience is not merely looked upon as one where vaginal intromission is the ultimate endpoint. This tends to allay performance anxiety and improve sexual performance.

C. Hormonal and Pharmacologic Therapy

Hormonal supplementation with adjunctive testosterone is often helpful when the testosterone level is in the low normal range or below normal. The normal range of serum testosterone is quite large, and a short trial of testosterone injections is not an unreasonable approach. In our experience testosterone seems to have its major effect on libido rather than erectile function. It should be given by the intramuscular route as oral absorption is quite variable. Naturally, it is contraindicated in the patient with prostate cancer.

Yohimbine, an α-adrenergic antagonist, has been reported to have a beneficial effect on sexual functioning in humans. A study in male rats demonstrated increased mounting behavior, improvement in initial heterosexual encounter, and induction of copulatory behavior in sexually inactive rats. The data suggest a central effect rather than a predominantly peripheral one.

Isoxsuprine may improve erectile function via a peripheral stimulation of β-adrenergic receptors.

D. Pharmacologic Injection Program

Neurologic stimulation initiates penile erection by inducing hemodynamic alterations in the corporal erectile tissue. It has been proposed that released postganglionic neurotransmitter substances such as acetylcholine or vasoactive intestinal polypeptide may result in relaxation of the smooth muscle in corporal arterioles as well as relaxation of the smooth muscle surrounding corporal lacunae. Pharmacologic agents that result in vascular and nonvascular smooth muscle relaxation may mimic the action of physiologic neurotransmitter substances when injected into the corporal bodies. The net effect of increasing arterial blood inflow to the erectile tissue and decreasing drainage from the corporal lacunae is an accumulation of corporal blood volume and an increase in intracavernosal pressure. If the intracavernosal pressure exceeds 90 mm Hg, there is sufficient rigidity for vaginal penetration.

It is now possible for patients to self-administer a combination of papaverine and phentolamine by direct injection into the corpora to initiate erection for intercourse. This is a rational option for patients with neurologic impotence whose penile tissue and blood supply are normal. It may also be effective in patients with minimal vascular disease. Intracavernosal pharmacologic erection should prove to be a useful diagnostic tool as well, perhaps indicating the degree of vascular impairment as a component of erectile dysfunction. Patients with refractory psychogenic impotence may also be helped. Sensation, emission, ejaculation, and orgasm do not seem to be interfered with. Test dosing is employed to achieve an erection lasting 1 to 3 hours.

E. Neurostimulation

Eckhard described the innervation of the dog penis in 1869 and was the first to show that electrical stimulation of the nerves from the sacral roots produced erection in this animal model. Habib in 1967 produced erection with sacral root stimulation in man, an event subsequently reproduced on purpose and by accident (as a byproduct of attempts to produce bladder emptying) by many others. Electrical stimulation centrally can produce erection, and stimulation more peripheral to the pelvic plexus can do likewise. Several research projects are currently attempting to develop clinically applicable neurostimulation units to allow for erection in individuals with neurologic disease. Such equipment would also be useful diagnostically.

VI. SURGICAL TREATMENT

A. History

In 1668, de Graaf injected the hypogastric artery in cadavers and concluded that erection was caused by venous stasis induced by perineal muscle contraction. In 1889, Brown-Sequard injected extract of dog testes into himself and noted an increase in sexual performance and a decrease in constipation. In 1903, Ancel and Bouin described an increase in sexual activity in rabbits after ligation of the vas deferens. Lydston at the University of Illinois in 1908 reported 100 ligations of the dorsal vein of the penis. Half of the patients were cured of their sexual dysfunction. He believed that the operation caused transient enlargement of the penis from obstruction of venous outflow, which acted to increase the patient's self-confidence.

In 1918, Voronoff felt that youth could be renewed by grafting the interstitial cells of monkeys into man. That same year Lespinasse grafted slices of human cadavar testes into impotent recipients. In 1922, Stanley performed 1000 testicular substance implants on 656 patients at San Quentin. He used goats, rams, and deer and reported alleviation of impotence as well as acne, senility, and tuberculosis. In 1920, Steinach advocated bilateral vasectomy for sexual rejuvination. Three years later Macht and Teagarden reported the first controled study of vas ligation in rats and showed no improvement.

In 1935, Lowsley and Bray reported excellent results in 31 of 51 patients by ligating the dorsal vein of the penis and plicating the ischiocavernosis and bulbocavernosis muscles. In 1936, Borgoras used a rib implantation to simulate erection. In 1948, Bergman wrote that ribs curved in 18 months and eventually resorbed. The stage was set for modern prosthetic surgical techniques. All that was needed was the technology to develop a nonreactive substance that could be safely implanted.

B. Indications

Surgery is indicated in cases of organic impotence not amenable to treatment with nonsurgical techniques and in psychogenic impotence where conventional therapy has failed and the patient and psychotherapist concur.

C. Vascular Procedures

Patients with vascular impotence secondary to arterial occlusion amenable to bypass may be considered for vascular reconstruction. At the present time this seems to be most successful in young patients with vascular occlusion on a traumatic basis. Although numerous techniques have been described, anastomosis of the inferior epigastric artery to the internal pudendal, common penile, dorsal, or cavernosal artery has yielded the best results in this country.

D. Prosthetic Surgery

Penile prostheses currently available for implantation can be divided into two major categories: rigid and semirigid prostheses and inflatable prostheses (Figs. 1–3). The rigid

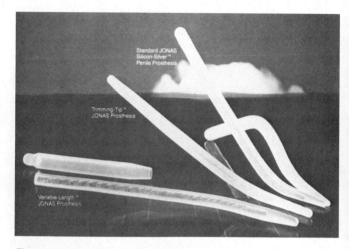

Figure 1. Jonas malleable prosthesis with silver wires within body of device to allow for stability in up and down position.

and semirigid devices are paired flexible or malleable rods composed of medical-grade silicone elastomer. When implanted they provide the patient with a permanent degree of penile rigidity suitable for vaginal penetration and sexual intercourse. The inflatable penile prosthesis is hydraulically operated. Original models are comprised of four parts: a reservoir placed in the abdomen extraperitoneally, a pump placed in the scrotum, and paired cylinders placed in the corporal bodies. Newer inflatable models are self-contained and consist only of the corporal cylinders. Inflatable devices provide for both an erect and flaccid state.

Patients must understand that to place any prosthesis, the normal erectile tissue must be hollowed out and destroyed. If the prosthesis must be removed for any reason, the patient will never be able to attain a normal erection. Because placement of a prosthesis is essentially "burning your bridges," it is a step not to be taken lightly. Nev-

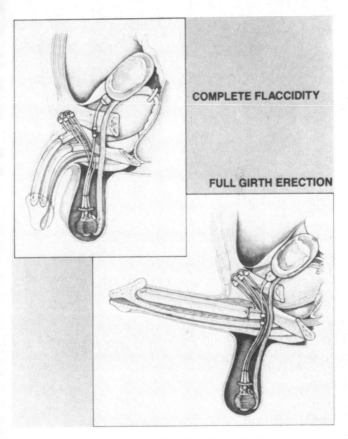

COMPLETE FLACCIDITY

FULL GIRTH ERECTION

Figure 2. Mentor inflatable penile prosthesis.

ertheless, when a patient suffers from organic impotence, it is often the best and/or only treatment alternative. A prosthesis does not affect sensation, emission, ejaculation, or orgasm. It enables vaginal penetration. Regardless of type of device, there is a 1% incidence of infection (5%

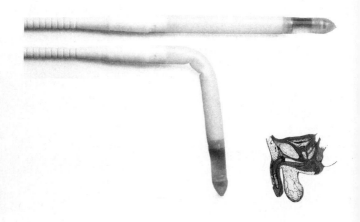

Figure 3. Flexiflate inflatable cylinders that are self-contained.

in diabetics) requiring removal of the foreign body for proper treatment. Often the prosthesis can be replaced at another time. There is a 1% incidence of discomfort severe enough to require removal. The mechanical malfunction rate of the inflatable variety is now somewhere around 3 to 5% in the 1st year.

VII. CONCLUSIONS

The advent of safe, reliable penile prosthetic devices has done more than anything in history to revolutionize the treatment of erectile dysfunction. New techniques in diagnosis and treatment are reported almost every year. The scientific study of impotence and its treatment is one of the most rapidly expanding frontiers of urology. At this point in time, almost any patient who presents with sexual dysfunction can be helped.

BIBLIOGRAPHY

Clark, JT, Smith ER, Davidson JM: Enhancement of sexual motivation in male rats by yohimbine. Science 225:847–849, 1984.

Hanno PM: Priapism. AUA Update Series, lesson 20, volume III, 1984.

Krane RJ, Siroky MB, Goldstein I (eds): Male Sexual Dysfunction. Boston: Little, Brown, 1983.

Masters WH, Johnson VE: Human Sexual Inadequacy. Boston: Little, Brown, 1970.

Morales A, Surridge DHC, Marshall PG, Fenemore J: Nonhormonal pharmacological treatment of organic impotence. J Urol 128:45–47, 1982.

Newman HF, Northup JD: Problems in male organic sexual physiology. Urology 21:443–450, 1983.

Van Arsdalen, KN, Wein AJ: Drugs and male sexual dysfunction. AUA Update Series, lesson 34, volume III, 1984.

Van Arsdalen KN, Wein AJ, Hanno PM, Malloy TR: Erectile failure following pelvic trauma: A review of pathophysiology, evaluation, and management, with particular reference to the penile prosthesis. J Trauma 24:579–585, 1984.

Wagner G, Green R: Impotence. New York: Plenum, 1981.

Wein AJ, Van Arsdalen KN, Hanno PM, Levin RM: Physiology of male sexual function. In Rajfer J (ed): Urologic Endocrinology. Philadelphia: W.B. Saunders, 1985.

Zilbergeld B: Male Sexuality. New York: Bantam, 1978.

Zorgniotti AW, Lefleur RS: Auto-injection of the corpus cavernosum with a vasoactive drug combination for vasculogenic impotence. J Urol 133:39–41, 1985.

18

Male Fertility and Infertility

Keith N. Van Arsdalen

I. INTRODUCTION

A. The Problem

1. Approximately 25% of couples will become pregnant after 1 month of trying to conceive. However, only 80% of couples will be pregnant by the end of 1 year.
2. Approximately 15 to 20% of couples will therefore have difficulty achieving pregnancy.
3. During the evaluation of the above couples, a male factor alone may be found in approximately 30% of couples and both a male and female factor in an additional 20% such that a male factor may be involved in the infertility problem in approximately one-half of the cases studied.
4. Unfortunately, the longer the period of infertility, the less likely is the chance of successful treatment and ultimately achieving pregnancy.

B. Chapter Plan—Topics to Be Considered Below

1. Reproductive Anatomy and Physiology
2. Evaluation of the Infertile Male
3. Classification of Male Infertility Problems
4. Treatment Modalities

II. REPRODUCTIVE ANATOMY AND PHYSIOLOGY

A. Gross Anatomy

1. The male reproductive system is well understood from a gross anatomic standpoint and includes the following

components: testes and seminiferous tubules, efferent ductules and rete testes, the epididymides, the vasa deferentia, the ejaculatory ducts, the seminal vesicles, the prostate, and the penis and urethra.

2. From the standpoint of infertility, it is important to consider these components as part of a larger system, i.e., the hypothalamic–pituitary–gonadal axis, and also it is important to look at the components histologically to better define and understand the physiology of the male system.

B. Reproductive Hormonal Axis (Fig. 1)

1. Components
   a. Extrahypothalamic central nervous system
   b. Hypothalamus
   c. Pituitary
   d. Testes
   e. Gonadal steroid sensitive end-organs
2. Functions
   a. Normal male sexual development
   b. Maintenance of secondary sexual characteristics
   c. Male sexual behavior
   d. Sperm production and maturation

C. Extrahypothalamic Central Nervous System

1. The extrahypothalamic central nervous system is responsible for a variety of stimulatory and inhibitory influences on fertility.
2. The pathways of olfaction and vision are well-defined in this regard for experimental animals but the pathways in man are unknown and the effects are less clear.
3. In particular, in man, the effects of stress of both a physical and/or emotional nature are probably mediated through this system, but again the mechanisms are unknown.

D. Hypothalamus—GnRH

1. The hypothalamus is the center of integration for neuronal and humoral messages. The anterior and ventromedial nuclei are most important with regard to male fertility.

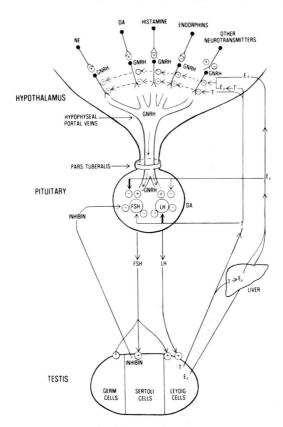

Figure 1. Feedback and stimulatory relationships within the hypothalamic pituitary–testicular axis. NE, norepinephrine; DA, dopamine; GnRH, gonadotropin-releasing hormone; T, testosterone; E$_2$, estradiol; LH, luteinizing hormone; FSH, follicle-stimulating hormone. *(From Vigersky RA: Pituitary–testicular axis. In Lipshultz LI, Howards SS (eds): Infertility in the Male. New York: Churchill Livingstone, 1983, chap 2, p. 20.)*

2. The hypothalamus is responsible for production of gonadotropin-releasing hormone (GnRH) as the primary releasing substance involved in male sexual function.

3. Multiple factors control GnRH secretion into the hypothalamo–hypophyseal portal system.

E. Pituitary—LH and FSH

1. The effect of GnRH is production and release of luteinizing hormone (LH) and follicle-stimulating hormone (FSH) from the pituitary.

2. Both LH and FSH are glycopeptides with two molecular chains. They share a common alpha chain and have their specificity determined by a unique beta chain.

3. LH and FSH are both secreted episodically. LH is rapidly metabolized, causing wide swings in its concentration within the bloodstream as determined by radioimmunoassay techniques. FSH is more slowly metabolized, resulting in a more constant level within the bloodstream.

4. The testes are the primary target organs for LH and FSH.

F. The Testes

1. Microscopic Anatomy—Two Main Elements
   a. Seminiferous tubules comprise the bulk of each testicle and are responsible for sperm production.
   b. The interstitium is the area between the seminiferous tubules and contains the blood vessels, the lymphatics, and the Leydig cells that are responsible for the production of testosterone.

2. Leydig Cells
   a. Leydig cells contain membrane receptors that bind LH, resulting in a reorientation of the cytoskeleton and increased enzyme activity.
   b. LH stimulation results in the conversion of cholesterol to testosterone.

3. Testosterone
   a. After production, testosterone diffuses into the plasma or into the lumen of the seminiferous tu-

bules. In the plasma it is bound to testosterone–estrogen-binding globulin. Within the seminiferous tubules, testosterone is bound to androgen-binding protein.

b. Depending upon the target tissue, testosterone may be active as testosterone alone or it may be reduced to dihydrotestosterone by the enzyme 5-α reductase.

c. Testosterone is responsible in part for sexual differentiation, maturation and behavior, spermatogenesis, and gonadotropin regulation.

4. Seminiferous Tubules—Sertoli Cells

a. The Sertoli cells contain membrane receptors that bind FSH, resulting again in a variety of enzyme changes within the cell and reorientation of the cytoskeleton for production of a variety of substances.

b. The primary secretory products from the Sertoli cells include Müllerian inhibiting factor in the fetus, androgen-binding protein, transferrin, and inhibin.

c. The Sertoli cells appear to be responsible for regulating the microenvironment within the seminiferous tubule. They are responsible for fluid secretion into the lumen, phagocytosis, steroid metabolism (in part), and regulation of sperm production and movement.

d. The Sertoli cells are also responsible for establishing the blood–testis barrier. This is a morphologic barrier created by the tight junctions between the Sertoli cells as well as a physiologic barrier that is maintained by active transport. The Sertoli cells further divide the developing germ cells into two compartments, i.e., a basal compartment for immature sperm-forming cells and a luminal compartment for the germ cells that are undergoing maturation. The importance of the blood–testis barrier in this regard is to provide an immunologically privileged site for the mature spermatozoa, as these mature cells have specific antigens that are not recognized as "self" by the body's immune system.

5. Seminiferous Tubules—Germ Cells
    a. LH, FSH, and testosterone all appear to be necessary for spermatogenesis to proceed normally.
    b. The Sertoli cells, as noted above, may ultimately be responsible for the regulation of this process.
    c. There are a variety of basic cell types that exist, including spermatogonia, the primary spermatocytes, secondary spermatocytes, spermatids, and spermatozoa. There are actually 13 subtypes that are recognized histologically. Spermatids and spermatozoa have a haploid complement of chromosomes.
    d. The process of spermatogenesis takes approximately 74 days for completion.
    e. Spermiogenesis is the process of maturation from a spermatid to a spermatozoan. The processes that occur here include condensation of the nuclear chromatin, formation of the acrosome, shedding of the residual material from the sperm, and formation of a tail.

G. Feedback Mechanisms (Fig. 1)
1. GnRH, LH, and FSH are generally felt to be responsible for driving the production of testosterone and spermatozoa as noted above. There are also feedback mechanisms, however, that regulate the production and release of these substances. This system works in a similar fashion to a thermostat and heater unit within one's home.
2. LH Regulation
    a. Testosterone and estradiol are the major negative feedback substances that control the formation and release of LH.
    b. Testosterone therefore regulates its own production and release by acting on the pituitary and the hypothalamus.
    c. Estradiol is produced within the testicle and also converted within the liver from testosterone. It oc-

curs in lesser amounts within the bloodstream but is more potent in action. The site of regulation is also at the level of the pituitary and the hypothalamus.

3. FSH Regulation
   a. Testosterone and estradiol are also important as noted above.
   b. In man there also appears to be an additional substance produced within the seminiferous tubules that regulates FSH production and release. This substance has been termed inhibin and recent evidence suggests that it is produced by the Sertoli cells.
4. There also appears to be a variety of "short feedback loops" and a variety of other modulating substances that may act to more finely tune this system.

H. Testicular Transport

1. As noted above, movement from the basement membrane to the lumen and release into the lumen of the seminiferous tubules appears to be controlled by Sertoli cells.
2. The movement of the spermatozoa from the testis to the epididymis is controlled by four factors:
   a. Fluid pressure generated within the seminiferous tubule.
   b. Myoepithelial contractions of the seminiferous tubules.
   c. Contraction of the tunica albuginea of the testis.
   d. Cilia within and contraction of the wall of the efferent ductules.
3. The spermatozoa enter the epididymis in an immature state.

I. Epididymal Functions

1. Transport and Storage
   a. The spermatozoa traverse the length of the epididymis in approximately 12 days. This process is governed by regular slow contractions of the muscular wall in a fashion similar to intestinal peristalsis.

    b. Approximately 700 million sperm are stored within the epididymides and the vasa deferentia. Approximately 60% of these are stored within the tails of the epididymides.

    c. At the time of emission and ejaculation, regular coordinated contractions of the tails of the epididymides and the vasa deferentia occur as mediated by the sympathetic nervous system propelling sperm into the urethra.

2. Sperm Maturation

    a. The chemical composition of the intraluminal fluid and of the spermatozoa changes significantly as one traverses the three anatomic portions of the epididymis.

    b. A variety of membrane changes with regard to permeability and antigenicity also occur.

    c. Motility and fertilizing capacity are gained during the trip through the epididymis.

    d. The final process of maturation, referred to as sperm capacitation, actually takes place after the sperm have been ejaculated and come in contact with the female reproductive tract. Fertilizing capacity lasts approximately 48 hours within the female internal genitalia.

J. Semen Composition

1. The bulk of the fluid appears to be from the accessory ducts, with the spermatozoa adding a negligible amount to the total volume.

2. Prostatic Fluid

    a. The prostatic fluid is usually found in the first part of the ejaculate and contributes approximately one-third of the total volume.

    b. The products specifically from the prostate include liquefaction factors (seminin), zinc, citric acid, acid phosphatase, and spermine. The latter substance when oxidized to aldahydes produces the characteristic odor of semen.

3. Seminal Vesicle Fluid

    a. The seminal vesicle fluid is usually found in the second part of the ejaculate and contributes approximately two-thirds of the total volume.

b. The specific substances added by the seminal vesicles include coagulation factors, prostaglandins, and fructose.

III. EVALUATION OF THE SUBFERTILE MALE

A. Fertility History

1. Present Marital History
   a. Duration
   b. Contraceptive methods and length of time used
   c. Length of time trying to conceive
   d. Number of pregnancies including miscarriages and therapeutic abortions—this gives some idea of possible ability to conceive

2. Previous Marital History and Relationships
   a. Patient—duration and number of pregnancies if attempted to conceive.
   b. Wife/partner—duration and number of pregnancies if attempted to conceive.
   c. Previous marriages and divorces are common. Potential fertility problems may be suspected if one partner had previously attempted to conceive without success. However, one must remember that the ability to conceive is a phenomenon involving both partners and therefore is determined by the current couple.

3. Sexual History
   a. Frequency of intercourse and masturbation. Overly frequent (daily) or too infrequent ejaculation (particularly around the time of ovulation) may adversely affect the couple's ability to conceive.
   b. Libido, potency, and sexual technique. One must determine if the desire and ability to have intercourse are adequate.
   c. Ejaculation. One must be certain that ejaculation can occur deep within the vagina. Severe problems with premature ejaculation may preclude proper deposition of sperm.
   d. Dyspareunia and use of lubrication. Difficulty with adequate natural vaginal lubrication may result in painful intercourse for either partner. Often ac-

cessory lubricants are used that are commonly spermicidal.

   e. Understanding of the ovulatory cycle. It is important that the couple understand when ovulation occurs and what this means regarding timing of intercourse.

4. Genitourinary History

   a. Testicular descent. Unilateral or bilateral cryptorchidism may both be associated with decreased spermatogenesis. With unilateral maldescent, even the contralateral, normally descended testical may not have normal sperm production.

   b. Sexual development and onset of puberty

   c. Infectious problems. Venereal, nonvenereal, mumps (at the time of puberty or later), recent febrile illness, or other infectious problems that directly involve the genitalia or the duct system may be associated with a significant amount of scarring and subsequent fertility problems. Viral infections and other febrile illnesses not specifically involving the genitalia may also be related to decreased spermatogenesis and lowered sperm counts. This may be noted for a period of 3 months or longer following one of these episodes.

   d. Trauma or torsion. Each may injure the duct system or result in ischemic damage to the seminiferous tubules.

   e. Exposure to chemicals. A variety of drugs and some recently discovered industrial compounds may be associated with abnormal semen analyses.

   f. Exposure to heat. Prolonged exposure to high temperatures may adversely affect spermatogenesis. It is presumed that hot tub baths, saunas, or steam rooms on a regular basis for long periods of time may have significance in this regard although this is by no means proven at the present time.

   g. Exposure to radiation. Ionizing radiation, particularly that used for radiation therapy, may destroy sperm-forming cells; the spermatogonia are particularly radiosensitive.

5. Previous Infertility Evaluation
   a. Patient. A history of previous semen analyses and medical or surgical treatment is certainly important with regard to determining prognosis and additional therapeutic modalities that may be instituted.
   b. Wife/partner. It is always wise to have some idea what type of fertility evaluation the patient's partner has undergone in the past or is undergoing at the present time. Obviously, conception is a phenomenon that involves two people and if for some physiologic or anatomic reason, an irreversible problem exists in one of the partners, a successful outcome is not likely. There is no reason that the evaluation of each partner cannot be carried out simultaneously although the evaluation of the male should be completed with regard to history, physical examination, and semen analyses prior to any of the invasive procedures required for a complete evaluation of the female partner.

B. **General Medical History**
   1. Medical Illnesses
      a. A variety of medical problems such as diabetes and hypertension or the treatment of these disorders with a variety of drugs may adversely affect erectile and ejaculatory function and subsequently fertility.
      b. Other problems such as liver disease and renal failure are also adversely associated with sexual function but may also result in abnormal metabolism and excretion of the sex steroids, hence interfering with the regulatory mechanisms involved with spermatogenesis.
   2. Surgical History
      a. Inguinal herniorrhaphy, particularly when performed on a young child and when performed bilaterally, may be associated with injury to the vas deferens in a significant number of patients.
      b. Surgery on the ureter, bladder, bladder neck, or urethra may result in problems with emission and/or ejaculation.

    c. Retroperitoneal surgery and other major pelvic procedures may also result in failure of emission and/or problems with retrograde ejaculation. Young males with testicular cancer are now being cured with a great deal of success. Many with non-seminomatous tumors are treated with retroperitoneal lymphadenectomy and subsequently have fertility problems due to absent ejaculation from either failure of emission or retrograde ejaculation.

3. Current and Past Medications
   a. A variety of drugs and chemotherapeutic agents may adversely affect sperm production and/or sperm function. The adverse affects are often reversible upon discontinuing the medication.
   b. These medications are listed in Table 1.
4. Occupation and Habits
   a. Occupation and stress. The effects of stress as encountered daily in our society is poorly quantitated with regard to fertility. Most patients, however, ask about this but it is extremely unlikely that they would change their job or style of living and therefore the effects of stress may in fact be a moot point.
   b. The active ingredients in cigarettes, marijuana, coffee, tea, and alcohol have all been demonstrated

TABLE 1. DRUGS AND CHEMICALS WITH POTENTIAL ADVERSE FERTILITY EFFECTS

Alcohol	MAO inhibitors
Alkylating agents (Ex: Cyclophosphamide)	Marijuana
Arsenic	Medoxyprogesterone
Aspirin (large doses)	Nicotine
Caffeine	Nitrofurantoins
Cimetidine	Phenytoin
Colchicine	Spironolactone
Dibromochloropropane (pesticide)	Sulfasalazine
Diethylstilbestrol (DES)	Testosterone
Lead	

in laboratory studies to be potentially gonadotoxic. The susceptibility of a given patient to these substances is difficult to quantitate.

5. Family History

a. The fertility status of the patient's siblings may be of interest in identifying familial problems.

b. In utero exposure to DES may result in testicular, epididymal, and penile abnormalities, as well as abnormal semen analyses.

C. Physical Examination

1. *General Examination*. This aspect of the physical examination looks at the patient's body habitus and secondary sexual characteristics. In particular, one looks at the pattern of hair distribution and observes for the presence or absence of gynecomastia. Evidence of general endocrine disorders may also be noted on this aspect of the physical examination.

2. Examination of the Genitalia

a. The examination of the genitalia is the most important aspect of the physical examination with regard to a male fertility evaluation. This should be performed in a systematic fashion, taking care to attempt to palpate and observe all the areas listed below.

b. Penis. The size of the penis and the location of the meatus are important in assuring delivery of spermatozoa deep within the vagina at the time of ejaculation.

c. Testes. The location, size, and consistency of the testes should be noted. The testes should be located within the scrotum in a dependent position. Testicular size is particularly important in that the bulk of the testicle is composed of seminiferous tubules that are involved in sperm production. The size of the testes can be compared to each other as well as to normal values by measuring the length and width of the testicle or by attempting to quantitate the volume by comparing the patient's testicles to plastic models of known volumes. The normal testicle in the adult should be greater than 4 cm in length and greater than 2.5 cm in width. Each testicle should be of a firm consistency.

d. Epididymides. The epididymides should be examined for size and consistency. The obstructed epididymis feels enlarged and soft. The epididymis that is scarred from either trauma or infection may be hard and irregular. Part of the epididymis may be missing in association with congenital absence of the vasa deferentia.

e. The vasa deferentia. Each vas deferens is clearly palpable as a distinct firm, cord-like structure in the scrotum.

f. The spermatic cords. Each spermatic cord should be compared for size and consistency. In this regard, the patient should be examined in the standing and supine positions and should be asked to perform the Valsalva maneuver while standing. This will accentuate differences in blood volume contained within the cord in patients with varicoceles. The internal spermatic veins and the veins of the pampiniform plexus fill while standing, and this filling may be increased while the Valsalva maneuver is performed. In the supine position, these veins drain more easily and hence the varicocele is not palpable. Other abnormalities involving the spermatic cord including hydroceles and/or spermatoceles may be detected during this part of the examination.

g. The inguinal region. The inguinal canals may be palpated following examination of the spermatic cord looking for evidence of inguinal hernias. In addition, the inguinal regions should be inspected to determine if previous surgery performed in this area may have injured the vasa deferentia or testicular blood supply.

h. Rectal examination. A general rectal examination should be performed, taking care not to miss any lower gastrointestinal pathology. The rectal examination is useful from a fertility standpoint to examine the prostate and the seminal vesicles. The prostate should be small, firm, and benign in consistency without tenderness or evidence of inflammation. The seminal vesicles are generally not palpable under normal conditions but may be palpable with obstruction of the ejaculatory ducts.

D. Semen Analyses

1. *Collection.* Generally at least two semen analyses are needed to establish a baseline for any given patient. If a discrepancy exists between the results of the two studies, then a third or perhaps even a fourth specimen may be required. An interval of at least 1 week is recommended between the semen analyses and each is collected with a 2- to 3-day period of abstinence. The specimen is generally collected by masturbation into a clean, dry, glass container and then is examined within 2 hours. If the specimen is collected at the patient's home, great care must be taken to keep it near body temperature during transportion to the laboratory.

2. *Minimal Standards of Adequacy.* It is generally agreed upon by workers in the field that the values noted in Table 2 represent the minimal standards of adequacy for a semen analysis.

TABLE 2. SEMEN ANALYSIS: MINIMAL STANDARDS OF ADEQUACY

On at least two occasions:	
Ejaculate volume	1.5–5.0 ml
Sperm density	>20 million/ml
Motility	>60%
Forward progression	>2 (scale 1–4)
Morphology	>60% normal
And:	
No significant sperm agglutination	
No significant pyospermia	
No hyperviscosity	

(From Lipshultz LI, Howards SS: Evaluation of the subfertile man. In Lipshultz LI, Howards SS (eds): Infertility in the Male. New York: Churchill Livingstone, 1983, chap 9, p. 191.)

3. *Additional Physical Parameters.* A variety of other properties are generally examined during the time of a routine semen analysis. These include the following:
   a. Color. The semen is generally grayish white in color with an opalescent character.
   b. Coagulation. This occurs almost immediately after ejaculation.
   c. Liquefaction. This occurs 5 to 25 minutes following ejaculation.
   d. Viscosity. This parameter refers to the fluid state of the semen after coagulation and liquefaction have taken place. The viscosity of the semen at this time is normal if it is possible to pour the semen in a drop by drop fashion.
   e. pH. pH is normally in the range of 7.4 to 7.6.
   f. Fructose. As noted above, fructose is specifically produced by the seminal vesicles. It is important to check the semen for fructose in cases of azoospermia and when the ejaculate volume is less than 1 ml. Absence of fructose in the semen suggests absence of the vasa deferentia and seminal vesicles, ejaculatory duct obstruction, or dysfunction of the seminal vesicles.

E. **Other Laboratory Tests**
   1. *Urinalysis.* This test is useful to rule out infection of the lower genitourinary tract and associated glandular structures, particularly the prostate.
   2. *Endocrine Evaluation.* Serum LH, FSH, and testosterone levels are checked as a routine in our laboratory. In combination, these tests will detect and differentiate hypogonadism due to either hypothalamic/pituitary failure or testicular failure. It can be argued that initially only an FSH level is necessary and if this is abnormal, then LH and testosterone can be checked.
   3. It is important to also be aware of other tests regularly recommended in the past that now appear to be unnecessary on a routine basis. These include tests of thyroid and adrenal function, prolactin levels, and buccal

smears or karyotypes. These tests can be saved for specific indications.

4. Tests of Sperm Function
    a. Mucus penetration test. This is a test of sperm function that determines how the spermatozoa move through a standard mucus median. Variations of this also exist where cross-penetration assays are established that compare the patient's sperm and his partner's cervical mucus to donor sperm and donor cervical mucus.
    b. Hamster egg penetration test. This is a cross-species assay that assesses the ability of human spermatozoa to penetrate zona-free hamster eggs. This is primarily an experimental tool at this time; its clinical usefulness is now being determined.

IV. CLASSIFICATION OF ABNORMALITIES

A. General Information

1. A variety of classification schemes have been developed in an attempt to categorize fertility problems. One of the most useful schemes is based upon the findings on semen analyses with initial classification of the problem into one of four categories: all parameters normal; azoospermia; a single abnormal parameter; and multiple abnormal parameters. This classification is discussed below, particularly with reference to the algorithm on the accompanying pages. This scheme was originally proposed and subsequently refined by Dr. Larry Lipshultz (Fig. 2).

2. *Distribution of Semen Abnormalities.* Based upon an earlier study at the Hospital of the University of Pennsylvania, the abnormal semen analyses were distributed such that azoospermia was found in 8% of the cases, a single abnormal parameter was found in 37% of the cases, and all parameters were abnormal in 55% of the cases. Among the single abnormal parameters, isolated abnormalities with motility accounted for the majority of these cases.

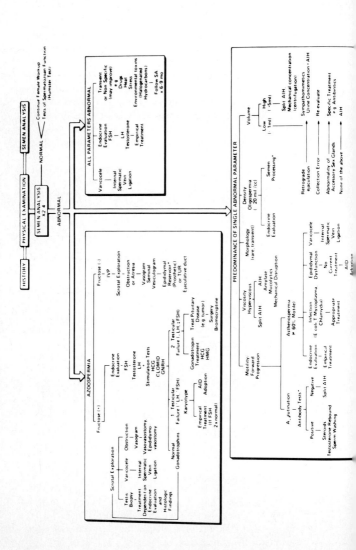

HISTORY → PHYSICAL EXAMINATION → SEMEN ANALYSIS

SEMEN ANALYSIS X 4

NORMAL → Continue Female Work-up
Tests of Spermatozoan Function
(Hamster Test)

ABNORMAL

ALL PARAMETERS ABNORMAL

Varicocele
Internal Spermatic Vein Ligation

Endocrine Evaluation
FSH
LH
Testosterone
Empirical Treatment

Transient or Non Specific (may improve)
e g
Drug
Heat
Stress
Environmental toxins (Halogenated Hydrocarbons)
Follow SA x 6-9 mo

AZOOSPERMIA

Fructose (-)

Scrotal Exploration

Testis Biopsy
Varicocele
Internal Spermatic Vein Ligation

Treatment
Dependent on Endocrine Evaluation and Histologic Findings

Obstruction
Vasogram
Vasovasostomy
Epididymovasostomy

Normal Gonadotrophins

1 Testicular Failure (LH ; FSH)
Karyotype
Empirical Treatment (if FSH 2 x normal)

2 Testicular Failure (LH ; FSH)
Gonadotropin Treatment
HCG
HMG

AID
Adoption

Fructose (+)
IVP
Scrotal Exploration

Obstruction or Atresia
Vasogram
Seminal Vesiculogram

Epididymal Reservoir*
(Prosthetic)

Ejaculative duct

Endocrine Evaluation
FSH
Testosterone
LH
Stimulation Tests
HCG
CLOMID
GNRH

Treat Pituitary Disease (e g tumor)
Surgery
Bromocriptine

PREDOMINANCE OF SINGLE ABNORMAL PARAMETER

Motility Forward Progression

A_zoination

Antibody Tests*

Positive

Steroids
Testosterone Rebound
Sperm Washing

Negative

Split AIH

Endocrine Evaluation

Empirical Treatment

Viscosity Hyperviscous

Split AIH

AIH
Amylase
Mucolytics
Mechanical Disruption

Asthenospermia (> 60% Motile)

Infection (E. coli, T Mycoplasma, Chlamydia)

Appropriate Treatment

AID
Adoption

Morphology (rare transient)

Endocrine Evaluation

Epididymal Dysfunction

No Current Treatment

Density Oligospermia (20 mil /cc)

Varicocele
Internal Spermatic Vein Ligation

Volume

Low (1ml)

Retrograde ejaculation
Collection Error
Abnormality of Accessory Sex Glands
None of the above

Semen Processing*

High (5ml)

Split AIH
Mechanical concentration (centrifugation)

Sympathomimetics
Urine Concentration + AIH
Re-evaluate
Specific Treatment e g Antibiotics
AIH

450

B. All Parameters Normal

1. When two semen analyses are normal and the history and physical examination is not suggestive of a fertility problem in the male, further evaluation of the female partner is then recommended.

2. If the evaluation of the female partner is also found to be normal, and the couple still has not conceived, then the tests of sperm function noted above, i.e., the mucus·penetration and hamster egg penetration tests, may be useful particularly with regard to prognosis.

C. Azoospermia (Fig. 3)

1. The results of the fructose test and the levels of gonadotropins determine what additional evaluation and treatment is necessary.

   a. The LH, FSH, and testosterone levels can differentiate primary testicular failure versus secondary testicular failure from either pituitary or hypothalamic dysfunction.

   b. If the FSH level is greater than two times normal, this is essentially equivalent to a "medical biopsy" and obviates the need for a surgical biopsy. A level this high generally indicates irreversible testicular damage.

2. After ruling out a major endocrine abnormality, a major differential diagnosis is ductal obstruction versus testicular failure.

   a. Fructose test negative. Three possibilities exist in the azoospermic patient with normal hormone studies and a negative fructose test. These include congenital bilateral absence of the seminal vesicles and vasa deferentia, bilateral ejaculatory duct obstruction, and a rare type of retrograde ejaculation with scant initial antegrade ejaculation of semen containing no sperm or fructose.

Figure 2. Composite algorithm of all possible steps needed to evaluate any abnormal patterns defined by the semen analysis. *(From Lipshultz LI, Howards SS: Evaluation of the subfertile man. In Lipshultz LI, Howards SS (eds): Infertility in the Male. New York: Churchill Livingstone, 1983, chap 9, p. 194.)*

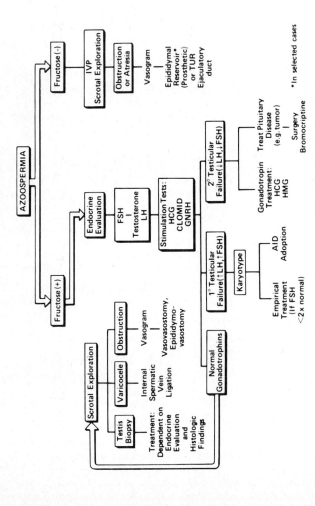

Figure 3. Algorithm for the azoospermic patient. *(From Lipshultz LI, Howards SS: Evaluation of the subfertile man. In Lipshultz LI, Howards SS (eds): Infertility in the Male. New York: Churchill Livingstone, 1983, chap 9, p. 195.)*

    b. Fructose test positive. A positive fructose test rules out obstruction of the ejaculatory duct and severe dysfunction of the seminal vesicles but it does not give any indication of the patency of the ductal system from the level of the rete testis through the vas deferens to the level of the ejaculatory duct itself. Therefore, if the fructose test is positive in the patient with azoospermia, it does not differentiate ductal obstruction from testicular failure.

    c. Testicular biopsy. A testicular biopsy is necessary in the azoospermic patient who is fructose positive. The microscopic examination of the testicular biopsy will indicate whether spermatogenesis is progressing normally, indicating ductal obstruction beyond the testis, or whether spermatogenesis is abnormal or arrested, suggesting that the azoospermia is secondary to a primary testicular defect.

    d. If the testicular biopsy indicates the presence of spermatogenesis and spermiogenesis, then a scrotal exploration and vasography is subsequently indicated. A vasogram is performed by injecting contrast material through one vas deferens to determine its patency. If patency is demonstrated, then exploration of the epididymis is required to determine the site of obstruction. A microscopic vasoepididymostomy is necessary to correct an intraepididymal obstruction. If no spermatozoa are detected in the tubules of the epididymis, then intratesticular ductal obstruction is presumed to be the cause for the azoospermia.

D. Isolated Abnormal Parameter on Semen Analysis (Fig. 4)

1. Decreased Motility and Forward Progression

    a. This is the most common isolated abnormality that may be found within this category. The sperm may function poorly on an individual basis and this slow movement has been referred to as asthenospermia. This may be secondary to endocrine dysfunction, infection of the accessory ducts, the

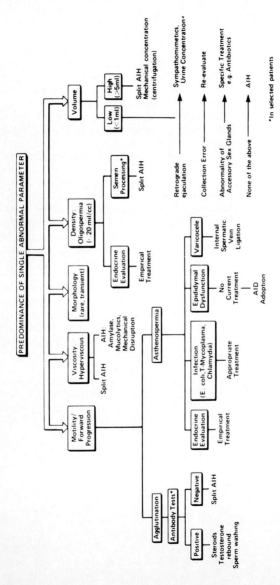

Figure 4. Algorithm for evaluating subfertile patients demonstrating the predominance of a single, isolated abnormal parameter in the seminal fluid. (*From Lipshultz LI, Howard SS: Evaluation of the subfertile man. In Lipshultz LI, Howards SS (eds): Infertility in the Male. New York: Churchill Livingstone, 1983, chap 9, p. 199.*)

presence of a varicocele, or epididymal dysfunction. Specific therapy is available for the first three problems noted. Unfortunately, epididymal dysfunction at the present time is poorly understood and essentially represents an untreatable diagnosis of exclusion at this time.

b. Sperm motility and forward progression may also be adversely affected by the presence of antisperm antibodies that result in agglutination, i.e., clumping or immobilization of the spermatozoa. Special tests are now available to determine the presence and levels of antisperm antibodies in both the semen and the blood. A variety of therapeutic modalities have been tried to remedy this situation. The most popular method now in use is short-term immunosuppression with steroids.

2. *Oligospermia.* Decreased sperm numbers as an isolated problem may be secondary to endocrine dysfunction or idiopathic in nature. Occasionally the absolute number of sperm is relatively normal but the number of sperm per milliliter may appear to be low due to the presence of a large ejaculatory volume.

Treatment of low sperm counts may be pursued in two directions. One may attempt to stimulate the testes with a variety of drugs in an attempt to increase the output of spermatozoa (see later section on idiopathic infertility). One may also attempt to utilize the spermatozoa that are present by concentrating them by mechanical means into a smaller volume and using these concentrated spermatozoa for artificial insemination. A variety of techniques are available for intracervical and intrauterine insemination. In addition, experimental studies are now underway that utilize in vitro fertilization techniques to deal with this problem.

3. *Abnormal Morphology.* An isolated problem with morphology is very unusual. Fortunately, when this is found, it may be a transient abnormality that is self-correcting in many cases, as there is no other known method of treatment.

4. Abnormal Semen Volume
   a. Large ejaculate volume. A volume greater than 5 ml may result in dilution of the spermatozoa and possibly even apparent oligospermia. Use of the split ejaculate or mechanical concentration of the spermatozoa with artificial insemination was noted above.
   b. Decreased ejaculatory volume. One should always check with the patient in cases of a low ejaculatory volume to be certain that all of the specimen was collected in the container. Once a collection abnormality has been ruled out, it is essential to be certain that the patient does not have retrograde ejaculation, infection of the accessory sex glands, or endocrine dysfunction. The presence of retrograde ejaculation can be confirmed by the finding of large quantities of spermatozoa in the postejaculatory urine sample. Sympathomimetic drugs with α-adrenergic activity may be useful in reversing this problem in some patients. In others, it may be necessary to obtain, wash, and inseminate sperm that are collected in the post ejaculatory urine sample. Endocrine abnormalities and infections may be treated with the appropriate hormones and antibiotics.
5. *Hyperviscosity*. Problems with hyperviscous semen may occasionally be encountered. A check of the split ejaculate may be useful, as the first portion may be less viscous than the second portion and therefore may be used for artificial insemination. Mechanical disruption of the sample as well as the use of amylase vaginal suppositories have been described.

E. **Multiple Parameters Abnormal on the Semen Analysis (Fig. 5)**
1. Diffuse abnormalities of all or many of the seminal parameters is the most common pathologic pattern identified. Once again, determination of the LH, FSH,

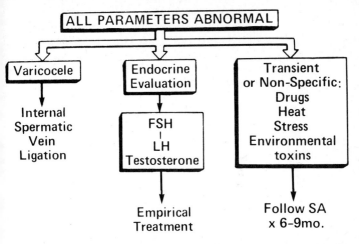

Figure 5. Algorithm for evaluating patient with impairment of all parameters of semen quality. *(From Lipshultz LI, Howards SS: Evaluation of the subfertile man. In Lipshultz LI, Howards SS (eds): Infertility in the Male. New York: Churchill Livingstone, 1983, chap 9, p. 198.)*

and testosterone levels are essential to rule out an endocrine abnormality.

2. One must also keep in mind, particularly when evaluating the male for the first time, that stress, infections, and other nonspecific environmental factors such as heat, drugs, and toxins to which the patient was exposed in the previous months may produce a transient abnormality of all seminal parameters. Therefore, when other specific factors cannot be identified by the history or physical examination, it is often wise to follow these patients for an additional 6 to 12 months to determine if the abnormalities will correct themselves. If after this period of time spontaneous correction has not occurred, nonspecific therapy can be instituted as discussed below.

3. Varicocele(s)

   a. A varicocele is simply a dilated, varicose internal spermatic vein producing fullness, dilatation, and poor drainage of the pampiniform plexus. A varicocele may be found in 10 to 20% of males in the general population but is often found in 35 to 40% of men presenting with infertility problems. Historically, the repair of varicoceles was based on case reports of oligospermic and azoospermic males who became normospermic and whose wives became pregnant following varicocele ligations.

   b. Varicoceles are classified according to size as either large, medium, or small. Large varicoceles can be seen as a "bag of worms" beneath the scrotal skin. Medium varicoceles are not evident to inspection but are readily detected by palpation. Small varicoceles can only be identified by noticing an impulse in the scrotum with the Valsalva maneuver or by noticing a difference in the size and fullness of the spermatic cord when the patient moves from the standing to the supine position. It has been stated that 78% of varicoceles occur on the left only, 2% occur on the right only, and 20% are bilateral.

   c. The exact mechanism through which the varicocele exerts its detrimental effect is not completely clear; the leading theory is that increased intrascrotal temperature occurs, producing abnormal spermatogenesis and spermiogenesis. An increased number of immature and tapered forms are noted to be associated with decreased sperm motility and varying degrees of oligospermia.

   d. Treatment of a varicocele involves one of two surgical approaches or transvenous angiographic identification and embolization of the involved internal spermatic veins. The standard approach to treatment has been either an inguinal or a retroperitoneal approach to the internal spermatic veins with ligation of the dilated venous structures. Newer interventional angiographic techniques and catheters have made it possible to selectively catheterize the internal spermatic veins and introduce a variety of substances, including sclerosing solutions, balloons, and stainless-steel coils that occlude these veins from the inside.

e. The results of varicocele ligation from a large number of series indicates approximately a 70% improvement in semen quality associated with a 40% pregnancy rate. With counts greater than 10 million sperm per milliliter, the improvement and pregnancy rates are significantly better than if the initial counts are less than 10 million sperm per milliliter. Both the surgical and the angiographic techniques for occlusion of the varicoceles have a 5 to 10% failure rate with persistence and/or recurrence of the varicocele noted during the course of follow-up. Pregnancies when they occur, generally are noted 6 to 9 months postvaricocelectomy.

F. Empirical Treatment of Idiopathic Infertility

1. Second only to the large number of patients who are found to have varicoceles, those with idiopathic infertility account for the next largest group of patients. In fact, the nonresponders to varicocele ligation probably also belong in this category. Essentially idiopathic infertility refers to the group of men who have an abnormal parameter or parameters on the semen analysis, with an essentially normal history, physical examination, and screening hormone analysis. The etiology of the abnormal semen quality is unclear and probably only reflects our incomplete knowledge with regard to normal fertility and associated fertility problems.

2. *Nonpharmacologic Treatment Modalities.* A variety of nonpharmacologic treatment modalities have been suggested but their efficacy has not been demonstrated. These include the following:

   a. Vitamins/diet. Specific vitamins and changes in dietary habits have not been associated with improved semen quality and fertility.

    b. Changing from jockey shorts to boxer shorts. Most males have already performed this maneuver prior to being evaluated in the Infertility Clinic with persistence of their problem.

    c. Prostatic massage

    d. Antibiotics for "occult infection"

    e. Varicocelectomy for the "occult varicocele"

3. Drug Therapy for Idiopathic Infertility

    a. The use of human menopausal gonadotropin (hMG, Pergonal), essentially FSH, the use of human chorionic gonadotropin (hCG, APL), essentially LH, or the combination of hMG and hCG have not resulted in significant improvement in sperm counts of men with idiopathic infertility or in a significant number of pregnancies in the various studies.

    b. Testosterone rebound has also been tried without success. This method utilizes complete suppression of spermatogenesis with exogenous testosterone followed by discontinuation of therapy after the patient's sperm counts have been reduced to zero. It is hoped that the recovery of spermatogenesis will be greater than prior to therapy. However, there is no physiologic basis for this or evidence to support that this will occur; in fact, it is clear that a percentage of patients so treated will remain azoospermic.

    c. Clomiphene citrate is an antiestrogen that has been used in a nonspecific fashion for idiopathic infertility. The scientific rationale for its use is based upon this drug's ability to block the negative feedback of estradiol on the hypothalamic–pituitary axis, presumably resulting in increased levels of LH and FSH. Some promise has been demonstrated using this drug, with overall improvement in the semen analysis noted in approximately 50% of patients and pregnancies occurring in 25 to 30% of patients. Although this is promising, it must be remembered that the baseline pregnancy rate without treatment in these patients is really unknown and in fact may approach these same values.

V. CONCLUSION

Our knowledge of normal reproductive physiology and the microanatomy of the male genitourinary tract has certainly improved recently. We are now able to better define many of the processes that result in the transformation of an immature spermatogonium into a mature spermatozoan with motility and fertilizing capabilities. There is still a great deal of knowledge to be gained in this regard, however, and our major difficulty in treating fertility problems at the present time is still our incomplete knowledge of normal reproductive physiology with regard to many subtle events and the ways to determine if these events are altered. Historical factors, the physical examination, and the semen analyses help us to define and classify a variety of abnormalities based on what we are able to observe grossly. A variety of specific treatment modalities are available for specific problems; however, a large number of patients still remain in the idiopathic category requiring empirical therapy. Although this therapy may be based on scientific grounds, the overall pregnancy rate may not be much higher, if at all higher, than the baseline pregnancy rate without treatment. These problems affect 15 to 20% of couples trying to conceive, and hopefully the research that is now being performed will allow these couples to lead fuller lives.

ACKNOWLEDGMENT

I would like to express my gratitude to Dr. Larry Lipshultz for teaching me about fertility and infertility. In helping to shape my approach to male infertility problems, his presence and contributions are still felt in the Male Fertility Section of the Hospital of the University of Pennsylvania.

BIBLIOGRAPHY

Amelar RD, Dubin L, Walsh PC: Male Infertility. Philadelphia: W. B. Saunders, 1977.

de Vere White R (ed): Aspects of Male Infertility. Baltimore: Williams & Wilkins, 1982.

Lipshultz LI, Howards SS: Infertility in the Male. New York: Churchill Livingstone, 1983.

19

Sexually Transmitted Diseases

Ruth Hanno

I. MAJOR SEXUALLY TRANSMITTED DISEASES (Tables 1 through 3)

A. Syphilis[1]

1. Etiology—spirochetal organism *Treponema pallidum*
2. Clinical
   a. Primary syphilis
      (1) Chancres are caused by direct inoculation of *Treponema pallidum* through intact mucous membranes during sexual contact.
      (2) Occur most commonly on mucous membranes abraded during sexual contact (glans penis, labia).
      (3) About 5% of chancres are extragenital and are commonly seen on the lips, tongue, tonsils.
      (4) Chancres occur in urethral meatus in 1 to 3% of patients with primary syphilis but endourethral chancres are rare.[1] When present, endourethral chancres produce discharge and induration. Urethroscopy is necessary for visualization. Unilateral or bilateral inguinal adenopathy is present in most cases.[1]
      (5) Chancre appears 10 to 90 days after inoculation (average 21 days) and heals without scarring in 2 to 12 weeks.[1]
      (6) Chancres are usually 1 to 2 cm in diameter and are often multiple. They appear as shallow ulcerations with noninflamed margins. The base

TABLE 1. SEXUALLY TRANSMITTED DISEASES—ETIOLOGY

Major Diseases	Etiology
Syphilis	*T. pallidum*
Gonorrhea	*N. gonorrhoeae*
Chancroid	*H. ducreyi*
Lymphogranuloma venereum	*C. trachomatis*
Granuloma inguinale	*C. granulomatis*
Herpes simplex genitalis	Herpes simplex virus Type II
Minor Diseases	**Etiology**
Condyloma acuminata	Human papilloma virus
Nongonococcal urethritis	*C. trachomatis; U. urealyticum*
Trichomoniasis	*T. vaginalis*
Pediculosis pubis	*P. pubis*
Scabies	*S. scabiei*
Molluscum contagiosum	Pox virus
Candidasis	*C. albicans*

                may be clean or crusted. Lesions are usually painless.

    (7) Lymphadenopathy is often present and may be unilateral or bilateral. Anal chancres, chancres on the lower two-thirds of the vulva, and cervical chancres drain to deep lymph nodes and inguinal lymphadenopathy is absent in these cases.[1]

  b. Secondary syphilis

    (1) Secondary lesion usually occurs 4 to 8 weeks after primary lesion but may be concurrent.

    (2) The rash is usually widespread and symmetrical and involves the palms and soles in 80% of patients. Lesions are variable and may be macular, papular, scaly, or pustular. They are usually erythematous.

    (3) Vegetative lesions of the intertriginous surfaces (condyloma lata) are frequent and appear as grouped vegetative moist papules that must be distinguished from the verrucoid papules of condyloma acuminata.

    (4) Mucous patches are raised, erythematous, centrally eroded papules about 1 cm in diame-

TABLE 2. DIFFERENTIAL DIAGNOSIS OF GENITAL ULCERS

	Clinical Appearance	Adenopathy	Laboratory Confirmation
Syphilitic chancre	Base clean; border indurated	Present, unilateral, or bilateral	Positive darkfield or serology
Chancroid	Ragged ulceration with undermined border; contiguous skin often involved	Usually present	Smear reveals gram negative rods in chains ("school of fish" pattern)
Granuloma inguinale	Red granulomatous plaque	Rare	Smear or biopsy reveals cytoplasmic inclusions (Donovan bodies in histiocytes on Giemsa stain)
Lymphogranuloma venereum	Primary lesions (vesicle or papule) are evanescent and usually not observed at time patient presents	Unilateral, often suppurative	Rising compliment fixation titers
Herpes simplex	Grouped vesicles on an erythematous base, later erode and crust over	Common in primary infection; rare in recurrences	Tzanck smear reveals viral giant cells; culture from vesicle should be positive
Traumatic	Usually a superficial erosion in areas of friction from sexual acts, i.e., penile shaft, labia minora	Only if secondary infection is present	None

TABLE 3. TREATMENT OF MAJOR SEXUALLY TRANSMITTED DISEASES

Syphilis	Primary, secondary and latent <1 year: IM penicillin G Benzathine, 2.4 mu Penicillin-allergic patients—tetracycline 500 mg po q.i.d. for 15 days or erythromycin 500 mg po q.i.d. for 15 days latent >1 year: IM penicillin G Benzathine, 2.4 mu weekly for 3 weeks Penicillin allergic patients—tetracycline 500 mg po q.i.d. for 30 days
Gonorrhea	Uncomplicated urethritis, endocervicitis, proctitis or pharyngitis: 4.8 mu aqueous procaine penicillin IM with 1 g oral probenecid. if oral therapy is preferred, tetracycline 500 mg q.i.d. for 7 days or ampicillin 500 mg q.i.d. for 7 days Penicillin-allergic patients—spectinomycin hydrochloride 2 g IM
Chancroid	Erythromycin 500 mg po q.i.d. for 10 days or until ulcers heal Trimethoprim/sulfamethoxazole D.S. (169/800 mg) b.i.d. for 10 days or until ulcers heal
Lymphogranuloma venereum	Tetracycline 500 mg q.i.d. for 2 weeks or Doxacycline 100 mg b.i.d. for 2 weeks or Erythromycin 500 mg q.i.d. for 2 weeks or Sulfamethoxazole 1 g b.i.d. for 2 weeks
Herpes simplex	Acyclovir: Primary episode: 200 mg 5 times daily for 10 days Secondary episode: 200 mg 5 times daily for 5 days

ter that occur on the oral or genital mucosa in secondary syphilis.

(5) Patchy alopecia occurs in less than 5% of patients with secondary syphilis.[1]

(6) Skin and mucosal lesions are accompanied by systemic symptoms in 50% of patients. Sore throat, malaise, headache, fever, myalgias, hoarseness, and weight loss are common.

(7) Bilateral symmetrical lymphadenopathy is common.

(8) Lesions of secondary syphilis resolve, with or without treatment, in 2 to 10 weeks.[1]

3. Laboratory
   a. Primary syphilis
      (1) Darkfield examination should be done on any patient with a genital ulceration or suspicious extragenital lesions.
         (a) Wipe lesion of superficial debris.
         (b) Abrade base with gauze and squeeze serous fluid onto slide.
         (c) Cover slip and examine for spirochetes under darkfield microscope.
         (d) Darkfield of oropharyngeal lesions is not advised since it is difficult to distinguish *Treponema pallidum* from indigenous saprophytic spirochetes.
      (2) VDRL or RPR (nontreponemal blood tests) should be obtained at initial visit and weekly for 1 month. Nontreponemal blood tests are positive in about 50% of patients with primary syphilis.
      (3) FTA-ABS or MHA-TP (treponemal blood tests) are positive in about 90% of patients with primary syphilis and can be obtained in patients with suspicious lesions in which VDRL or RPR remain negative.
   b. Secondary syphilis
      (1) Darkfield examination of condyloma lata and genital mucous patch is often positive.
      (2) VDRL is highly reactive in over 90% of cases.

(3) Positive VDRL should be confirmed with FTA-ABS since the latter is a more specific test.
4. Treatment[2]
   a. Intramuscular penicillin G benzathine, 2.4 million units at a single session, is the treatment of choice for primary and secondary syphilis.
   b. Patients who are allergic to penicillin should be treated with oral tetracycline 500 mg q.i.d. for 15 days or erythromycin 500 mg q.i.d. for 15 days.
   c. The Jarisch–Herxheimer reaction occurs several hours after treatment in many patients treated for syphilis. It is a reaction to lipopolysaccharides suddenly released from degenerating treponemes. Patients experience fever, chills, arthralgias, myalgias, and nausea. Symptoms subside within 24 hours.
   d. VDRL titers return to nonreactive 1 year after treatment in almost all patients adequately treated for primary syphilis and in 75% of patients with secondary syphilis.[1] Two years after treatment almost all patients should have nonreactive serologic tests. If serology remains high, treatment may be inadequate or reinfection may have occurred.

B. Gonorrhea[3]
   1. Etiology—gram-negative diplococcus *Neisseria gonorrhoeae*
   2. Clinical
      a. Male genitalia
         (1) Gonococcal urethritis presents as dysuria accompanied by a profuse, usually purulent urethral discharge.
         (2) Anterior urethritis usually lasts 2 to 3 weeks but may persist longer. Extension to the posterior urethra, seminal vesicles, or epididymis may occur.[3]
      b. Female genitalia
         (1) Primary site of infection is usually the endocervix with secondary infection or coloniza-

tion of the urethra or rectum. The vagina itself is not infected.

(2) Yellow-white non-odorous discharge may be present but infection is often assymptomatic.

(3) Ascending infection causes gonococcal salpingitis characterized by diffuse pelvic pain, fever and malaise.

c. Other manifestations

    (1) Gonococcal proctitis—often asymptomatic although mucopurulent or bloody anal discharge may occur.

    (2) Pharyngitis—often asymptomatic but may be responsible for hematogenous dissemination.

    (3) Disseminated gonococcemia—scattered discrete pustulovesicular lesions, most commonly on the extremities and joint spaces. Arthralgias and/or arthritis are frequently present.

3. Laboratory

  a. Culture appropriate site (urethra, cervix, anus, pharynx) on Thayer–Martin media.

  b. Gram stain of smear reveals gram-negative intracellular diplococci.

4. Treatment[2]

  a. Standard treatment for uncomplicated urethritis, endocervicitis, proctitis, or pharyngitis is 4.8 million units of aqueous penicillin G procaine intramuscularly (IM) accompanied by 1 g oral probenecid.

  b. If oral therapy is preferred, use ampicillin 500 mg q.i.d. for 7 days or tetracycline 500 mg q.i.d. for 7 days. Ampicillin can also be given in a single dose of 3.5 g accompanied by 7 g oral probenecid.

  c. In penicillin-allergic patients or penicillin-resistant infections, spectinamycin hydrochloride 2 g IM may be administered.

  d. To assure adequate treatment, repeat cultures should be obtained 3 to 7 days after treatment. In addition, anal cultures should be obtained from women since standard treatments may fail to eradicate anal infections. In men with continued urethral symptoms, smears should be done to detect treatment failure or reinfection. If smears are negative, symptoms may be attributable to postgonococcal urethritis (see ''Nongonococcal Urethritis'' below).

C. Chancroid[4]
1. Etiology—gram-negative rod *Haemophilus ducreyi*
2. Clinical
    a. Initial lesion is a papule that becomes a pustule that then ulcerates. Lesions are located on the external genitalia.
    b. Patients present with shallow ragged ulcerations with undermined borders. The base is often necrotic. Autoinoculation is frequent, with ulcerations developing on contiguous skin.
    c. Adenopathy is common.
3. Diagnosis
    a. Smear reveals gram-negative rods in chains (''school of fish'' pattern).
    b. Culture may be positive on appropriate medium (enriched chocolate agar containing vancomycin).
    c. Often diagnosis is made on clinical grounds when syphilis and herpetic ulcers are ruled out.
4. *Treatment.* Erythromycin 500 mg orally q.i.d. or trimethoprim/sulfamethoxazole double strength tablet (160/800 mg) b.i.d. Treatment should be continued for at least 10 days or until lesions have healed.

D. Lymphogranuloma Venereum
1. Etiology—*Chlamydia trachomatis* Types I, II, III
2. Clinical
    a. A vesicle or papule develops 3 days to 3 weeks after contact. This disappears over a few weeks, usually by the time the patient presents.
    b. One to two weeks later, enlarged inguinal nodes are noted (usually unilateral).
    c. The lymph nodes suppurate and chronic draining sinus tracts develop.

      d. Rectal strictures from anorectal node involvement can be seen.

      e. Systemic symptoms (fever, chills, malaise, arthralgias) sometimes develop.

  3. *Diagnosis.* Complement fixation titers should show a fourfold increase after 4 weeks. The titer is usually greater than 1:16.

  4. Treatment

      a. Tetracycline 500 mg orally q.i.d. for at least 2 weeks is the treatment of choice.

      b. Alternative regimens are doxycycline 100 mg b.i.d., erythromycin 500 mg orally q.i.d., or sulfamethoxazole 1 gram b.i.d. Treatment should continue for at least 2 weeks.

      c. Surgical intervention may be needed for late sequelae such as strictures or fistulas. In general, incision and drainage of nodes is contraindicated.

E. Granuloma Inguinale

  1. Etiology—gram-negative bacterium *Calymatobacterium granulomatosis*

  2. Clinical

      a. Sexual transmission of granuloma inguinale is not proven and the disease is not considered as highly contagious as the other major sexually transmitted diseases.

      b. The initial lesion is a papule that erodes, producing a velvety, red, granulomatous plaque that gradually extends to contiguous anogenital skin.

      c. Scarring often develops in chronic cases. Squamous cell carcinoma can be a late complication in the chronically inflamed skin.

  3. Laboratory

      a. Intracytoplasmic inclusion bodies (Donovan bodies) are seen in histiocytes on Wright or Giemsa stain of smears of crushed fresh biopsy material.

      b. Giemsa stain of fixed skin biopsy material shows similar findings.

  4. *Treatment.* Tetracycline 500 mg q.i.d. for 2 to 4 weeks or streptomycin 1 gram q.i.d. for 1 week.

F. Herpes Simplex Genitalis[5]

1. Etiology—herpes simplex virus Type II (HSV-2), a linear double-stranded DNA-containing virus. Herpes simplex virus Type I (HSV-I) may occasionally cause genital infections.

2. Clinical
   a. Primary lesion
      (1) Usually occurs on the genitalia after puberty via sexual contact.
      (2) Incubation period varies between 3 and 14 days (average 5 days).
      (3) Lesions appear as grouped vesicles on an erythematous base. The vesicles erode, producing shallow ulcerations that heal without scarring in 2 to 3 weeks.
      (4) Fever and adenopathy are common.
      (5) Lesions are usually found on the shaft or glans of the penis in males and the vulva, cervix, or vagina in females. Lesions are less commonly seen on the buttocks and thighs.
   b. Secondary lesions
      (1) Due to reactivation of latent infection or reinfection.
      (2) Fifty to eighty percent of patients will suffer a recurrence within 3 months of their initial infection and less than 10% of patients will experience more than four such episodes per year for the first 2 years.[5]
      (3) Secondary lesions are similar to primary ones except the duration and severity are less and accompanying fever and adenopathy are rare.
      (4) The frequency and severity of recurrence tend to decrease with time in most patients.

3. Diagnosis
   a. Tzanck smear of base of a fresh vesicle (Giemsa stain) reveals multinucleated giant cells. This is useful as a rapid bedside test, although false negatives are not uncommon.
   b. Culture requires 48 to 72 hours and is the most accurate form of diagnosis.

4. Treatment
   a. Topical acyclovir may be useful in primary herpes simplex infections to decrease duration of pain, itching, viral shedding, and healing time. It should be applied six times daily.
   b. Topical acyclovir has *not* been shown to either prevent the transmission of the infection or to decrease the rate of recurrent herpes simplex infection. It probably should *not* be prescribed for recurrent HSV-2 infections since its efficacy is not established and the potential for acquired resistance to the drug might present a problem in the future.
   c. Oral acyclovir, 200 mg 5 times daily for 10 days for primary herpes; 200 mg 5 times daily for 5 days for recurrent herpes, may reduce duration of acute infection and diminish healing time. It is rapidly replacing the topical agent.

II. MINOR SEXUALLY TRANSMITTED DISEASES (Table 4)

A. Condyloma Acuminata

1. Etiology—subtype of human papilloma virus (HPV-6 most common)
2. Clinical
   a. Soft, flesh-colored verrucous papules that may coalesce into cauliflower-like masses.
   b. Occur on penis, female genitalia, and perianal areas.
3. *Diagnosis.* Usually recognized clinically, although biopsy can be done on equivocal cases and serology might be useful to rule out condyloma lata of secondary syphilis.
4. Treatment
   a. External genital and perianal condylomata
      (1) Podophyllin (10 to 20%) in compound tincture of benzoin is applied to the warts and washed off thoroughly in 1 to 4 hours. Warts are treated weekly. Alternate therapy should be used if

TABLE 4. TREATMENT OF MINOR SEXUALLY TRANSMITTED DISEASES

Condyloma accuminatum	External genital or perianal: Podophyllin (10–20%) in tincture of benzoin applied topically and left on 1–4 hours. Repeat treatment weekly if needed for 4–6 weeks. Alternative therapy—cryotherapy, electrosurgery, or scissor or curette excision Urethral: intraurethral 5% 5-Fluorouracil or thiotepa
Nongonococcal urethritis (except trichomonal)	Tetracycline 500 mg q.i.d for 7 days or Doxycycline 100 mg b.i.d. for 7 days or Erythromycin 500 mg po q.i.d. for 7 days
Trichomoniasis	Metrinidazole 2 g po in one dose or Metrinidazole 250 g t.i.d. for 7 days
Pediculosis pubis	Lindane 1% (Kwell) lotion or cream—cover involved areas, leave in place 8–12 hours, wash off
Scabies	Lindane 1% (Kwell) lotion applied neck down, leave on 12 hours. Repeat application in 7 days (optional) Alternative therapy—crotamiton cream—apply all over daily for 2 consecutive days 6% precipitated sulfur in petrolatum—apply all over daily for 3 consecutive days
Candidiasis	Topical clotrimazole, miconazole, or nystatin—apply b.i.d. until clear

there is no response to podophyllin therapy in 4 to 6 weeks. Alternative therapies include cryotherapy, electrosurgery, or scissor or curette excision.
  b. Urethral condylomata
    (1) Urethroscopy should be done to detect urethral condylomata in men with recurrent meatal warts.
    (2) Intraurethral 5% 5-fluorouracil or thiotepa may be effective treatment; podophyllin should not be used in the urethra.

B. Nongonococcal Urethritis (NGU)[6]
  1. Etiology
    a. Forty to fifty percent of cases may be caused by *Chlamydia trachomatis*.
    b. Twenty to twenty-five percent of cases may be caused by *Ureaplasma urealyticum*.
    c. *Trichomonas vaginalis* may be an etiologic factor in some cases.
  2. Clinical
    a. Men
      (1) Incubation period of 2 to 3 weeks.
      (2) Urethral discharge scant watery to copious and purulent.
      (3) Dysuria and frequency are common.
      (4) Fifty to seventy percent of men with Reiter's syndrome have NGU.
      (5) NGU occurs in 30 to 60% of heterosexual men with gonococcal urethritis treated with drugs other than tetracycline.
    b. Women
      (1) Mucopurulent cervicitis and urethral infections common.
      (2) Ascending infection causes endometritis and salpingitis.
  3. Diagnosis
    a. Confirmation of urethritis and exclusion of gonococcal infection.
      (1) Five or more neutrophils per 1000x oil immersion field urethral smear.

        (2) No gram-negative diplocci on smear or negative gonococcal culture on Thayer–Martin medium.

    b. Culture for *C. trachomatis.*

    c. Wet smear of discharge may reveal *T. vaginalis.*

  4. Treatment[2]

    a. Tetracycline 500 mg orally q.i.d. for 7 days or doxycycline 100 mg orally b.i.d. for 7 days.

    b. If tetracyclines are contraindicated or not tolerated, use erythromycin 500 mg orally q.i.d. for 7 days.

    c. In *T. vaginalis* infections—Metrinidazole 2 g in one dose or 250 mg t.i.d. for 1 week.

C. Pediculosis Pubis

  1. Etiology—*Phthirius pubis,* the "crab" louse

  2. Clinical

    a. Contracted by adults through sexual intercourse; occasionally may be transmitted via clothing, bedding, toilets.

    b. Usually involves pubic area but other hairy areas (axillae, eyelashes) may be involved.

    c. Appear as yellow–grey dots clinging to the skin. In some areas red specks are seen on the skin representing the louse excrement. Maculae cerulae are blue skin macules due to penetration of the louse into the upper skin layer, leading to punctate bleeding.

    d. Nits are seen as white dots attached to the hairs,

  3. *Laboratory.* Lice are recognizable grossly, or under a magnifying lens, or on low-power microscopic preparation.

  4. *Treatment.* Lindane 1% lotion (Kwell) apply to involved areas, leave on 8 to 12 hours, one application only.

D. Scabies

  1. Etiology—itch mite *Sarcoptes scabie var hominis*

  2. Clinical

    a. Intense itching, most severe at night, is the main symptom.

    b. Pruritic papules, papulopustules, and crusted lesions are seen most commonly in the web spaces of the fingers, the penis, around the nipples, and on the flexor aspects of the wrist. Other common areas of involvement may be the extensor aspects of the arms and legs and the abdomen. A distinctive lesion is the burrow which is a linear channel just underneath the skin with a grey speck at one end.

  3. *Laboratory.* Scrapings of suspicious lesions show the mite on low power microscopic preparation.

  4. Treatment

    a. Lindane lotion 1% (Kwell) is applied neck down, left on for 12 hours, and then showered off. Application may be repeated in 7 days. Clothing and bed linen must be thoroughly laundered at the same time. Family contacts should also be treated.

    b. If itching persists after two treatments, therapy with topical steroids and antihistamines can be used. Patients should not be treated with Kwell unless treatments were done improperly or microscopic evidence of scabies is again demonstrated. Kwell itself can be irritating to the skin and overtreatment may cause an irritant dermatitis.

    c. Alternative therapy (precipitated sulfer or crotamiton cream) can be used in children and pregnant women.

E. Molloscum Contagiosum

  1. Etiology—pox virus

  2. *Clinical.* Dome-shaped papules, 2 to 6 mm, with central umbilication are most commonly seen in children on the face and other exposed areas. They can be spread by any close contact, but sexual transmission is often responsible for adult genital lesions.

  3. Laboratory

    a. Incision of papule reveals white waxy core.

    b. Smear of contents of papule reveals swollen epithelial cells.

    c. Skin biopsy is diagnostic.

        4. *Treatment*. Curettage, electrodesiccation, or cryosurgery are effective.

F. Candidiasis
1. Etiology—yeast organism *Candida albicans*
2. Clinical
    a. Men
        (1) Red, edematous, pruritic skin, often with peripheral pustules, seen on glans penis, frequently in uncircumsized and/or diabetic males.
    b. Women
        (1) Vaginal involvement common with tender, pruritic mucosa and profuse creamy-white discharge.
        (2) Seen more commonly in diabetic women and women on long-term antibiotic therapy for acne.
3. *Laboratory*. Culture or smear demonstrates *C. albicans*.
4. Treatment
    a. Skin infections
        (1) Clean areas well with soap and water followed by a thin film of antifungal cream—clotrimazole, miconazole, or nystatin—b.i.d.
        (2) Circumcision may be needed for chronic balanitis in uncircumsized men.
    b. Vaginal
        (1) Antifungal vaginal suppositories (clotrimazole, nystatin) daily for 1 week.
        (2) Correction of underlying factors (diabetes control, discontinuation of oral contraceptives or antibiotics).

REFERENCES
1. Chapel TA: Primary and secondary syphilis. Cutis 33:47–53, 1984.
2. Centers for Disease Control: Sexually Transmitted Diseases Treatment Guidelines 1982. Morbid Mortal Weekly Rep 31(25):355–605, 1982.

3. Harrison WD: Gonorrhea. Cutis 33:51–61, 1984.
4. Felman YM, Nikitas JA: Update on chancroid. Cutis 31:602–609, 1983.
5. Ryan ML: Herpes genitalis. Michigan Drug Lett 1(7), 1982.
6. Bowie WR: Etiology and treatment of nongonococcal urethritis. Sex Trans Dis 5(1):27–33, 1978.

20

Disorders of the Adrenal Gland

Joseph A. Jacobs
Nathan P. Goldin

I. ADRENAL EMBRYOLOGY

A. Cortex

1. During the 4th week of embryonal life, mesothelial buds along the upper third of the mesonephron form and later coalesce to form the fetal cortex.

2. The fetal cortex is larger than the kidney by the 4th month but then begins to regress.

3. The adult cortex is connected to the superior pole of the kidney. This permanent cortex differentiates into three zones by the 2nd year of life.

B. Medulla

1. The neural crest gives rise to sympathetic primordial cells (sympathogonia).

2. Sympathogonia ultimately give rise to mature ganglion cells and chromaffin endocrine cells. The latter penetrate into the proliferating adrenal cortical primordium at approximately the 7th week of fetal life.

3. Most other paraganglia regress after the medulla becomes functional. The most common exception is the preaortic organ of Zuckerkandl.

C. Clinical and Surgical Implications

1. Ectopic adrenal glands with cortex and medulla have been found from the cranium to the pelvis.

2. Accessory cortical tissue has been found in continuity with the genital portion of the mesonephric blastema (i.e., ovary, testis, epididymis).
3. Extramedullary chromaffin tissue (residual paraganglion tissue) can be found in the retroperitoneum and periaortic areas. These sites must be considered during explorations for pheochromocytoma.
4. Adrenal Anomalies
   a. Unilateral agenesis of the adrenal is often associated with ipsilateral renal agenesis or hypoplasia. In renal ectopy the adrenal is orthotopic.
   b. Renal fusion (i.e., horseshoe kidney) is associated with adrenal fusion.
5. The gland at term is very vascular and friable, and thus there is a high incidence of hemorrhage in the newborn.

II. ANATOMY

A. Appearance
1. The adrenal glands are small, yellowish, triangular structures, medial and superior to the upper pole of each kidney and contained within separate envelopes of perinephric (Gerota's) fascia.
2. Adrenal weight ranges from 5 to 10 g but varies considerably with stress.
3. The right adrenal is pyramidal and the left appears more as a crescent.

B. Vasculature
1. Arteries and veins do not course together (unlike in other organs).
2. The adrenal has an extraordinarily rich vascular supply (7 ml/mg/min) from three sources:
   a. Superior adrenal (from inferior phrenic)
   b. Middle adrenal (from aorta)
   c. Inferior (from renal artery) forms vascular arcade around gland.

3. Venous drainage is more variable than arterial supply.
   a. The main adrenal vein courses through the medulla and cortex.
   b. The right adrenal vein is short and enters directly into the vena cava.
   c. The left adrenal vein is longer and enters the left renal vein.
   d. On each side, veins accompany branches of the phrenic artery and also leave the cortex to join the vena cava and the splanchnic, splenic, and pancreatic veins to reach the portal system.
   e. There are more frequent accessory adrenal veins from the right adrenal gland to the inferior vena cava, making right adrenalectomy more hazardous.

C. Innervation
1. Mainly sympathetic (T10–L1); stimulation results in release of medullary hormones.
2. Most fibers are postganglionic (via splanchnic chain) and synapse directly with chromaffin cells.

D. Contiguous Anatomic Relationships
1. Right
   a. Liver superiorly
   b. Inferior vena cava medial
   c. Kidney and renal vessels lateral
   d. Inferior diaphragmatic crus and pleural reflection posterior
   e. Duodenum anterior
2. Left
   a. Pleura and diaphragm posterior
   b. Posterior wall of stomach, tail of pancreas, tail of spleen anterior

E. Steroid Production
1. The zona glomerulosa produces aldosterone and is regulated by angiotensin II (Fig. 1).
2. The inner layers (fasiculata and reticularis), which secrete cortisol and sex steroids, are dependent on pitui-

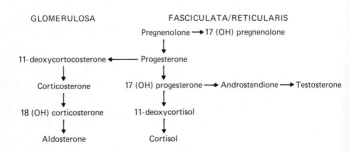

Figure 1. Functional differences between the ACTH-dependent zones of fasciculata/reticularis and the renin-dependent zona glomerulosa.

tary adrenocorticotropic hormone (ACTH) for control of growth and secretions. The release of ACTH is controlled by corticotropin hormone from the hypothalamus.

3. The medulla is the site for production of epinephrine and norepinephrine.

III. PHYSIOLOGY

A. Biosynthesis of Steroids (Fig. 2)

B. Control of Mineralocorticoid Secretion (Fig. 3)

1. Control is closely related to the juxtaglomerular apparatus (JGA) of the kidney.
2. The juxtaglomerular cells are part of the renal afferent arteriole just before it gives rise to the glomerular capillary.
3. The macula densa is a portion of the distal tubule lying adjacent to the JGA, which has osmoreceptors for serum sodium.
4. Renin is released by the juxtaglomerular cells in response to stress, changes in blood pressure and blood volume, and changes in urinary sodium as sensed by the macula densa.
5. Renin acts on its substrate to release angiotensin I, which is converted to angiotensin II.

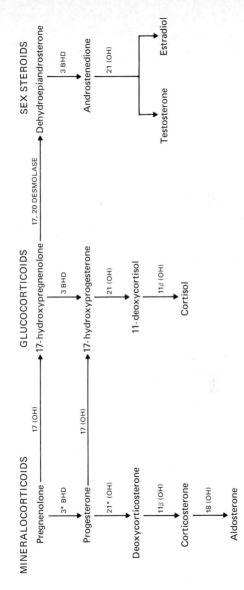

Figure 2. Adrenal steroidogenesis. BHD, β-Hydroxysteroid dehydrogenase; OH, hydroxylase.

485

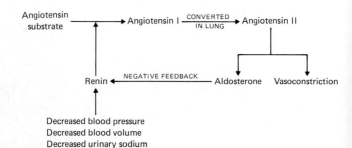

Figure 3. Renin–angiotensin–aldosterone interaction. Reduced blood pressure in the afferent arteriole of the kidney results in renin release from the juxtaglomerular cells. Renin acts on angiotensin to release angiotensin I, which is converted to angiogensin II in the lung, and this activates aldosterone secretion from the zona glomerulosa. Aldosterone stimulates sodium retention by the renal tubule, leading to increased blood pressure and decreased renin secretion.

6. Angiotensin II is the most potent naturally occurring vasoconstrictor. It is formed in the lung by the conversion of angiotensin I and then stimulates the release of aldosterone by the zona glomerulosa.

7. Aldosterone stimulates sodium retention by the renal tubule, leading to increased blood pressure and diminished renin secretion.

C. Regulation of Glucocorticoid Secretion

1. Normally 15 to 30 mg of cortisol is secreted daily. This can be increased to over 200 mg/day during periods of stress.

2. Pituitary ACTH is inhibited by rising concentrations of cortisol.

3. Inhibition of cortisol synthesis (i.e., with metyrapone, which blocks 11β hydroxylase) causes increases in ACTH.

4. Effects of glucocorticoids include
   a. Induction of gluconeogenesis and lipolysis
   b. Stabilization of lysozomal membranes
   c. Decreased inflammatory response
   d. Decreased numbers of lymphocytes and eosinophils

D. Mechanism of ACTH and Steroid Hormone Action

1. ACTH binds on cell surface receptor sites and increases cyclic adenosine monophosphate (AMP).
2. Steroids penetrate cells and bind with receptor proteins. The resulting receptor steroid complex is translocated to the nucleus affecting messenger RNA and, thus, protein synthesis.

E. Adrenal Medulla

1. The adrenal medulla is the site of biosynthesis of catecholamines. Tyrosine undergoes decarboxylation to form dopa, dopamine, and, finally, norepinephrine and epinephrine (Fig. 4).
2. The conversion of norepinephrine to epinephrine is promoted by phenylethanolamine-*N*-methyl transferase (PNMT), which is induced by the high levels of glucocorticoids in the medullary venous blood. Thus, epinephrine is the main catecholamine of the adrenal medulla. Extraadrenal chromaffin tissue, lacking the enzyme, produces mainly norepinephrine.

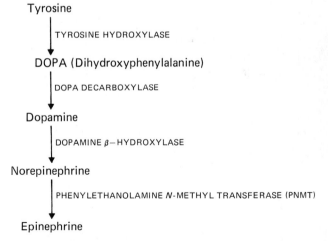

Figure 4. Biosynthetic pathway for production of catecholamines in the adrenal medulla.

IV. PATHOLOGY

A. Adrenogenital Syndrome (see also Chapter 23)

1. *Definition.* All cases of sexual precocity and hetero-sexual abnormalities due to adrenocortical dysfunction are grouped under one descriptive term—the adrenogenital syndrome. This can be subdivided into two classes:
   a. Prenatal—congenital adrenal hyperplasia (CAH)
   b. Postnatal—two types
      (1) Prepubertal—virilization
      (2) Postpubertal—heterosexual development

B. Congenital Adrenal Hyperplasia

1. Most common disorder of adrenal function in childhood
2. Most common cause of ambiguous genitalia
3. Recognized in females three times as often as males
4. Caused by a partial deficiency of one or more enzymes necessary for production of cortisol. Diminished cortisol production results in elevation of ACTH levels, thus increasing the production of cortisol precursors and androgens.
5. There are four clinical syndromes based on isolated enzyme deficiencies: (Fig. 2)
   a. 21 hydroxylase deficiency
      (1) Most common type (95% of all cases of CAH)
      (2) Produces virilism
      (3) More easily recognized in females because of more obvious genital abnormalities.
      (4) Diagnosis confirmed by demonstrating increased levels of progesterone and 17 hydroxyprogesterone with decreased cortisol levels.
      (5) In the most severe form there is markedly decreased aldosterone. This can be fatal due to severe salt wasting.
   b. 11 hydroxylase deficiency
      (1) Produces virilism and hypertension related to increased levels of androgens and deoxycorticosterone, respectively

      c. 3β hydroxydehydrogenase deficiency
- (1) Causes ambiguous genitalia in both males and females.
- (2) Can be accompanied by hypertension or salt-wasting.
- (3) Very rare and sometimes fatal

      d. 17 hydroxylase deficiency
- (1) Very rare
- (2) Produces hypertension but no virilism
- (3) Usually recognized after puberty and treatable with prednisone and sex hormones.

6. Therapy
- a. Primary goal to replace deficient cortisol and mineralcocorticoids. This reduces ACTH levels and precursors of cortisol.
- b. Sexual abnormalities in the female including hypertrophied clitoris and fused labia can be treated with surgery.

C. Cushing's Syndrome

1. *Definition.* Clinical and metabolic disorder resulting from excess glucocorticoids, especially cortisol.
2. Described in 1932 by Harvey Cushing.
3. Occurs most frequently in young adults and is four times more common in women.
4. Causes
- a. Adrenocortical neoplasm secreting cortisol—can be adenoma or adenocarcinoma
  - (1) Accounts for 25% of cases of Cushing's syndrome
  - (2) More commonly benign than malignant
  - (3) Causes suppression of ACTH and thus non-tumorous adrenal tissue is atrophic
- b. Nonpituitary (ectopic) secretion of ACTH—most frequently seen with small cell cancer of lung
- c. Excess pituitary secretion of ACTH (Cushing's disease)
  - (1) Seventy to seventy-five percent of cases
  - (2) Due to basophilic or chromophobe pituitary adenoma

5. Symptoms and Signs
    a. Physiognomy
        (1) Central obesity (truncal distribution)
        (2) Rounded (moon) face
        (3) Prominent fat deposits in the supraclavicular and suprascapular areas (buffalo hump)
    b. Skin
        (1) Striae found in two-thirds of the patients
        (2) Thin skin with easy bruisability, slow wound healing, and ecchymosis
        (3) Superficial fungal and bacterial infections
        (4) Acne
        (5) Hirsutism in females without virilization
    c. Reproduction
        (1) Amenorrhea in females
        (2) Impotence (due to low testosterone) in males
    d. Musculoskeletal
        (1) Growth arrest in children
        (2) Osteoporosis
        (3) Pathologic fracture
        (4) Muscle wasting
    e. Renal/Cardiovascular
        (1) Hypertension, edema, and, sometimes, congestive heart failure
        (2) Hypokalemia and occasionally hypochloremia with metabolic alkalosis
        (3) Urolithiasis—due to calcium mobilization from bone
    f. Hematologic. Erythrocytosis, granulocytosis, lymphopenia, eosinopenia
    g. Metabolic—Carbohydrate Intolerance
        (1) Ninety percent have abnormal glucose tolerance test
        (2) Twenty percent have diabetes mellitus
    h. Psychologic. Mental disturbances ranging from depression to major psychoses appear frequently
6. *Diagnosis*. Requires evidence of a maintained increase in cortisol secretion, loss of diurnal variation, and loss of pituitary adrenal feedback control. The best evidence of this diagnosis is from demonstration that the

feedback control is abnormal. This is done with a low-dose dexamethasone suppression test (Fig. 5A).

a. Low-dose dexamethasone (0.5 mg every 6 hours) will suppress the level of cortisol in normal patients but not in those with Cushing's syndrome.

b. Increased cortisol, free cortisol in the urine, or measurement of 24-hour urinary hydroxycorticoids can also confirm the diagnosis, but, are not as definitive or specific.

c. In patients with documented Cushing's syndrome, the causative adrenal lesion can be ascertained by a high-dose dexamethasone suppression test (Fig.

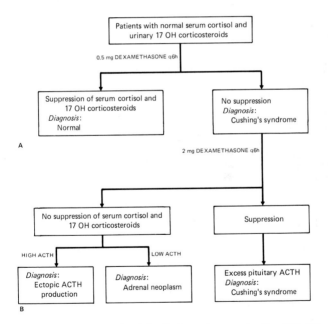

Figure 5. A. Clinical diagnosis of Cushing's syndrome, using low-dose dexamethasone suppression test. **B.** Differential of causes of Cushing's syndrome, using high-dose dexamethasone suppression test.

5B). High-dose dexamethasone (2 mg every 6 hours) will suppress plasma cortisol and urinary free cortisol in patients with Cushing's disease (excess pituitary ACTH) but not in those with ectopic (ACTH) production or adrenal neoplasm. These two latter conditions are differentiated on the basis of ACTH level; high in ectopic production and low in patients with adrenal tumors.

7. *Treatment.* Objectives in Cushing's syndrome are to reduce cortisol levels to normal, remove any tumors, and prevent secondary hormonal insufficiencies.

   a. Cushing's disease. May be treated with transsphenoidal resection of the adenoma or, in children, with pituitary radiation. Also, can use Mitotan (o.p'DDD), a drug that selectively affects the zona fasciculata and reticularis and does not affect aldosterone secretion. In the past, bilateral adrenelectomy was often performed.

   b. Ectopic ACTH production sites are usually unresectable. If unresectable, then use metyrapone, a drug that can partially block cortisol synthesis. Bilateral adrenalectomy is not an acceptable therapeutic alternative.

   c. Adrenal neoplasm is treated with surgical resection.

D. Primary Aldosteronism (Conn's Syndrome)

1. *Definition.* Autonomous, hypersecretion of aldosterone unrelated to renin.

2. Found in 1% of patients with hypertension.

3. Females predominate 2:1 over males.

4. All clinical consequences are related to sodium retention and potassium secretion.

5. Characterized by arterial hypertension, hypokalemia, alkalosis, muscle weakness, and polyuria. In patients with hypertension and unprovoked hypokalemia, 50% will have primary aldosteronism.

6. Etiology is usually a small, unilateral, solitary cortical tumor (85%), but there are increasing reports of bilateral tumors. Rarely, an adrenocortical carcinoma is responsible.

7. Laboratory Findings
   a. A low renin and elevated aldosterone levels
   b. No decrease in aldosterone following a sodium load
   c. Hypokalemia
   d. Must rule out Cushing's syndrome with plasma cortisol and urinary free cortisol levels
8. Radiologic studies for localization are not consistently helpful.
   a. CT scan is the best of available modalities.
   b. Adrenal arteriography, venography, and selective adrenal vein catherization can be hazardous and should be reserved for those cases that cannot be defined by less invasive methods.
9. Treatment
   a. Surgical treatment of tumor by unilateral adrenalectomy is best treatment.
   b. For poor-risk patients or those with bilateral disease, treatment should be with spironolactone, 100 to 200 mg/day.
10. *Secondary Aldosteronism*. Represents a physiologic response to any stimulus that increases renin (i.e., dehydration, shock, congestive heart failure, chronic liver disease).
    a. Hypokalemia is not as prominent as in primary aldosteronism.
    b. Renin levels are increased.
    c. Treatment is directed to the underlying disease process.
11. Bartter's syndrome consists of diffuse juxtaglomerular hyperplasia with increased renin and secondary aldosteronism

E. Tumors of the Adrenal Cortex
1. *Types*. Adenoma, carcinoma, hamartoma, cysts, and metastatic carcinoma.
2. Small benign nodules are very common, occurring in as many as one-third of all adults.
3. Tumors are often malignant if mass is sufficiently large to be symptomatic. Diagnosis based on histology tends to vary with different observers.

4. *Symptoms*. Mass effect may be asymptomatic until large enough to cause necrosis, hemorrhage, or impingement on adjacent organs.

5. *Diagnosis*. Often seen on intravenous pyelography because of inferior and lateral displacement of kidney. Also, ultrasound and computerized tomography have increased the diagnostic accuracy.

6. Age ranges from 4th to 7th decade

7. Adrenal Cysts
   a. Increasingly found because of routine ultrasound and computed tomography (CT) scans of the abdomen.
   b. Autopsy incidence is 0.6% and both glands are equally affected.
   c. Types
      (1) Parasitic cysts—5%
      (2) Epithelial cysts (usually cystic adenoma) 10%
      (3) Endothelial cysts (usually lymphangiomatous) 45%
      (4) Pseudocysts—40% usually caused by hemorrhage (i.e., after birth trauma)
   d. Symptoms. Often related to displacement of kidney or intestine when cyst is large.
   e. Diagnosis
      (1) Ultrasound or CT scan are the best modalities.
      (2) Cyst puncture with analysis of cyst fluid and "cystography" have not yet proven to be reliable in distinguishing benign from malignant cysts.
      (3) In children, must rule out cystic Wilms' tumor and neuroblastoma.
      (4) Arteriography and venography are sometimes helpful.
   f. Treatment
      (1) Benign cysts should be removed only for relief of symptoms.
      (2) Operative goal is to preserve the ipsilateral kidney.
      (3) If cyst is difficult to remove, then it can be marsupialized.

8. Adrenocortical Carcinoma
   a. General
      (1) Very rare—0.25% of all cancer deaths
      (2) Age range—20 to 50 years
      (3) Females diagnosed earlier (due to virilization)
      (4) Eighty percent are functional tumors
      (5) Most frequent clinical manifestations are virilization and/or Cushing's syndrome.
   b. Syndromes of functional adrenal carcinoma
      (1) Isosexual precocity in male children
      (2) Virilization in females
      (3) Cushing's syndrome (When it occurs in a child, adrenal carcinoma is the most frequent cause. In the adult, adrenal hyperplasia is much more common.)
      (4) Aldosteronism—usually in benign tumor
      (5) Hypoglycemia—rare
      (6) Combination of Cushing's syndrome and virilization most frequent disorder
      (7) Feminizing syndromes in males
         (a) Age range—25 to 50 years
         (b) Gynecomastia most frequent sign
   c. Radiologic diagnosis
      (1) Intravenous pyelography (IVP), ultrasound, and CT scan
      (2) Adrenal venography rarely necessary
      (3) More recently, skinny needle biopsy using either ultrasound or CT guidance has established a diagnosis in over 80% of cases
   d. Laboratory findings
      (1) High levels of urinary 17-ketosteroids are always suggestive of adrenal carcinoma
      (2) Increased urinary dehydroepiandrosterone
      (3) Increased urinary 17-hydroxycorticoids and free cortisol
      (4) Stimulation with ACTH or suppression with dexamethasone does not significantly change steroid output.
   e. Metastases
      (1) Most common sites are lung, liver, and lymph nodes

   (2) Direct spread to kidney and retroperitoneum

 f. Treatment

   (1) Primarily radical surgical removal of the lesion through a thoracoabdominal approach. Preoperative preparation with cortisol is essential.

   (2) Local recurrences are frequent and should also be removed surgically.

   (3) Chemotherapy (with o,p'DDD) reserved for patients who are poor surgical risks or have metastases

    (a) Toxic effects seen in 90% of patients, mostly neuromuscular and gastrointestinal (GI).

    (b) Must be accompanied by glucocorticoid and mineralocorticoid administration.

   (4) Radiotherapy is useful only for bony metastases, which are rare

 g. Survival

   (1) For all cases: 2 years, 50%; 3 years, 25%; 5 years, 10%

   (2) For advanced lesions, average survival is about 8 months.

F. Adrenal Insufficiency

 1. Addison's Disease (Primary Adrenal Cortical Insufficiency)

  a. Etiology

   (1) Idiopathic atrophy—probably of autoimmune origin

   (2) Granulomatous destruction (TB or fungal)

   (3) Exogenously administered glucocorticoids

   (4) Infiltrative disease (amyloid, metastatic cancer)

  b. Pathogenesis. Depends on relative deficiency of cortisol, aldosterone, and adrenal androgens.

   (1) Cortisol deficiency—signs and symptoms

    (a) Increased ACTH causes increased MSH melanocyte stimulating hormone (MSH), causing skin pigmentation.

- (b) Decreased appetite and lethargy
- (c) Shock with minor stress
- (2) Aldosterone deficiency
  - (a) Sodium wasting, increased potassium
  - (b) Volume depletion, decreased cardiac output
- (3) Androgen deficiency
  - (a) In males, of no consequence
  - (b) In females, decreased axillary and pubic hair
- c. Diagnosis. ACTH test—no increase in serum cortisol following IV infusion of ACTH
- d. Treatment
  - (1) Chronic replacement
    - (a) Only cortisol and aldosterone need to be replaced. Treatment is lifelong.
    - (b) Requirements fluctuate.
    - (c) Normally need 30 mg hydrocortisone and 0.1 mg aldosterone (given as 0.1 mg fluorocortisone, florinef) per day.
    - (d) Replace during stress, 200 to 500 mg hydrocortisone per day.
  - (2) Acute replacement (Addisonian crisis)
    - (a) Treat volume depletion with normal saline. Usually there is a deficit of 20% of extracellular fluid volume.
    - (b) Hydrocortisone, 100 mg/L of saline.
    - (c) Treat hyperkalemia as needed.
    - (d) Rule out infection as a precipitating cause.
2. Adrenal Insufficiency Secondary to Pituitary Failure
   - a. Etiology
     - (1) Pituitary tumor, infarction, infection, histiocytosis, surgical resection, radiation
     - (2) Injury to the hypothalamic–pituitary axis
   - b. Pathogenesis
     - (1) Diminished ACTH levels cause decreased cortisol and androgen release.
     - (2) Aldosterone secretion is not affected.

      c. Clinical manifestations
        (1) Sodium deprivation is better tolerated than in Addisonian patients.
        (2) Can be associated with other end organ dysfunction, such as hypothyroidism or hypogonadism, and visual field defects from impingement on the optic chiasm.
      d. Diagnostic findings
        (1) Low serum cortisol and urinary 17-ketosteroids, which increase to normal with exogenous ACTH
        (2) Hypothyroidism with hypogonadism
      e. Treatment
        (1) Glucocorticoid replacement
        (2) Treatment of other end organ dysfunction
   3. Drugs (i.e., Dilantin, amphotericin, aminoglutethimide) cause "adrenal" insufficiency by altering the extradrenal metabolism of cortisol.

G. Pheochromocytoma

   1. Most common adrenomedullary tumor
   2. Very rare; no age or sex predilection
   3. Five percent familial, usually as part of multiple endocrine neoplasia
   4. Can arise wherever chromaffin cells are located
      a. Eighty-five percent are located in the adrenal gland.
      b. Seventy percent are discrete unilateral tumors.
      c. Fifteen percent are outside of adrenal gland, usually below the diaphgram.
      d. Ten percent are located in multiple sites.
   5. Pathologic Aspects
      a. Only feature diagnostic of malignancy is development of metastases.
      b. Approximately 5% are truly malignant.
      c. The majority of these lesions are functional.
      d. Metastases go to bones, lung, liver, and spleen.
      e. Malignant tumors tend to be large (1 to 16 cm).

     f. Histology (three types)—epithelial, pleomorphic, and spindle cell.

       (1) No relationships between cell type and malignant potential.

       (2) Diagnostic feature of tumor tissue believed to be pheochromocytoma is the ability to change to a dark brown color in a dichromate solution.

6. Clinical Manifestations
   a. Hypertension (over 90%) episodic as often as sustained
   b. Abdominal mass or pain
   c. Excessive perspiration
   d. Hypermetabolism. Elevated basal metabolic rate, hyperglycemia, and elevated plasma free fatty acids.
   e. Associated diseases: Cholelithiasis, neurofibromatosis.

7. Biochemical Testing
   a. Twenty-four-hour urine for catecholamines, VMA, and metanephrine. Five percent of patients will have false negative results.
   b. These assays are not accurate if the patient is taking α-blockers (i.e., Aldomet), an MAO inhibitor, or sympathomimetic amines (found in most nose drops).

8. Radiologic Testing
   a. IVP, CT scan, arteriogram, bone survey (to detect lytic metastases).
   b. For extraadrenal tumors, use venography with blood sampling to detect elevated catecholamine levels.
   c. Radiologic localization is appropriate only after biochemical diagnosis is made.

9. Preoperative Management
   a. Treatment with α-blockers (i.e., phenoxybenzamine, 30 to 60 mg/day) for 7 to 10 days is recommended.

    b. β-Blockade with propanolol, 30 to 60 mg/day,
      should be given for 3 days prior to surgery to
      reduce the incidence of arrhythmias.
   10. Operative Considerations
    a. Innovar is the preferred anesthetic.
    b. Transabdominal incision is preferrable because:
      (1) Seven percent have multiple tumors.
      (2) Ten percent have extraadrenal tumors.
      (3) All chromaffin tissue must be explored.
    c. Site of tumor should be explored last to minimize
      changes in blood pressure.
    d. If tumor is bilateral, try to leave part of one
      cortex.
   11. Follow-up
    a. Survival at 5 years
      (1) Ninety-six percent if benign
      (2) Forty-four percent if malignant
    b. A majority of patients are normotensive following
      definitive surgery.

BIBLIOGRAPHY

Budd DC: Cysts of adrenal gland. Ann Surg 45(10):649–652, 1979.
Dluhy RG, Gittes RF, Harrison JH: The adrenals. In Harrison JH (ed): Camp-
 bell's Urology, ed 4. Philadelphia: W.B. Saunders, Vol. 3, 1979, pp 2559–
 2640.
Dunnick NR: CT in adrenal tumors. Am J Roentgenol 132(1):43–46, 1979.
Glenn JF (ed): Symposium on adrenal diseases. Urol Clin of North Am 4(2),
 June 1977.
Javadpour N: Adrenal neoplasma. Curr Prob Surg 1:1–52, 1980.
Palubinskas AJ: Localization of pheo. Radiology 136(2):495–496, 1980.
ReMine W: Current management of pheo. Ann Surg (179):740–746, 1974.
Richie J: Carcinoma of adrenal cortex. Cancer 15:1957–1964, 1980.
Scott HW: Pheo-dx and management. Ann Surg 183(5):587–593, 1976.
Siehavizzo J: Supra-renal mass, differential diagnosis. Urology 18(6):625–
 632, 1981.
Stewart BH: Localization of pheo by CT. N Engl J Med 299(9):460–461,
 1978.
Sullivan J: Adrenal cortical Ca. Urol 120(6):660–665, 1978.
Teply JF: Pheochromocytoma. Am J Surg 140(1):107–111, 1980.
Zaitoon MM: Adrenal cortical tumors in children. Urology 12(6):645, 1978.
Zornoza J: Percutaneous biopsy of adrenal tumors. Urology 18(4):412, 1981.

21

Urologic Aspects of Renal Transplantation

Bruce Malkowicz
Leonard Perloff

Approximately 22,000 Americans develop end-stage renal disease each year, and the number of kidneys transplanted in the United States is expected to reach 15,000 to 18,000 per year in the near future. Although major technical obstacles have been overcome, strict attention to detail is still mandatory in every phase of the transplantation process from initial evaluation of the donor and recipient through the surgical procedure and into the long-term treatment of varied, and often serious, complications.

I. RECIPIENT EVALUATION

A. Etiology of End-Stage Renal Disease

1. Fifteen percent of end-stage renal disease is caused by urologic syndromes (Table 1).
2. Infectious causes include chronic pyelonephritis or infected nephrolithiasis.
3. Chronic obstructive uropathy includes neurovesical dysfunction, ureteropelvic junction narrowing, or retroperitoneal fibrosis.

B. General Preoperative Considerations

1. Up to 25% of transplant candidates may have previously undetected urologic abnormalities, the majority of which involve the lower tracts and may be secondary to prolonged catheter drainage from pre-

TABLE 1. UROLOGIC CONDITIONS LEADING TO CHRONIC RENAL FAILURE

Chronic pyelonephritis	Urethral valves
Chronic infection secondary to nephrolithiasis	Retroperitoneal fibrosis
Neurovesicular dysfunction	Ureteropelvic junction obstruction

    vious transplant attempts or prior urologic instrumentation.
2. Minimal preoperative symptoms can be exacerbated after restoration of renal function with successful transplantation.
3. Urodynamics are indicated in potential recipients and may have particular value in prospective diabetic patients.
4. Reconstructive procedures such as transurethral resection of the prostate or creation of ileal conduits should be performed prior to transplantation.

C. Pretransplant Nephrectomy
1. The procedure is performed selectively due to increased morbidity and mortality ranging from 2 to 16%.
2. Loss of vascular access, wound infection, pneumothorax, and prolonged ileus comprise the majority of morbidity (Table 2).
3. The procedure provides *no* advantage with regard to allograft survival and frequency of urinary tract infections.

TABLE 2. COMPLICATIONS OF PRETRANSPLANT BILATERAL NEPHRECTOMY

Thrombosed vascular access	Intraabdominal abscess
Inadvertent injury to spleen	Prolonged ileus
Pneumothorax	Operative death
Wound infection	

TABLE 3. INDICATIONS FOR PRETRANSPLANT NEPHRECTOMY

Absolute	Relative
Renin-mediated hypertension	Excessive proteinuria
Persistent infection	Hypertension
Infected stones	Goodpasture's disease
Persistent bleeding	Extremely large polycystic kidneys
Malignancy	

4. Transplant patients with native kidneys benefit from erythropoietin production, improved vitamin D metabolism, and fluid balance.
5. Absolute indications for pretransplant bilateral nephrectomy include (Table 3):
   a. Uncontrolled hypertension
   b. Persistent infection or infected stones
   c. Persistent bleeding
   d. Renal malignancy
6. Relative indications for nephrectomy:
   a. Severe hypertension
   b. Goodpasture's syndrome
   c. Heavy proteinuria
   d. Extremely large polycystic kidneys
7. Abdominal, flank, and posterior approaches have all been employed. The last approach has had the least morbidity and mortality.
8. The posterior approach is not indicated if the native kidneys are very large, bilateral reflux exists, or adjunctive procedures, e.g., splenectomy, are required.

D. Polycystic Kidneys
1. These patients comprise 5.5% of transplant populations.
2. These patients are usually older than average recipient (43 to 45 years old).
3. No significant difference is seen with respect to overall patient or graft survival.
4. Patient mortality usually due to bacterial sepsis.

II. DONOR CONSIDERATIONS

A. Living Donor Evaluation

1. This includes urinalysis, urine culture, 24-hour creatinine–protein determination, intravenous urography, and an aortogram (Fig. 1).
2. Small renal cysts or unilateral fibroplasia do not rule out using a kidney for a graft.
3. A single renal artery is preferred.
4. The left kidney is usually taken to obtain larger renal vein.

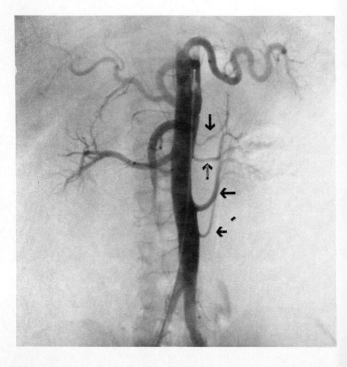

Figure 1. Aortogram demonstrating multiple renal arteries to the left kidney (*arrows*) of a prospective living related donor.

5. The right kidney is used as graft when donor is female of child-bearing age for this one is at higher risk for hydronephrosis during pregnancy.
6. Flank incision with very wide margins of dissection is employed.
7. Procedure carries 15 to 40% complication rate; prolonged ileus, pneumothorax, wound infection, and death (<0.1%).
8. Long-term donor morbidity minimal.

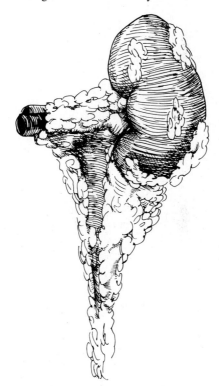

Figure 2. Specimen demonstrating preservation of hilar and periureteral structures via wide dissection of kidney.

B. Cadaver Donors

1. The majority of renal allografts are from this source.
2. Donor criteria:
   a. Brain death
   b. Age 1 to 55
   c. Normal pre-morbid renal function
   d. Absence of systemic sepsis, hypertension or neo-plasia outside CNS
3. Only 1 to 2% of hospital deaths meet these criteria and only 20% of these patients eventually become organ donors.
4. Wide margins of dissection are employed; the ureteral sheath is left undisturbed (Fig. 2).
5. Graft preservation is accomplished by cold storage or pulsatile perfusion, with good results obtained if transplant is performed within 48 hours.
6. Warm ischemia time (<2 minutes) is the major determinant of immediate graft function.

III. URINARY TRACT RECONSTRUCTION

A. General Considerations

1. Methods for reconstruction include ureteropyelostomy, ureteroureterostomy, and endo- or extravesical ureteroneocystostomy.
2. Transvesical approaches were avoided in early transplant attempts but mortality and morbidity are much higher when ureteropyelostomy or ureteroureterostomy is used as the method of primary reconstruction (Table 4).
3. In such reconstructive procedures urinary tract fistulae are the major complication while obstruction accounts for only 2% of the morbidity and no mortality.

TABLE 4. COMPLICATION RATE OF VARIOUS URINARY TRACT RECONSTRUCTIVE PROCEDURES

	Complications	Mortality
Ureteroneocystostomy	10%	22%
Ureteropyelostomy	21%	38%
Ureteroureterostomy	17%	13%

4. Ureteropyelostomy is a favored and effective alternative in secondary reconstruction following a urologic complication.

B. Ureteroneocystostomy

1. Contemporary series have a 0 to 9% fistulazation rate with ureteroneocystostomy. Obstruction comprises 0 to 6.5% of complications. Many fewer deaths are reported with these techniques than in the past (0 to 10% mortality in patients with fistulas).
2. A Politano–Leadbetter variation of the procedure is favored in most centers (Fig. 3).
3. Extravesicular ureteroneocystostomy, a variation of

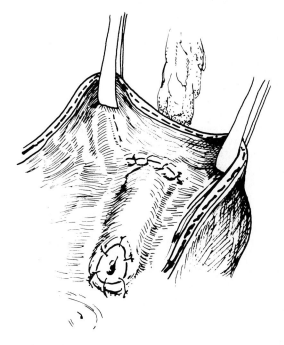

Figure 3. Allograft ureter implantation by a standard intravesicular ureteroneocystostomy. (Modification of Politano-Leadbetter.)

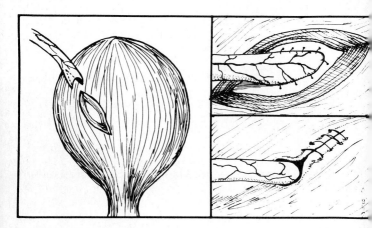

Figure 4. Extravesicular ureteroneocystostomy. (Modification of Litch.)

the Litch method, is also employed by many groups (Fig. 4).

4. Fistula formation for both techniques ranges from 1 to 5%.
5. Obstruction occurs in 1 to 2% of endovesicular procedures and 1 to 4% in extravesicular procedures; the latter may be due to implanting the ureter into the mobile bladder dome, resulting in kinking.
6. Extravesical approach is more expedient and requires less bladder dissection, thus decreasing the likelihood of a lymphocele and also avoiding a large vesicotomy.

C. Complicated Reconstruction

1. In complicated patients ileal diversion, ileocystocecoplasty, pyelovesicostomy, cystosigmoidoplasty, Boari flap, and psoas hitch reconstruction have been employed with good results.
2. Diversion is reserved for irreversible lower tract obstruction or severely damaged small capacity bladders.
3. Intact, nonfunctional bladders can be managed with clean, intermittent catheterization.

4. More elaborate urinary tract reconstructions have a higher incidence of bacterial colonization, but urosepsis can be controlled with bacterial suppression.

IV. UROLOGIC COMPLICATIONS

A. General

Urologic complications occur in 1 to 15% of transplant series and are responsible for a major proportion of allograft failures (Table 5).

B. Fistula

1. The most common and most difficult of complications to manage.
2. Fistulas usually occur within first 30 postoperative days; they can involve any part of urinary tract.
3. Calyceal fistulas are rare (5%) and caused by segmental renal infarction secondary to occlusion.
4. Ureteral fistulas are the most common and occur at the ureteropyelostomy suture line or ureterovesicular junction of ureteroneocystostomy (Fig. 5).
5. Ureteric injury, ischemia, immunosuppression, and rejection contribute to fistula formation.
6. Vesicular fistulas account for 5 to 30% of fistulas, and occur with greater frequency in previously operated bladders.
7. Clinical manifestations similar to rejection:
   a. Pain and swelling about allograft
   b. Oliguria/anuria

TABLE 5. MAJOR UROLOGIC COMPLICATIONS OF TRANSPLANTATION

Extravasation	Obstruction
Pyelocaliceal	Ureteric stenosis
Ureteral	Lymphocele
Vesicular	Hematoma
	Ureteropelvic junction obstruction
	Ureteric fibrosis
	Calculus
	Spermatic cord compression

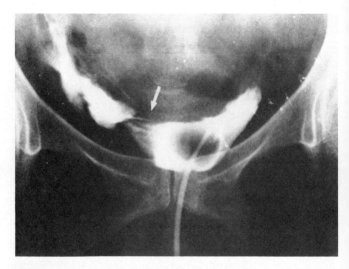

Figure 5. Urinary tract fistula (*arrow*) at ureteroneocystostomy site as demonstrated by cystography.

    c. Scrotal or labial edema
    d. Hypertension, fever
    e. Rising serum creatinine
  8. Best diagnostic information is obtained with nuclear scans and cystography; percutaneous antegrade pyelography, intravenous (IV) urography, and ultrasound are also helpful.
  9. Immediate surgery is the traditional approach to fistula management and still the best therapy for acute fistulas.
 10. Invasive nonsurgical techniques have aided treatment and obviated the need for emergency surgery in chronic or infected fistulas.
 11. Nephrostomy drainage or ureteral stent placement allows for diversion of urinary flow, correction of patient's fluid and electrolyte balance, and performance of surgery under stable conditions.

12. Calyceal and vesicular fistulae can close with drainage alone.
13. Standard therapy for chronic ureteral fistula is ureteropyelostomy—joining the patient's native ureter with the transplanted renal pelvis, after native nephrectomy.

C. Obstruction
1. Accounts for 25 to 33% of all urologic complications in the transplant population; morbidity and mortality are considerably less than that of fistulas.
2. Time course is acute or chronic (reported as late as 5

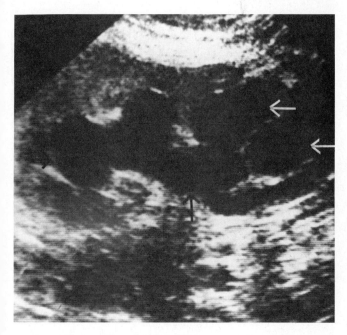

Figure 6. Ultrasound of renal allograft revealing dilatation of the collecting system secondary to ureteral obstruction.

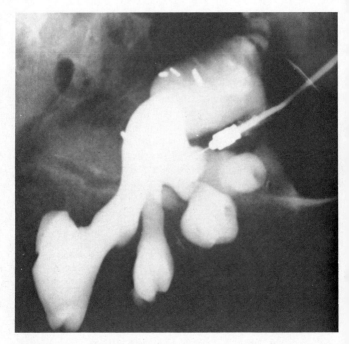

Figure 7. Obstruction of allograft collecting system demonstrated by percutaneous antegrade pyelography.

years postoperatively), and may be indistinguishable from chronic rejection.

3. Ultrasound and renal scans are of great value in initial diagnosis with antegrade pyelography providing the most anatomic information (Figs. 6 and 7).

4. Potential complications of antegrade studies include transient gross hematuria (10%), renovascular injury, or perforation of intraperitoneal viscera; in most series little morbidity is noted.

5. Definitive repair is usually accomplished by reimplantation of the ureter, native nephrectomy, and ureteropyelostomy.

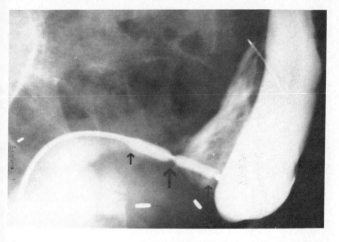

Figure 8. Antegrade percutaneous transluminal ureteroplasty of a high-grade allograft ureter stenosis. Small arrows point to limits of balloon; narrowing is seen at large arrow.

      6. Percutaneous balloon dilatation is employed in some instances (Fig. 8).

      7. Rare causes of obstruction include ureteral torsion, abscess, fungus balls, urolithiasis, and compression by the spermatic cord.

D. Lymphocele

    1. Lymphoceles occurred in 1 to 18% of patients in transplant series, although most recent reports show an incidence of less than 3%.

    2. They are many times asymptomatic but may obstruct the urinary tract (Fig. 9).

    3. Etiology—disruption of renal lymphatics and lymph channels along iliac vessels.

    4. Presentation may be acute with pain and swelling of incision site accompanied by external genitalia or ipsilateral lower extremity edema. More often lymphoceles are found in routine evaluation for deteriorating renal function.

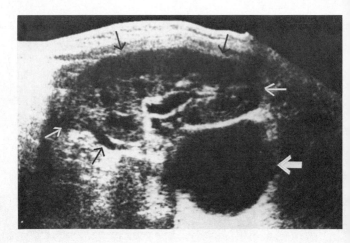

Figure 9. Ultrasonogram of a lymphocele adjacent to a renal allograft (*large arrow*) small arrows point to outline of kidney.

     5. Best treated with transabdominal peritoneal marsupialization.
     6. Prevention best accomplished by meticulous ligation of host lymphatics. Ligation of renal lymphatics is also advocated.

  E. Reflux
     1. Vesicoureteric reflux occurs in 10 to 30% of most recent series and has a questionable effect on allograft survival.
     2. In one large series, 25% of grafts demonstrated reflux and 48% of those eventually failed. The majority of these failed grafts demonstrated membranoproliferative glomerulonephritis, but this has not been seen in other series.
     3. Antireflux and simple ureteroneocystostomies have demonstrated similar low rates of reflux.
     4. In general, reflux accompanied by bacteriuria contributes to graft dysfunction.

F. Urinary Tract Infection (UTI)

1. Most common urologic complication; reported to occur in 50 to 75% of patients. In posttransplant diuretic phase repeat cultures of 1×10^3 per ml may be defined as infection.
2. Of these, 9 to 17% develop persistent infections.
3. *Escherichia coli* is the predominant pathogen in most series.
4. Recatheterization, patient age greater than 40, and sex (female predominance) appear to contribute to the development of infection.
5. Though usually benign, UTIs rank as the primary cause of bacteriuria and major source of many deep-wound infections.
6. Early infections, infections caused by organisms other than *E. coli,* and infection during acute rejection or acute tubular necrosis have been associated with poor graft survival and an increase in septic complications.
7. The role of antibiotic prophylaxis is not well defined.

V. SEXUAL DYSFUNCTION

A. General

1. In chronic uremia this is thought to be related to an imbalance in the hypothalamic–pituitary–gonadal axis as well as peripheral and autonomic neuropathy.
2. Gonadal changes include germ cell aplasia with hypospermatogenesis, oligospermia, and impaired motility (Table 6).
3. After transplant, testosterone and zinc levels return to near normal, not so in dialysis patients.
4. Follicle-stimulating hormone (FSH), luteinizing hormone (LH), and prolactin levels are variable but tend to remain high in both groups.

TABLE 6. SEXUAL DYSFUNCTION SECONDARY TO UREMIA

Germ cell aplasia	Impaired motility
Hypospermatogenesis	FSH, LH, and prolactin elevation
Oligospermia	Testosterone depression

5. Though not fully understood, an exaggerated pituitary response to gonadotropin releasing factors may be responsible for these elevated hormone levels.
6. Several studies show that transplant recipients have a better level of sexual function than dialysis patients and that the majority of transplant patients with long-term graft survival return to preuremic levels of sexual activity.
7. After transplant sperm counts rise but are rarely over 30 million per milliliter (>80 million per milliliter is standard for normal). Transplant patients have been reported to father children but a significant amount of irreversible gonadal damage appears to accompany chronic uremia.

B. Impotence
1. Classically 10% of first transplant recipients and 65% of second transplant recipients were impotent.
2. This was attributed to bilateral ligation of internal iliac arteries and further confirmed with penile blood pressure measurements and nocturnal penile tumescence testing.
3. End-to-side anastomosis of renal artery to external iliac artery is recommended for recipients receiving second graft.
4. Surgical correction of impotence via insertion of penile prosthesis is discouraged since poor healing and infection are more common in immunosuppressed patients.
5. Revascularization procedures have also been described.

C. Testicular and Scrotal Complications
1. Traditionally the spermatic cord was transected for better exposure during surgery.
2. This approach is accompanied by complication rate of up to 70%.
3. Majority of complications were hydroceles but testicular atrophy and frank necrosis were described and the procedure has been abandoned.

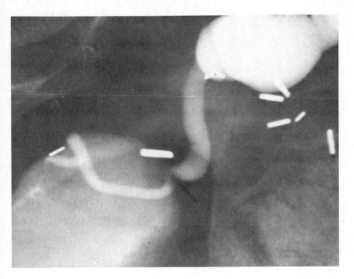

Figure 10. Antegrade pyelogram demonstrating obstruction of allograft collecting system secondary to spermatic cord compression. Obstruction completely relieved by mobilization of cord.

4. Epididymitis occurs occasionally and is due to intra-operative retraction on the vas deferens or prolonged catheter drainage.

5. The spermatic cord is also capable of causing ureteral obstruction. This has been reported with anterior and posterior placement of the ureter (Fig. 10).

VI. PEDIATRIC TRANSPLANTATION

A. General

1. Children comprise 8% of the renal transplant population.

2. Patient survival is high (70 to 85%), with 60% graft survival at 4 years (Table 7).

3. End-stage renal disease is urologic in origin in 20 to 25% of cases.

TABLE 7. PEDIATRIC RENAL TRANSPLANTATION

Eight percent of transplant population
Graft and patient survival superior or equal to adults
Modification in surgical technique required
Urologic complications similar to adults
Few recipients exceed 10th percentile of normal stature posttransplant

4. Major anomalies include posterior urethral values, vesicoureteral reflux, ureterovesicular or ureteropelvic obstruction, and neurogenic bladder dysfunction with or without myelomeningocele.

B. Reconstruction
1. Technical modifications are necessary for the accomodation of an adult renal graft.
   a. Graft placed in retrocecal position.
   b. Anastomosis usually to great vessels or common iliac vessels.
   c. For a child less than 8 kg, a pediatric renal graft is usually needed.
2. Patients do well with conduits but all efforts are made to employ the recipient's bladder.
3. Small capacity prolonged defunctionalization and trabeculation of the bladder does not necessitate supravesicular diversion.

C. Complications
1. Occur in 10 to 30% of recipients.
2. Urinary extravasation is the most common complication.
3. Thirty to sixty percent of recipients develop UTIs.
4. Despite normal allograft function few children exceed the 10th percentile of normal stature.

D. Infant Transplantation
1. Infants present a great technical challenge but have exhibited excellent graft survival.
2. Major etiologies of renal failure include renal dysplasia and congenital nephrotic syndrome.

VII. RENAL LITHIASIS, GRAFT RUPTURE, AND MALIGNANCY

A. Renal Lithiasis

1. A rare complication of transplantation; slightly over 20 cases reported.
2. Calcium phosphate and struvite stones most common.
3. Secondary hyperparathyroidism often present.
4. Total parathyroidectomy with autografting is the major treatment for persistent hypercalcemia or recurrent stone formation.
5. Indications for graft surgery include:
   a. Infection
   b. Enlarging stones
   c. Deteriorating allograft function

B. Allograft Rupture

1. Very rare complication less frequent in recent years.
2. Etiology obscure and associated with severe rejection, obstruction, and renal vein thrombosis.
3. Graft salvage unusual, but when successful, long-term graft salvage has occurred.

C. Neoplasia

1. Relative risk of neoplasia is 80 times that of nonuremic controls.
2. Most are lymphoid or epidermoid in nature.
3. Genitourinary tumors are rare but those reported include:
   a. Renal adenocarcinoma
   b. Transitional cell carcinoma of the bladder
   c. Squamous cell carcinoma of the penis
   d. Nephrogenic adenoma

BIBLIOGRAPHY

Corriere JW Jr, et al: The ureteropyelostomy in human renal transplantation. J Urol 110:24–26, 1973.

Goldstein I, Cho SI, Olsson CA: Nephrostomy in renal transplantation. J Urol 126:159–163, 1981.

Greenberg SH, et al: Ureteropyelostomy and ureteroneocystostomy in renal transplantation: Postoperative urological complications. J Urol 118:17–19, 1977.

Howard RJ, Simmons RL, Najarian JS: Prevention of lymphoceles following renal transplantation. Ann Surg. 184:166–168, 1976.

Masur H, Cheigh JS, Stubenbord WT: Infection following renal transplantation: A changing pattern. Rev Infect Dis 4:1208–1219, 1982.

Mathew TH, Kincaid-Smith P, and Vikraham P: Risks of vesicoureteric reflux in the transplant kidney. N Engl J Med 297:414–418, 1977.

Normann E, Fryjordet A, Halvorsen S: Stones in renal transplants. Scand J Urol Nephrol 14:73–76, 1980.

Novick AC, et al: Results of renal transplantation in children. J Urol 124:787–789, 1980.

Penn I, Starzl TE: Malignant tumors arising de novo in immunosuppressed organ transplant recipients. Transplantation 14:407–417, 1972.

Salvatierra O Jr, et al: Urologic complications of renal transplantation can be prevented or controlled. J Urol 117:421–424, 1977.

Waltzer WC: Sexual and reproductive function in men treated with hemodialysis and renal transplantation. J Urol 126:713–716, 1981.

Waltzer WC, et al: Urinary tract reconstruction in renal transplantation. Urology 16:233–241, 1980.

22

Renovascular Hypertension

John W. Francfort
Ali Naji

I. INCIDENCE

A. **It is estimated that 25 million hypertensive patients** are currently being treated in the United States.

B. **Less than 5%** have a surgically correctable etiology.

C. **Renovascular hypertension (RVH) is present** in 2% of all patients with high blood pressure, is the most common cause of surgically treatable high blood pressure, and is produced by a critical stenosis of the renal artery.

II. HISTORICAL

A. **In 1836, Bright** was the first to associate hypertension and renal disease.

B. **The classic experiments of Goldblatt** in 1934 clearly demonstrated that ischemia localized to the kidneys was sufficient to elevate blood pressure, which, in its early stages, was unaccompanied by decreased renal function.

C. **In 1937, Butler** cured high blood pressure through nephrectomy in a 7-year-old boy with pyelonephritis.

D. **Clinical evidence of the validity of Goldblatt's experiment** came in 1938 when Leadbetter and Burkland cured sustained diastolic hypertension in a 5-year-old boy by nephrectomy. Pathologic examination of the renal artery from this kidney revealed a lumen severely occluded by a mass of smooth muscle outlined by an elastic lamella representing fibromuscular hyperplasia (FMH).

E. Evidence linking atherosclerotic obstruction of the renal arteries to hypertension was described in 1937 by Moritz and Oldt, who described severe vessel obstruction in an

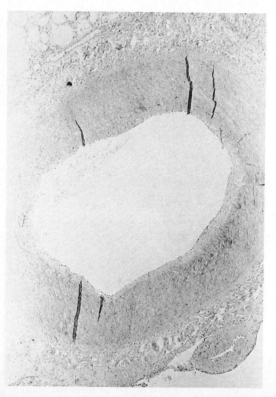

Figure 1. These are photomicrographs of histologic cross sections of two renal arteries. **A.** This section represents the histologic appearance of an unobstructed renal artery.

autopsy series of chronic hypertensives.

F. **Ultimately, it was the development of translumbar arteriography** in the 1950s that opened the door to large scale investigation and clinical correction of renovascular hypertension.

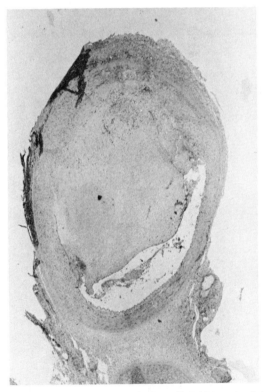

Figure 1. B. This section depicts a renal artery with a high-grade obstruction secondary to atherosclerosis.

III. PATHOLOGY

A. General
1. Significant stenosis of the renal artery as demonstrated by Goldblatt is necessary to produce RVH.
2. The specific etiology of the narrowing may be related to atherosclerosis, fibromuscular disease (FMD), renal artery thrombosis or embolism, dissecting aortic aneurysm, arteriovenous fistula, trauma, Takayasu's arteritis, or renal artery aneurysm.
3. Over 90% of all lesions can be classified into two groups, however: atherosclerotic or fibromuscular renal artery stenosis.
4. Bilateral stenosis is present in over 50% of RVH patients, occurring more frequently in the FMD group than in those with atherosclerosis.

B. Etiology
1. Atherosclerosis is by far the most common cause. The plaques generally originate in the renal artery (Fig. 1). However, they may also extend into the orifice of that vessel from an aortic atheroma. Poststenotic dilatation is a common feature.
2. Fibromuscular disease, the second most common lesion producing RVH has been subdivided anatomically into four subgroups.
   a. Intimal fibroplasia describes a lesion produced by a circumferential accumulation of fibrous tissue at or above the internal elastic membrane.
   b. Medial fibroplasia consists of narrowing produced by unorganized fibrous tissue.
   c. Fibromuscular hyperplasia, also an enlargement of the tunica media, consists of a mixture of fibrous tissue and smooth muscle that causes lumenal stenosis (Fig. 2).
   d. Subadvential fibroplasia produces a severe stenosis characterized by a dense collection of collagen in the outer portion of the media.

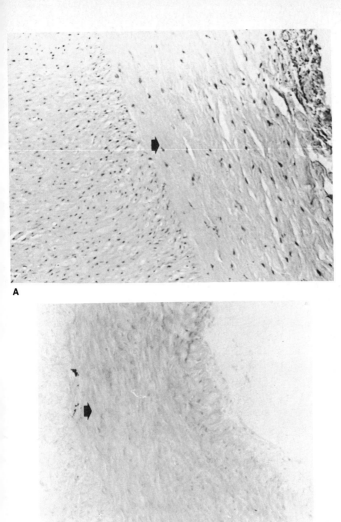

Figure 2. These high-power photomicrographs demonstrate the appearance of a (**A**) normal renal artery and tunica media (*arrow*). **B.** The vessel with fibromuscular hyperplasia of the tunica media demonstrates overgrowth of the fibrous tissue and smooth muscle of that layer (*arrow*).

525

C. Location
1. Atherosclerotic Plaques
    a. Typically occupy the proximal one-third of the renal artery.
    b. They more frequently involve the left side.
2. Fibromuscular Lesions
    a. Characteristically these are found in the distal two-thirds of the renal artery.
    b. They occur more commonly in the right renal artery.

D. Age
1. *Atherosclerotic lesions.* These generally occur between the 5th and 7th decades of life.
2. Fibromuscular Lesions
    a. Most frequently identified in younger patients in the 2nd and 3rd decades of life.
    b. Although infrequent in childhood, fibromuscular lesions are the most common cause of RVH in the 1st decade of life.

E. Sex
1. Atherosclerotic plaques are significantly more common in older men.
2. Fibromuscular lesions occur more frequently in young women.

IV. PATHOPHYSIOLOGY OF RENOVASCULAR HYPERTENSION

A. General
1. The renin–angiotensin–aldosterone system is important in maintaining blood volume, blood pressure, and total body sodium.
2. Hemorrhage, sympathetic tone, posture, and renal artery sodium are known factors that alter renin release.

B. **Function of the Renin–Angiotensin System**

 1. Renin is a proteolytic enzyme that is released from the granules of the juxtaglomerular apparatus (JGA) in response to changes in the pressure of the afferent arteriole.
 2. Renin is not a vasoconstrictor.
 3. Renin acts upon a protein in the plasma, angiotensinogen, to produce angiotensin I, which is then proteolytically converted by a plasma enzyme to angiotensin II, an extremely potent vasopressor.
 4. Angiotensin II also effects the release of aldosterone from the adrenal cortex, which potentiates sodium reabsorption and potassium excretion in the distal renal tubule.
 5. Therefore, in the face of decreasing afferent arteriolar pressure, the compensatory mechanisms cause immediate vasoconstriction and enhance sodium reabsorption to expand the plasma volume.

C. **Mechanisms of RVH**

 1. There appear to be at least two mechanisms producing hypertension in the setting of renal artery stenosis.
    a. Renin-dependent hypertension is documented in 90% of patients with high blood pressure and renal artery stenosis.
    b. It is well known that some individuals can become normotensive after surgical therapy even in the absence of elevated or lateralizing renin values. Current research is focusing on the role of prostaglandins as possible mediators of RVH in this small group of patients.
 2. Renin activity is increased in the renal vein when the kidney is perfused through a stenotic renal artery. Moreover, in most patients peripheral blood renin levels are also increased.
 3. Experiments reducing renal blood flow, but maintaining perfusion pressure, suggest that decreased renal flow per se will not elicit renin release.
 4. Of greater significance is a large pressure gradient across the renal artery lesion or a low diastolic blood

pressure, both of which correlate well with renin release.

5. Pharmacologic therapy designed to lower the blood pressure in patients with RVH interferes with this compensatory system designed to increase kidney perfusion pressure. This stimulates even more renin release and occasionally the hypertension cannot be controlled.

6. In patients who respond to antihypertensive agents the effected kidney may be inadequately perfused. This may explain the higher rate of renal failure and loss of renal mass in patients who are treated by medical therapy alone.

V. HISTORY AND CLINICAL PRESENTATION

A. **There are no distinctive clinical features** that enables one to make the diagnosis of RVH.

B. **Nevertheless there are suggestive findings** in both the history and physical examination that might lead one to suspect RVH.

1. Hypertension in young women and children.
2. Sudden onset of hypertension.
3. Severe hypertension after age 55.
4. The only finding on examination that appears to correlate well with RVH is an upper abdominal bruit. This bruit is audible in 40 to 50% of all patients with RVH and is more common in the presence of FMH.

VI. DIAGNOSTIC STUDIES

A. **General**

It is customary to screen hypertensive patients who have unusual presentations or who are refractory to medical regimens in order to identify those with surgically correctable causes. Although numerous procedures have been advocated to identify patients with RVH, many clinicians feel that the renal arteriogram and bilateral renal vein renin concentrations are the only important diagnostic tests in patients with suspected RVH.

B. Specific Tests
1. Laboratory Tests
   a. Serum blood urea nitrogen (BUN), creatinine, sodium, potassium, bicarbonate, chloride.
   b. Urinalysis with electrolytes.
   c. Secondary blood tests should include peripheral vein renins, measured when the patient is both salt and volume restricted and antihypertensive medications are decreased as much as possible.
2. Renal Biopsy
   a. Percutaneous renal biopsy has not been found to be very useful because of the nonspecific nature of the histologic picture produced by hypertension.
   b. Also poses a risk of bleeding from the biopsy site.
3. Renal Artery Pressure Gradients
   a. This has been associated with renal artery thrombosis on occasion.
   b. It is not as useful as renal vein renins in diagnosing RVH.
4. Radiologic Evaluation
   a. Excretory urogram
      (1) This eliminates the need for the evaluation of renal size by abdominal films or ultrasound and dispenses with the need for isotope renography.
      (2) The rapid-sequence intravenous pyelogram (IVP) may appear to be normal in the presence of bilateral stenosis of the segmental renal arteries.
      (3) Radiologic criteria suggesting RVH include
         (a) A difference in length between kidneys of more than 1 cm
         (b) Delayed pyelocalyceal appearance time (which reflects glomerular filtration)
         (c) Decreased concentration or prolongation in the early nephrogram (10 to 30 seconds) on the involved side
         (d) Underfilling of collecting system
         (e) Segmental renal atrophy
         (f) Notching of the upper ureter or renal pelvis by enlarged collateral vessels

(4) The utility of the IVP is lessened because of a 20% false-negative result. It is specifically for this reason that many clinicians advocate renal arteriography to identify patients with RVH. They feel that all patients with positive IVPs will need angiograms prior to surgery. Furthermore, they argue that no patient should be denied the benefit of cure based on a test with a poor specificity.

b. Arteriography

(1) The value of arteriography, properly per-

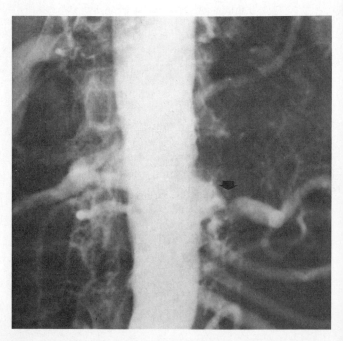

Figure 3. Aortogram of a 57-year-old female with severe hypertension that displays a significant proximal left renal artery stenosis consistent with atherosclerotic disease (*arrow*).

formed, is to evalute the anatomy of the renal artery.

(a) Multiple arteries to both kidneys are frequent.

(b) Atherosclerotic stenosis can be differentiated from FMD.

(c) Although other tests alluded to may indicate the presence of a unilateral abnormality, they cannot specify the site or type of lesion present.

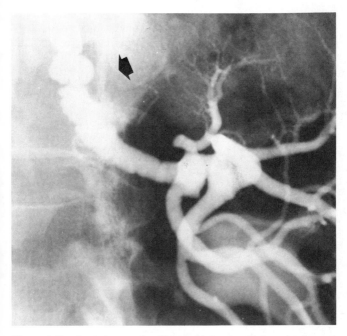

Figure 4. Renal arteriogram of a 60-year-old female with hypertension and postprandial pain who was found to have fibromuscular disease of both renal arteries as well as the superior mesenteric artery. The classic "string of beads sign" is demonstrated in the arteriogram.

(2) Atherosclerotic lesions are identified as stenotic areas in the proximal third of the artery (Fig. 3).

(3) Fibromuscular lesions occur in the distal two-thirds of the vessel and may produce the "string of beads" sign (Fig. 4).

(4) The low morbidity and rare mortality of this test have lead to its present widespread use.

c. Magnetic resonance imaging. It is probable that in the very near future the information now obtained by angiography will be elicited noninvasively with the magnetic resonance scanner. The image from this machine can detail clear three-dimensional re-productions of the abdominal aorta and the vascular supply to the kidney. Computer subtraction of the blood flow allows visualization of the vessel-lumen, delineating plaques or aneurysms as small as 5 mm in size. Because the only contraindications are patients with pacemakers or prosthetic valves and joints, this technology should eventually revolutionize vascular radiology.

VII. DIFFERENTIAL RENAL STUDIES

A. General

1. Although angiography permits the diagnosis of renal artery disease in the presence of hypertension, it does not confirm the diagnosis of RVH.

2. Widespread use of angiography has shown that renal artery stenosis may be present in the absence of hypertension. For this reason functional assessment of the impact of the stenosis on the kidney must be performed. Two tests are currently available.

B. Differential Renal Function Studies

1. Originally proposed by Howard with modifications by Stamey. These tests are only infrequently used today.

2. This test required catheterization of both ureters, prolonged collection of urine volumes and multiple sample analysis of specimens for volume, sodium concentration, osmolality, and reabsorption of filtered sodium and water.

3. Data from this test can be affected greatly by changes in blood flow, perfusion pressure, and glomerular filtration rate (GFR).

4. *Physiology.* Renal artery stenosis results in a reduction of the GFR, which permits greater sodium reabsorption in the proximal tubule and decreased delivery of sodium to the collecting ducts. Thus, urine from such a kidney has a dramatic decrease in volume and sodium concentration with a higher osmolality and creatinine.

5. *Results.* Although this test may be positive in 80% of patients with unilateral main renal artery stenosis, it is negative in patients with RVH secondary to a segmental renal artery lesion.

6. The involved procedure necessitating bilateral ureteral catheterization and possible infectious sequale has decreased the utility of this technique.

C. Renal Vein Renin Assays

1. Current diagnosis is now solely based on the results of renin assays in patients with angiographically demonstrable renal artery stenosis.

2. Renin samples are collected from the inferior vena cava and both renal veins by a catheter placed percutaneously in a retrograde fashion via a femoral vein.

3. The presence of lateralizing renin values of 1.5:1 or greater, in the presence of a low sodium diet is considered a positive test. A positive result, together with an elevated baseline peripheral renin level (>3.7 ng/ml), can be found in approximately 90% of patients who will respond to surgical correction.

4. A positive test has a high predictive value for RVH (90%).

5. It is interesting that in the small group of patients with severe hypertension, angiographically proven renal artery stenosis, and yet normal renin values, approximately 50 to 80% will respond to surgical intervention. Speculation as to the reason for this finding centers on the improper preparation of patients for the test. The lingering effects of antihypertensive agents, inaccurately placed catheters, and the failure to restrict

sodium intake have all been described. Alternatively the possibility of a nonrenin dependent mechanism for RVH remains consistent with present data. (See IV.C: Mechanisms of RVH.)

VIII. MEDICAL THERAPY

A. Goal

The goal of medical therapy is good hypertension control without deterioration of renal function.

B. Patient Indications

Considerations that favor a decision of medical therapy include:

1. Mild hypertension
2. Old age with severe associated cardiac, cerebrovascular or aortic disease
3. The presence of adequate blood pressure control with good renal function that remains stable

C. Methods of Medical Control

1. Control of dietary sodium and weight loss are important parts of hypertension control.
2. Diuretics are generally the first medications added.
3. Antihypertensive agents such as aldomet are generally added if the diastolic blood pressure remains above 100 mm Hg.
4. Multiple drug regimens including β-blockers, calcium-channel blockers, vasodilators, and, rarely, ganglionic blocking agents are often necessary to achieve blood pressure control. (The use of ganglionic blocking agents, while sometimes effective, usually prompts therapeutic intervention in the absence of extreme contraindications.)
5. The use of captopril, an angiotensin inhibitor, helps control the blood pressure of patients who are otherwise resistant to standard medical therapy.

IX. SURGICAL THERAPY

A. General

The goals of surgical intervention include the cure of hypertension and the preservation of functional renal tissue.

Innovative surgical techniques, preoperative correction of cardiac and stroke risk factors, and improved anesthesia delivery and monitoring has significantly lowered present day surgical risks.

B. Risks and Efficacy
1. Most centers now achieve mortality statistics of less than 1% for fibromuscular hyperplasia, less than 2% for atherosclerotic RVH, and a success rate of 90% in both groups.
2. Postoperatively normal blood pressure is found in 50% of patients.
3. Blood pressure is improved in another 40% of patients, allowing for a significant reduction in medications.

C. Renal Failure Reversibility
Recent results from patients undergoing surgical revascularization for deteriorating renal function, including the Cleveland Clinic series, show that over 90% of patients will have stabilized or improved function postoperatively, with over 75% of patients showing lower serum creatinines.

D. Patient Indications
1. Clearly, young patients, especially those with fibromuscular RVH, should undergo surgery to avoid medical treatment of long duration
2. The failure of medical therapy
3. The failure to tolerate medical regimens
4. The deterioration of renal function even in the presence of adequate blood pressure control

E. Preoperative Care and Evaluation
1. Surgical therapy consists of preoperative evaluation to identify patients with a high risk of a myocardial event or stroke. Selective arteriography and revascularization of these areas should be carried out in high-risk patients.
2. Antihypertensive medications are gradually discontinued 7 to 10 days prior to surgery for RVH.
3. One-third of patients with RVH have significant

intravascular volume deficits of 1 to 1.5 liters, which should be slowly replaced preoperatively.

F. Therapeutic Options

1. Aortorenal bypass involves the use of reversed saphenous vein or synthetic conduit anastamosed between the infrarenal aorta and the renal artery distal to the stenosis (Fig. 5). This procedure is most commonly utilized on patients with FMH, although it is also used for patients with atheromatous lesions.

2. Thromboendarterectomy employs the removal of the intraluminal atheroma through an arteriotomy in the

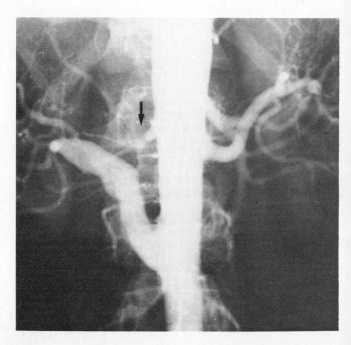

Figure 5. Arteriogram of a 40-year-old female, 10 years after revascularization with a right aortorenal bypass for renovascular hypertension. The origin of the stenotic right renal artery is still visible (*arrow*).

renal artery. Venous patch angioplasty is commonly used to close the opening and prevent narrowing of the vessel lumen.

3. The presence of severe atherosclerotic disease of the aorta has prompted some surgeons to use alternative operative approaches. For instance, splenorenal bypass to the left kidney has been used.

4. Renal autotransplantation is occasionally employed.

5. Intraoperative balloon dilatation, embolectomy, and nephrectomy are infrequently used procedures.

X. PERCUTANEOUS TRANSLUMINAL ANGIOPLASTY (PTA)

A. General

Historically, balloon dilatation of vascular lesions was first performed in 1964. Since that time renal angioplasties have been performed for RVH using a coaxial catheter system.

B. Patient Indications

Indications include all patients with RVH, both those considered for medical and surgical therapy.

C. Risks and Benefits

1. The risks of PTA are low, a mortality of 0.05% and a morbidity of 5%. The most common complications include acute renal failure, peripheral embolization, and vessel damage at the femoral artery catherization site (Fig. 6).

2. When balanced with a 2-year success rate of approximately 90% and a 50% cure rate, it is understandable why many clinicians feel that it is the therapy of choice for FMH (Fig. 7).

3. Although there is a consensus that it is the procedure of choice for all patients with FMH causing RVH, the success rate (70%) and cure rate (30%) is lower with PTA in patients with atherosclerotic lesions than with surgery (90% and 50%, respectively).

4. There exists one lesion that does not appear to be correctable by PTA. When aortic plaques are responsi-

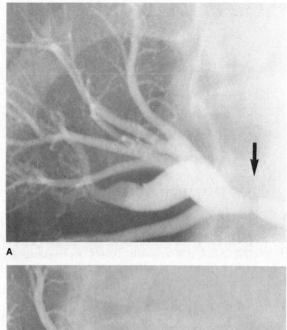

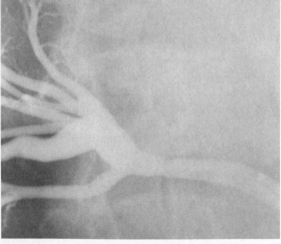

Figure 6. A. Arteriogram of a web-like lesion (*arrow*) in the right renal artery of a 17-year-old male with hypertension for 7 months. **B.** The lesion was subsequently treated by successful percutaneous transluminal angioplasty.

538

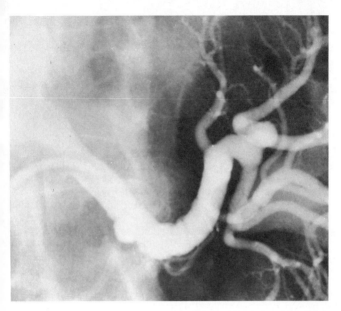

Figure 7. This angiogram shows the successful result of dilatation of a stenosis caused by fibromuscular disease. The predilatation film can be viewed in Figure 4.

ble for inflow obstruction either alone or in combination with a proximal renal artery lesion, the success rate of angioplasty is under 35% versus 90% for surgical therapy.

XI. MEDICAL VERSUS SURGICAL THERAPY

A. Prospective Medical Series

During the late 1970s controversy over the selection of medical or surgical therapy for patients with RVH began to abate as surgical morbidity, mortality, and results improved. Prospective medical studies have contributed to the preference for surgical intervention during the past decade. A series from the Mayo Clinic in 1973 prospectively followed 214 medically managed cases of combined atheromatous and fibromuscular renal artery stenosis. One hundred patients were referred to surgical therapy after the first 3 months because of a failure of medical management (82%) or because of exceedingly severe hypertension (18%). In spite of this, while the death rate at 7- to 14-year follow-up was 16% among surgical patients, it was 40% for those who continued on medical treatment. Moreover, 50% of surgically treated patients were normotensive without any medication. Mortality was most commonly caused by myocardial infarction, stroke, or renal failure— all known sequale of poorly controlled hypertension. A prospective study from Vanderbilt in 1981 confirmed these data in patients that were randomly selected and medically treated for RVH. Forty-five percent of patients had greater than a 25% increase in the serum creatinine and a greater than 25% decrease in glomerular filtration rate. Twelve percent went on to total arterial occlusion. These results occurred despite good blood pressure control in 90% of patients with deteriorating renal function.

B. Surgical Series

In 1975, the Hospital of the University of Pennsylvania published data on 38 patients with no operative mortality and an 88% success rate. Results showed that 95% of patients with lateralizing renal vein renins were cured. One-third of patients failed to lateralize and yet 85% of them were cured. Clearly the selection of these patients on the basis of clinical presentation and arteriographic findings were valid. Subsequent reports up to the present confirm that proper patient selection and meticulous technique results in success rates of 85 to 90%, with mortality under 1% in patients with FMH and under 2% in patients with generalized atherosclerosis. The Cleveland Clinic in 1981 reported such data on 100 consecutive revascularizations on patients with atherosclerotic renovascular disease. Patients at high risk of myocardial infarction and extracranial occlusive disease were identified preoperatively. Coronary bypass grafting or carotid endarterectomy was performed prior to renal revascularization in patients with significant extrarenal lesions demonstrated by angiography. Modification of the surgical approach to avoid severely atherosclerotic aortas by alternate revascularization procedures (splenorenal and hepatorenal bypass) undoubtedly contributed to the 90% success rate.

C. Angioplasty Series

The emergence of PTA in the last decade, first by surgeons intraoperatively and then by angiographers, has lowered the risk of morbidity and mortality even further. The risks to patients approach the mortality and morbidity of angiography (0.05% and 5%, respectively). The success rate approaches 90% in FMD and 70% in atherosclerotic RVH.

D. Conclusions

Overall, surgical therapy can cure hypertension in 50% of cases and lower the need for antihypertensive medication in another 40%, for an overall success rate of 90%. PTA provides success rates almost as high and is the treatment of choice for RVH secondary to FMD. These statistics, together with evidence suggesting a genuine prolongation of life due to better hypertension control and preservation of functional renal tissue, argue effectively for the aggressive therapy of patients with renovascular hypertension.

BIBLIOGRAPHY

Couch N, Sullivan J, Crane C: The predictive value of renal vein renin activity in the surgery of renovascular hypertension. Surgery 79:70, 1976.

Dean R, Kieffer R, et al: Renovascular hypertension: anatomic and renal function changes during drug therapy. Arch Surg 166:1408, 1981.

Hunt J, Strong C: Renovascular hypertension: Mechanisms, natural history and treatment. Am J Cardiol 32:562, 1973.

Mahler F, Probst P, et al: Lasting improvement of renovascular hypertension by transluminal dilatation of atherosclerotic and nonatherosclerotic renal artery stenosis. Circulation 65:611, 1982.

McCombs P, Berkowitz H, Roberts B: Operative management of renovascular hypertension. Ann Surg 182:762, 1975.

Novick A, Straffon R, et al: Diminished operative morbidity and mortality in renal revascularization. JAMA 246:749, 1981.

Starr D, Lawrie G, Morris G: Surgical treatment of renovascular hypertension. Arch Surg 115:494, 1980.

23

Intersex

William F. Tarry
Howard M. Snyder
John W. Duckett

I. NORMAL SEXUAL DIFFERENTIATION

A. Genotypic Sex
1. Defined by karyotype XX female, XY male
2. Short arm of Y chromosome normally contains HY antigen, which stimulates male gonadal differentiation

B. Gonadal Sex
1. Defined by biopsy-proven presence of testicular, ovarian, or both tissues
2. Dysgenetic gonads may histologically resemble neither testis nor ovary

C. Phenotypic Sex
1. Defined by the presence of recognizable external genitalia
2. Least helpful diagnostic feature
3. Presence or absence of functional phallus may be critical factor in assigning sex of rearing
4. Often most important factor to parents and child

D. Endocrine Factors
1. Endocrine state usually determined by **B** and determines **C**.
2. Testis produces:
   a. Testosterone, which is acted on by 5α-reductase to create 5-dihydrotestosterone, which is bound in

nucleus of tissue of external genitalia to lead to male external phenotypic differentiation. Internally, testosterone causes active Wolffian duct development to produce epididymis, seminal vesicles, and prostate.

  b. Müllerian regression factor (MRF), which suppresses development of internal Müllerian structures, fallopian tube, uterus, upper vagina.

3. In the absence of the effect of the testis, the external genitalia passively differentiate into the female phenotype and internal Müllerian structures develop.

4. In essence, intersex states can be thought of as abnormalities of gonadal differentiation or inadequate masculinization of a gonadal male or excessive masculinization of a gonadal female.

E. "Sexual Identity"

1. Psychological Considerations
  a. Sexual identity is not fixed until about 18 months of age.
  b. Uncertainty on part of parents may communicate itself to the child.
  c. Sexual identity can develop independent of physiologic sex as defined in A–D, or can fail to develop at all.
  d. Careful attention must be paid to questions and doubts of parents and children throughout childhood, with preparation for the events of puberty, which may be perceived as an illness when brought on by exogenous hormones.

2. Anatomic Considerations
  a. The status of the phallic structure is the overriding concern
    (1) Corporal bodies of reasonable dimension with potential for growth must exist for male sex of rearing to be considered.
    (2) Prominent phallus should be reduced *early* if female sex of rearing is chosen (see 1b,c).

II. CLASSIFICATION OF DISORDERS: BASED ON GONADAL HISTOLOGY

A. **Female Pseudohermaphrodite** (Genetic and Gonadal Female with Masculinized Phenotype)
   1. Adrenogenital syndrome: Endogenous Androgens (Most Common Intersex Problem). (See Fig. 1.)
      a. Pathophysiology: Enzymatic deficiency that leads to a variable block in the production of cortisol by the adrenal. Hypothalamic–pituitary feedback results in adrenal stimulation and accumulation of steroids above block with metabolic spillover of adrogenic by-products.
      b. 21-Hydroxylase deficiency is most common enzyme defect (90%), producing clinical salt wasting and dehydration in about half, and variable masculinization.
      c. 11β-Hydroxylase deficiency is much less common and leads to accumulation of deoxycorticosterone (DOC), a mineralocorticoid, and thus producing hypertension as well as a masculinized phenotype.
      d. 3β ol dehydrogenase deficiency is also rare and produces ambiguity in both sexes, although males are more severely affected; the adrenal insufficiency may be lethal in the newborn period.
   2. Exogenous androgens are a rare cause.
      a. Exposure to androgenic progestational agents during gestation
      b. Arrhenoblastoma
   3. Clinical Features (Variable)
      a. Enlarged clitoris sometimes equaling normal newborn male: suspect diagnosis no matter how much phallus resembles a penis if the *gonads are not palpable*.
      b. Fusion and rugation of labioscrotal folds sometimes with increased pigmentation
      c. Uterus and vagina always present. Vagina may enter urogenital sinus at any level; most commonly

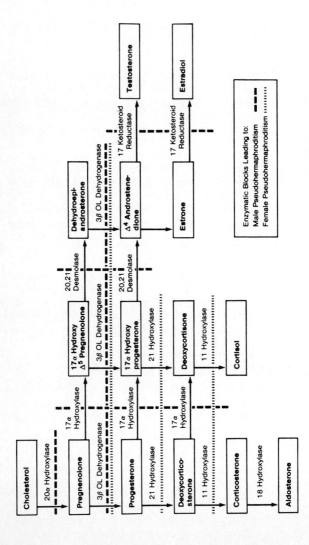

Figure 1. Androgenic steroids produced in both adrenal and testis. *(From Allen TD: Disorders of sexual differentiation. In Kelalis P, King L, Belman B (eds): Clinical Pediatric Urology, ed 2. Philadelphia: W. B. Saunders, 1984, vol II, p 908.)*

low near the perineal opening (which determines the type and age of vaginoplasty)

d. Autosomal recessive pattern of inheritance

B. True Hermaphrodite

1. Defined histologically by the presence of both testicular and ovarian tissue

   a. Each gonad may be all ovary or testis or a mix (ovotestis)

   b. Ovotestis may be arranged in a linear fashion or one gonadal type tissue may be contained within the other

   c. A deep linear biopsy of each gonad is required to establish the diagnosis

2. Rare, about 300 cases reported, more common in blacks

3. Clinical Features

   a. Sixty to seventy-five percent are sufficiently masculinized to have been raised as males, but 80% of these have hypospadias.

   b. Nearly all have a urogenital sinus, and most have a uterus.

   c. Internal sexual duct differentiation usually corresponds to the gonad on that side; those with ovotestis may have both epididymis and fallopian tube, but only 15% have a vas deferens.

   d. Gonads can be present at any level but generally only testes descend into scrotum (rarely, an ovotestis will).

   e. Eighty percent develop gynecomastia at puberty, 50% menstruate; fertility has been reported in both sexes, but is rare.

   f. Some familial cases (autosomal recessive); 51% are 46XX, 19% 46XY, and 30% mosaics or chimeras, but presence of some Y chromatin by translocation or nondysjunction seems to be necessary.

4. Management Considerations

   a. Diagnosis is established only after bilateral gonadal biopsy.

    b. In the absence of well-developed phallus, sex of rearing must be female. Female assignment more frequent now than in past.

    c. If the phallus is large and well virilized and there is descended normal testicular tissue, male gender assignment may be appropriate.

    d. Once sex of rearing is established, inconsistent gonadal tissue and internal sexual ductal tissue is removed and reconstruction as indicated is carried out.

    e. Gonadal malignancy is not common except in undescended testicular tissue.

C. Male Pseudohermaphrodite (Genetic and Gonadal Male with Inadequately Masculinized Phenotype—see Table 1)

  1. Inadequate Androgen Production

    a. Five possible enzymatic blocks lead to inadequate androgen production.

    b. Diagnosis is usually made only after gonadal biopsy, as endocrine assays to permit establishment of diagnosis are not clinically available in most centers.

    c. Phenotype varies from male with hypospadias to near normal female.

    d. Management depends on the degree of external genital development and responsiveness to testosterone.

  2. Inadequate Androgen Utilization

    a. Incomplete testicular feminization (incomplete male pseudohermaphroditism type 1)—a spectrum of X-linked recessive disorders with variable degrees of genital ambiguity.

      (1) Pathophysiology: incomplete effect of 5-dihydrotestosterone (5=DHT) to produce normal masculinization of the external genitalia

      (2) Reifenstein's syndrome describes a family with nearly adequately masculinized males; Lub's syndrome describes a family with very poorly masculinized males. All grades in be-

TABLE 1. DIFFERENTIAL DIAGNOSIS OF DEFECTS IN STEROID HORMONE SYNTHESIS THAT PRODUCE MALE PSEUDOHERMAPHRODITISM

Enzyme	Urinary 17-Ketosteroids	Urinary 17-Hydroxy-corticoids	Dominant Steroid Secreted	Coexisting Clinical Features
20,22-Desmolase	Low	Low	(?)Cholesterol	Adrenal insufficiency and salt wastage
3β-Hydroxysteroid dehydrogenase	Elevated	Low	Pregnenolone, dehydroepiandrosterone	
17-Hydroxylase	Low	Low	Progesterone	Hypertension
17,20-Desmolase	Low	Normal	17-Hydroxyprogesterone	
17β-Hydroxysteroid dehydrogenase	Elevated	Normal	Androstenedione	

(From Wilson JD, Walsh PC: Disorders of sexual differentiation. In Campbell's Urology, ed 4. Philadelphia: W. B. Saunders, 1979, p 1509, with permission.)

549

tween (such as Gilbert–Dreyfus syndrome) are also possible.

(3) Cryptorchid small testes with maturation arrest and sterility are common.

(4) Except in very virilized cases, male sexual assignment is inappropriate and a feminizing genitoplasty, orchiectomy, and a female gender assignment produces a more functionally satisfactory individual.

b. Complete testicular feminization is also X-linked.

(1) Pathophysiology: 5-DHT production is normal but it is not bound in cells of external genitalia secondary to absence or malfunction of the cytosol binding protein. Thus external genitalia passively develops into female phenotype. As testicular production of MRF is normal, there is suppression of fallopian tube, uterus, and upper vaginal development.

(2) Clinical features: phenotypic females with short blind ending vagina

(3) Present with amenorrhea or hernia (1 to 2% of inguinal hernias in phenotypic females). Identifying Müllerian structures (rectal exam or on vaginoscopy) will rule out testicular feminization.

(4) Incidence 1 per 20,000 to 1 per 64,000; behind gonadal dysgenesis and equal to congenitally absent vagina as cause of primary amenorrhea.

(5) Diagnosis requires gonadal biopsy.

(6) Removal of testes is mandatory due to high incidence of malignancy; pubertal feminization will occur with testis in place.

3. Inadequate testosterone to dihydrotestosterone conversion (5α-reductase deficiency, pseudovaginal perineoscrotal hypospadias, incomplete male pseudohermaphroditism type II is sex reversal syndrome)

a. Pathophysiology: deficiency of 5α-reductase leads to inadequate conversion of testosterone to 5-DHT and therefore failure of masculinization of external genitalia.

      b. This is an autosomal recessive trait.

      c. Clinical features: female phenotype in infancy with mild phallic enlargement, large utricle (pseudo-vagina), normal internal Wolffian structures with vas terminating in the utricle; if testes are left in place at puberty, severe virilization (probably due to direct action of testosterone), occurs, with sexual function as male possible.

      d. Diagnosis requires gonadal biopsy.

      e. Female sexual assignment with early orchiectomy is appropriate, as otherwise child must grow until puberty with inadequate male genitalia.

   4. Isolated Müllerian regression factor deficiency (hernia uteri inguinalis)

      a. May be X-linked or autosomal recessive.

      b. Clinical features: phenotypic male with unilateral cryptorchidism and contralateral inguinal hernia containing fully developed Müllerian structures.

      c. Fowler–Stephens orchidopexy may be required; uterus and vagina usually should be left, as vas may run in broad ligament.

D. Mixed Gonadal Dysgenesis (Second Most Common Intersex Disorder)

   1. This is very similar to dysgenetic male pseudohermaphroditism (bilateral dysgenetic gonads in XY infant).

   2. Cases usually have an XO in karyotype; testis on one side lacking germ cell elements and streak gonad opposite (resembling ovarian stroma histologically).

   3. Incompletely virilized external genitalia; incompletely developed female internal genitalia (uterus, vagina, and one fallopian tube usual).

   4. One-third of cases exhibit Turner's stigmata.

   5. Incidence of gonadoblastoma is 27% in mixed gonadal dysgenesis and 15% in dysgenetic male pseudohermaphroditism; tumor occurs prior to puberty occasionally.

   6. Early bilateral gonadectomy and female rearing is preferred, although male gender assignment may be ap-

propriate with very virilized phenotype and a scrotal
testis.

E. Gonadal Dysgenesis (Turner's Syndrome)

1. This should be distinguished from Noonan's syndrome
   (autosomal dominant affecting males and females with
   normal gonads and karyotype), mixed gonadal dysgenesis, and pure gonadal dysgenesis by XO or
   XO/XX genotype, absence of testis/virilization, and
   presence of stigmata (shield chest, low hairline, web-
   bed neck, cubitus valgus, short stature, sexual infantilism and renal malformations in 50%).
   a. Suspect in short female with horseshoe, ectopic, or
      absent kidney
2. Expression is variable, depending on exact chromosome content.
   a. Loss of part or all of one X or Y chromosome
      before first cleavage division results in isochrom-
      osome formation, translocation, etc.
3. All should be raised as female.
   a. Gonadectomy is indicated in those with a Y chro-
      mosome or virilization.

F. Pure Gonadal Dysgenesis

1. Phenotypic females with bilateral streak gonads, infantile uterus and tubes, sexual infantilism, normal
   height, no other anomalies, and 46XX or 46XY
   karyotype.
2. Clinical features indistinguihable from gonadal dysgenesis or mixed gonadal dysgenesis but X-linked and
   autosomal recessive inheritance has been demonstrated, providing compelling evidence that autosomal
   genes influence gonadal development and at least one
   Y gene is required for testicular differentiation.
3. Severe estrogen deficiency may be accompanied by
   osteoporosis.
4. Those with Y chromosome in karyotype develop dys-
   germinoma or gonadoblastoma in one-third of cases,
   which may produce secondary virilization.
5. Management
   a. All are raised as females.

     b. Gonadectomy is required when Y chromosome is in karyotype.

     c. Exogenous estrogen maintenance from puberty balanced with progestational hormones required. The combination reduces risk of endometrial malignancy, which can result from estrogen therapy alone.

G. Miscellaneous Disorders

1. A group of 46XY patients with predominantly female phenotype, and no functioning gonads, have been classified as testicular regression, gonadal agenesis, dysgenetic testes, or vanishing testis syndrome. Variations in internal and external development indicate that testosterone influence was lost very early in some (50 mm crown–rump length) and later in others.

2. Micropenis results from loss of androgen influence after complete differentiation (12 weeks); if central (hypogonadotropic hypogonadism), micropenis will enlarge with human chorionic gonadotropin (hCG). If no response to hCG or testosterone or if penis is minute, gender conversion to female should be considered.

3. Undescended testis and hypospadias (any level): up to one-third will have abnormal karyotype, usually a mosaic. Sterility is frequent.

III. EVALUATION OF AMBIGUOUS GENITALIA (TABLE 2, FIG. 2)

A. History

1. Family history of:
   a. Abnormal sexual development: unusual changes at puberty
   b. Unexplained infant deaths
   c. Sterility
   d. Amenorrhea
   e. Hirsutism

2. Genetics
   a. Similar disorder in aunt, uncle, or cousin suggests X-linked disorder

TABLE 2. USUAL CHARACTERISTICS OF THE CLASSIC INTERSEX STATES

Diagnosis	Karyotype	Gonad	Internal Ducts	External Ducts
Female				
Pseudohermaphrodite				
3β-ol-dehydrogenase deficiency	XX	Ovary	Müllerian	Mildly ambiguous
11β-Hydroxylase deficiency	XX	Ovary	Müllerian	Ambiguous
21-Hydroxylase deficiency	XX	Ovary	Müllerian	Ambiguous
Secondary to maternal androgens	XX	Ovary	Müllerian	Ambiguous
True hermaphrodite	XX, XY XX/XY, etc.	Ovary Testis	Müllerian and Wolffian	Ambiguous
Male				
Pseudohermaphrodite				
Hernia uteri inguinalis	XY	Testis	Müllerian and Wolffian	Cryptorchid male
20α-Hydroxylase deficiency	XY	Testis	Wolffian	Female
3β-ol-dehydrogenase deficiency	XY	Testis	Wolffian	Hypospadiac male
17α-Hydroxylase deficiency	XY	Testis	Wolffian	Female
17,20-Desmolase deficiency	XY	Testis	Wolffian	Ambiguous
17-Ketosteroid reductase deficiency	XY	Testis	Wolffian	Female
Lubs' syndrome	XY	Testis	Wolffian	Ambiguous (Female)
Gilbert–Dreyfus syndrome	XY	Testis	Wolffian	Ambiguous
Reifenstein's syndrome	XY	Testis	Wolffian	Hypospadiac male
Testicular feminization syndrome	XY	Testis	Wolffian	Female
Pseudovaginal perineoscrotal hypoapadias	XY	Testis	Wolffian	Female
Dysgenetic testes	XO/XY, etc.	Testis	Wolffian and Müllerian	Ambiguous
	XXY, XX, etc.	Testis	Wolffian	Variable
Mixed Gonadal Dysgenesis	XO/XY, etc.	Testis and Streak	Wolffian and Müllerian	Ambiguous
Gonadal Dysgenesis				
Turner's syndrome	XO, etc.	Streak	Immature Müllerian	Female
Pure gonadal dysgenesis · XX type	XX	Streak	Immature Müllerian	Female

Pubertal change	Fertility	Gonadal Malignancy	Sex Assignment	Comment
Feminization (if treated)	Yes (if treated)	No	Female	Severe salt wasting
Feminization (if treated)	Yes (if treated)	No	Female	Hypertension
Feminization (if treated)	Yes (if treated)	No	Female	Frequent salt wasting
Feminization	Yes	No	Female	
Tendency to virilization; gynecomastia	No	Rare	Variable	
Virilization	Rare	Rare	Male	
Unknown	No	No	Female	Severe salt wasting
Partial virilization with gynecomastia	No	No	Usually male	Severe salt wasting
Usually eunuchoid	No	No	Female	Hypertension
Unknown	No	No	Uncertain	
Partial virilization with gynecomastia	No	No	Female	
Feminization	No	No	Female	
Partial virilization with gynecomastia	No	No	Variable	Elevated Testosterone and LH
Virilization with gynecomastia	No	No	Usually male	
Feminization	No	Yes	Female	
Virilization	No	No	Female	
Virilization	No	Yes	Variable	
Partial virilization	No	No	Variable	
Usually Virilization	No	Yes	Variable	
Eunuchoid	No (one exception)	Usually No	Female	Webbed neck, shield chest, etc.
Eunuchoid	No	Usually No	Female	

(From Allen TD: Disorders of sexual differentiation. Urology 7. (Suppl 4): 4, 1976, with permission.)

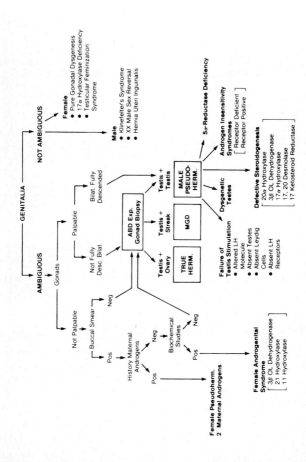

Figure 2. Flow sheet disorders of sexual differentiation. (From Allen TD: Disorders of sexual differentiation. In Kelalis P, King L, Belman B (eds): Clinical Pediatric Urology, ed 2. Philadelphia: W. B. Saunders, 1984, vol II, p. 914.)

       b. Consanguinity facilitates expression of autosomal recessive traits in siblings

   3. Maternal virilization during pregnancy or ingestion of any androgenic drugs

   4. In older patients, carefully note growth and development and menstrual history

B. Physical Examination

   1. Presence of gonad in scrotum or labioscrotal fold is most significant finding. Although in rare instances an ovotestis can fully descend, this usually indicates a testis is present.

       a. Excludes female pseudohermaphrodite, Turner's syndrome, and pure gonadal dysgenesis

   2. Areolar and labioscrotal hyperpigmentation are common in adrenogenital syndrome.

   3. Palpation of uterus or cervix on rectal examination in newborn indicates presence of internal Müllerian

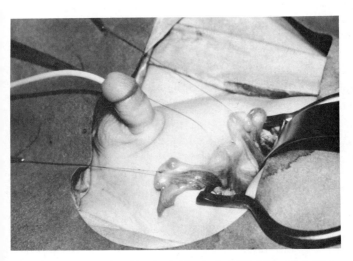

Figure 3. Internal anatomy of hernia uteri inguinalis (MRF deficiency) showing normal testis and associated Müllerian structures found in hernia sac.

structures and rules out male pseudohermaphrodites except bilateral dysgenetic testis syndrome.
   a. Patients with hernia uteri inguinalis do not have external genital ambiguity (Fig. 3).
4. Pubertal feminization, virilization, or infantilism are often diagnostic in older child.
5. Careful assessment of the phallus and the location of urethral and vaginal openings offer little diagnostic help but are the most important factors in gender assignment decisions, as the ability to produce a functional penis is critical to male gender assignment.
6. Note other anomalies, particularly Turner's stigmata.

C. Laboratory Studies
1. Genetic
   a. Karyotyping is readily available now and should be done routinely; Barr body analysis from buccal smear is little used today.
   b. Presence of mosaicism is significant and may only be demonstrated by examining multiple tissues (e.g., WBC, gonadal tissue, genital skin).
2. Biochemical
   a. Beware of interpreting studies within the first week of life, when urinary 17-ketosteroids and pregnanetriol are often modestly elevated.
   b. Both values are elevated in adrenogenital syndrome due to 11- or 21-hydroxylase deficiency.
   c. Specific tests to confirm each block can be determined from Table 2 and should be employed to reinforce diagnosis made on other grounds rather than ordered indiscriminately.

D. Radiography
1. Retrograde flush genitogram is performed by wedging blunt needle or syringe tip in urogenital sinus and infusing contrast under fluoroscopy to demonstrate urogenital sinus, urethra, bladder, vagina, and cervix or uterus.
   a. Helps in diagnosis as well as planning reconstruction

2. Upper urinary tract and internal genitalia may be assessed by ultrasound examination.
   a. Renal abnormality is common in Turner's syndrome.
   b. Ultrasound will demonstrate uterus in newborn if present and often can show gonad if normal sized testis or ovary is present.

E. Endoscopy and Exploratory Laparotomy
   1. Cystovaginoscopy augments finding of genitogram.
      a. Distance between bladder neck and vaginal entry into urogenital sinus important in determining what type of vaginoplasty will be required.
      b. Presence of cervix can be determined, indicating the presence of internal Müllerian sexual structures.
      c. Degree of virilization of posterior urethra can be assessed.
   2. Exploratory Laparotomy and Biopsy of Gonads
      a. Necessary in almost all cases, as gonadal histology is critical to diagnosis
      b. Unnecessary in only four conditions:
         (1) Adrenogenital syndrome: karyotype is 46XY and diagnosis is made biochemically
         (2) Exogenous virilization: karyotype is 46XY and history or maternal evaluation makes diagnosis
         (3) Turner's syndrome: 46XO karyotype with characteristic physical stigmata
         (4) Male pseudohermaphrodites with enzyme block in testosterone synthesis. In most cases, a gonadal biopsy is required because the biochemical assays are not routinely available.
      c. Biopsy should be deep, longitudinal, and include sample of all suspected gonadal tissue; only streaks should be removed prior to obtaining the results of permanent sections.
      d. Careful note should be made of Müllerian and Wolffian structures for diagnosis and for future reconstructive efforts.

IV. MANAGEMENT

A. Gender Assignment

1. The family should be dissuaded from the belief that the child has no proper gender.
   a. Initial statement should be that development is *incomplete* and further tests will reveal the appropriate gender.
   b. Expeditious evaluation and decision is vital.
   c. Family should *never* be told that their child is male but will be made female or vice versa; "true" sex does not exist, is *not* defined by chromosomal sex or gonadal sex alone. The goal is to produce an individual with a functional sexual role.
2. The overriding consideration for male gender assignment is always adequacy of a phallic structure.
   a. All patients with inadequate phallus should be raised as females.
   b. Patients with a large phallus must be evaluated thoroughly, as some will be female adrenogenitals and some true hermaphrodites that may be more appropriately raised as females.
   c. Fertility is usually not a consideration in gender assignment, as only adrenogenitals, some hernia uteri inguinalis, and (rare) true hermaphrodites can be expected to be fertile.
3. Definitive gender assignment (a poor term) must be made prior to age 18 months because sexual identity is established in the child by then. Gender conversion after the newborn period is usually a disaster for the family.

B. Reconstruction

1. Male reconstruction may require hypospadias repair, usually carried out between 1 and 2 years of age, orchidopexy, removal of inappropriate gonads, as well as internal Müllerian structures.
2. Gonadectomy applies to both sexes when gonadal tissue inappropriate to the assigned gender has been identified or the risk of malignancy exists.

    3. Female Reconstruction—Feminizing Genitoplasty

       a. Clitoral reduction is carried out as early in life as possible, as it is the presence of a large phallus that is most disturbing to parents who have been told they have a little girl.

       b. Vaginoplasty is required in many patients either to widen the introitus and separate it from the urethra, or to create an entire vagina de novo

          (1) Perineal flap vaginoplasty for a low entry vagina into the urogenital sinus can usually be carried out at the time of clitoral reduction in first months of life.

          (2) Pull-through type vaginoplasty for vagina entering urogenital sinus high near the bladder neck is usually postponed until child is older.

          (3) Substitution vaginoplasty (bowel or skin graft—McIndoe) is usually carried out when patient is ready to become active sexually.

    4. Psychologic and metabolic support require a team approach involving primary physicians, geneticists, endocrinologists, and psychiatrists; counseling regarding likelihood of involvement of subsequent siblings should be provided; metabolic care is a lifelong process in those patients requiring steroid supplements.

BIBLIOGRAPHY

Allen TD: Disorders of sexual differentiation. Urology 7 (Suppl 4), 1976.

Allen TD: Disorders of sexual differentiation. In Kelalis PP, King LR, Belman AB (eds): Clinical Pediatric Urology, ed 2. Philadelphia: Saunders, 1984, vol II.

Duckett JW: Hypospadias. In Walsh PC et al (eds): Campbell's Urology, ed 5. Philadelphia: W. B. Saunders, 1986, chap 47, pp 1969–1999.

Duckett JW, Caldamone AA: Anomalies of the urinary tract, bladder, and urachus. In King L, Kelalis P, Belman B (eds): Clinical Pediatric Urology, ed 2. Philadelphia: W. B. Saunders, 1984, vol II, pp 726–751.

Duckett JW, Snow BW: Disorders of the urethra and penis. In Walsh PC (ed): Campbell's Urology, ed 5. Philadelphia: W. B. Saunders, 1986, chap 48, pp 2000–2030.

Gonzalez ET, Woodard JR (eds): Symposium on Pediatric Urology. (Sections on Hypospadias, Exstrophy, Female Genital Reconstruction.) Urol Clin North Am 7:2, 1980.

Potter EL: Normal and Abnormal Development of the Kidney. Chicago: Year Book, 1972.

Rafjer J (ed): Cryptorchidism. Urol Clin North Am 9:3, 1982.

Snyder HM: Ureteral duplication, ureterocele and ectopic ureters. In Whitfield H, Hendry WH (eds): Textbook of Genitourinary Surgery. London: Churchill Livingston, 1985, pp 150–177.

Snyder HM, Retik AB, et al: Feminizing genitoplasty: A synthesis. J Urol 129:1024, 1983.

Stephens FD: Congenital Malformations of the Rectum, Anus, and Genitourinary Tract. Philadelphia: Praeger, 1983.

24

Pediatric Oncology

William F. Tarry
Howard M. Snyder
John W. Duckett

I. WILMS' TUMOR

A. General

1. First characterized by Max Wilms, 1899, first described by Rance, 1814
2. Seven new cases per million children per year in United States (350 cases per year)
   a. Eighty percent of all childhood solid tumors
   b. Eighty percent of all genitourinary (GU) cancers below age 15
   c. Seventy-five percent of patients between 1 and 5 years of age; peak incidence 3 to 4 years; 90% of cases before age 7
   d. Male-to-female ratio equal, 1% familial

B. Pathology—Embryology

1. Gross Pathologic Features
   a. Sharply demarcated, encapsulated
   b. Usually solitary
   c. Frequently hemorrhagic or necrotic
   d. True cyst formation rare
   e. Pelvis invasion rare; venous invasion 20%
   f. Extrarenal sites rare—retroperitoneum, inguinal, mediastinal, sacrococcygeal
2. Microscopic Features—Wide Spectrum
   a. Triphasic composed of metanephric blastema, epithelium (glomerulotubular), and stroma (mixoid,

563

occasionally differentiated into striated muscle, cartilage, or fat)

b. Unfavorable histology (UH) occurs in 10% of cases and in three types.

(1) Anaplasia: threefold variation in nuclear size with hyperchromism and mitoses

(2) Rhabdoid: uniform large cells with large nuclei, prominent nucleoli and eosinophilic cytoplasmic inclusions (fibrils), metastasize to brain, may not be metanephric

(3) Clear-cell sarcoma, "bone metastasizing tumors of childhood": vasocentric spindle cell pattern, may be malignant version of congenital mesoblastic nephroma (pure blastemal origin) and not a true form of Wilms' tumor

c. Favorable histology (FH) consists of all other types, tubular predominance being perhaps most favorable of all.

d. Multilocular cysts are benign tumors consisting of localized cluster of cysts with blastema and mature fibrous tissue in cyst walls; they are always unilateral, occur in adults as well, and may be variant of Wilms' tumor. Although they may be a precursor of Wilms' tumor, they are benign and local excision of the cysts is adequate treatment.

e. Congenital mesoblastic nephroma occurs in early infancy, is associated with polyhydramnios, resembles leiomyoma grossly, and histologically exhibits sheets of spindle-shaped uniform cells that appear to be fibroblasts; there is no capsule but when completely excised, it follows benign course; it may be hamartoma rather than variant of Wilms' tumor.

3. Genetics and Associated Anomalies

a. $11p$ chromosomal deletion and sporadic, not congenital, aniridia associated with 20% incidence of Wilms' tumor

b. $11p$ deletion common in tumor genotype; $12 + q$ also reported

    c. Trisomy 8 and 18, 45 XO (Turner's) and XX/XY mosaicism associated

    d. Sporadic (nonfamilial) aniridia associated; full syndrome includes early tumor (<3 years), other genitourinary (GU) anomalies, external ear deformities, retardation, facial dysmorphism, hernias, and hypotonia

    e. Hemihypertrophy (1 per 14,000 general population, 1 per 32 among Wilms' patients) along with other malignancies, i.e., adrenal carcinoma, hepatoblastoma, as well as pigmented nevi and hemangiomas

    f. Beckwith–Weidemann syndrome: visceromegaly involving adrenal, kidney, liver, pancreas, gonads; with omphalocele, hemihypertrophy, microcephaly, retardation, macroglossia; 10% develop a neoplasm of liver, adrenal, or kidney

    g. Musculoskeletal deformities in 2.9%, with 30-fold increase in neurofibromatosis incidence

    h. GU anomalies in 4.4%, including renal hypoplasia, ectopia or fusion, duplications, cystic diseases, hypospadias, cryptorchidism, pseudohermaphroditism

4. The nephroblastomatosis complex appears to be a precursor of Wilms' tumor and consists of persistent primitive metanephric elements beyond 36 weeks' gestation; it occurs in three forms.

    a. In superficial infantile form, entire kidney is replaced by blastema; infants present with massive nephromegaly and die shortly after birth; this is the rarest form.

    b. Multifocal juvenile form or nodular renal blastema (NRB) consists of gross or microscopic NRB nodules that may be sclerotic or glomerulocystic and papillary, usually in the subcapsular region or along the columns of Bertin.

    c. Wilms' tumorlet exhibits triphasic histology in nodules between 1 and 3.5 cm.

    d. Some component of nephroblastomatosis is present

in 100% of bilateral Wilms' patients, at least 40% of unilateral cases.

    e. May represent Wilms' tumor precursor in "two-hit" theory of oncogenesis of Knudson and Strong.

    f. NRB should be sought carefully, mobilizing and inspecting the contralateral kidney. Any area of abnormal color or a cleft should be biopsied; it does respond to chemotherapy, but the best program and the full therapeutic implications remain to be demonstrated.

C. Management of Wilms' Tumor

  1. Diagnosis and Management

    a. Three-fourths present with palpable abdominal mass, usually smooth and rarely crossing midline (in contrast to neuroblastoma).

    b. One-third present with abdominal pain, often associated with minor trauma and hemorrhage within tumor.

    c. Hypertension accompanies 25 to 60% of cases.

    d. Differential includes other tumors and hydronephrosis or cystic disease (see Table 1).

    e. The combination of intravenous pyelography and abdominal ultrasound will diagnose most Wilms' tumors, as well as evaluate the retroperitoneum, liver, and vena cava for extension of disease.

TABLE 1. CHILDHOOD TUMORS

Malignant tumors	Benign Abdominal Masses
Renal: renal cell carcinoma	Renal: renal abscess, multicystic dysplastic kidney, hydronephrosis, polycystic kidney, congenital mesoblastic nephroma
Neuroblastoma	
Rhabdomyosarcoma	
Hepatoblastoma	Mesenteric cysts
Lymphoma, Lymphosarcoma	Choledochal cysts
	Intestinal duplication cysts
	Splenomegaly

(From Snyder HM, D'Angio GJ, et al: Pediatric oncology. In Walsh P, Gittes RF, et al (eds): Campbell's Urology ed. 5. Philadelphia: W. B. Saunders, 1986, chap. 57, pp 2244–2296.)

    f. Four-view chest x-ray completes the metastatic workup.

    g. Angiography and cavography are rarely indicated; computerized tomography may be helpful with very extensive lesions.

    h. Complete blood count, urinalysis, serum creatinine and urea nitrogen levels complete the preoperative testing; urine catecholamines help rule out neuroblastoma.

2. Surgical Treatment

    a. Exploration is carried out as soon as the child is stable and the above studies are completed.

    b. Transverse abdominal incision provides adequate exposure in most cases; tip of 12th rib on involved side to lateral rectus border on opposite side.

    c. Exploration of the contralateral kidney with biopsy as needed should be carried out first; reflection of colon and complete mobilization of kidney are required for adequate visual and manual inspection of front and back surfaces of the kidney.

    d. Resectability depends largely on degree of attachment to liver, duodenum, pancreas, spleen, diaphragm, or abdominal wall; heroic extirpation involving major resection of these organs is not warranted.

    e. Unresectable lesions should be treated with chemotherapy and reexplored; usually the tumor may then be removed. Pretreatment of large tumors reduces the rate of intraoperative rupture but does not influence survival and may alter histology (FH vs. UH distinction). As the preoperative diagnostic error rate has been 5% in the United States, routine pretreatment has not been recommended.

    f. Beginning dissection along posterior abdominal wall inferiorly and great vessels medially with early ureteral ligation allows early exposure and ligation of renal vessels prior to mobilization of the mass.

    g. Biopsy of the tumor or localized operative spill does not upstage the tumor unless it is massive, in which case whole abdomen irradiation is needed to avoid an increased incidence of abdominal recurrence.

h. The adrenal is taken if the tumor involves the upper pole.

i. Gross assessment of nodes has a 40% false-positive and 10% false-negative rate, and thus routine biopsy of hilar and periaortic nodes is warranted; radical node dissection does not influence survival but may improve staging.

j. Remaining tumor in nodes or other organs should be marked with surgical slips to facilitate direction of radiation therapy.

3. Staging (see Tables 2 and 3)

a. A few changes from original National Wilms' Tumor Study (NWTS) staging have been made for

TABLE 2. NATIONAL WILMS' TUMOR STUDY GROUPING SYSTEM

Group	Features
I	Tumor limited to kidney and completely excised Surface of renal capsule is intact. Tumor was not ruptured before or during removal. There is no residual tumor apparent beyond margins of resection
II	Tumor extends beyond kidney but is completely excised There is local extension of tumor, that is, penetration beyond pseudocapsule into pararenal soft tissues, or para-aortic lymph node involvement. Renal vessel outside kidney substance is infiltrated or contains tumor thrombus. There is no residual tumor apparent beyond margins of resection.
III	Residual nonhematogenous tumor confined to abdomen Any of the following may occur: A. Tumor has ruptured before or during surgery, or biopsy has been performed B. Implants are found on peritoneal surfaces C. Lymph nodes are involved beyond abdominal paraaortic chains D. Tumor is not completely resectable because of local infiltration into vital structures
IV	Hematogenous metastases Deposits are beyond group III, affecting lung, liver, bone, and brain
V	Bilateral renal involvement either initially or subsequently

(From D'Angio GJ, et al: Cancer 47: 2302–2311, 1981.)

TABLE 3. NATIONAL WILMS' TUMOR STUDY 3 STAGING: DIFFERENCES FROM GROUPING SYSTEM[a]

Stage	Features
I	Same as Table 2, group I
II	Same as Table 2, group II except: A. Biopsy or local spillage of tumor may have occurred B. Lymph nodes may not be involved
III	Same as group III except: A. Lymph nodes at any level are involved B. There has been massive tumor spillage (local spills or positive biopsy specimens do not qualify)
IV	Same as group IV
V	Bilateral renal involvement at diagnosis

[a]Staging criteria are the same for tumors of favorable or unfavorable histologic pattern. Both staging and histologic type should be specified for all patients. (From Snyder HM. D'Angio GJ, et al: Pediatric oncology. In Walsh P, Gittes RF, et al (eds): Campbell's Urology ed. 5. Philadelphia: W. B. Saunders, 1986, chap 57, pp 2244–2296.)

NWTS-3, itemized in Table 3, based on data from NWTS-1 and NWTS-2.

   b. Staging is the same for both FH and UH; both stage and histology influence survival and must be specified for each patient.

4. Chemotherapy and radiation therapy are given in NWTS-3 according to Figure 1.

   a. RT is begun 1 to 3 days postoperatively.

      (1) Omitted in Stage I, FH

      (2) Flank 2000 rads, 1000 rads in infants

      (3) Whole abdomen 2000 rads

      (4) Kidney 1500 rads

      (5) Lung (both) 1200 rads

      (6) Liver 3000 rads (3 to 4 weeks)

      (7) UH higher doses, 1200 to 4000 rads whole abdomen depending on age

   b. Chemotherapy is begun when bowel function returns after laparotomy (see Table 4 for dosage schedule).

   c. Platelet and WBC counts, ECG (adriamycin) are closely monitored and therapy adjusted accordingly.

FAVORABLE HISTOLOGY

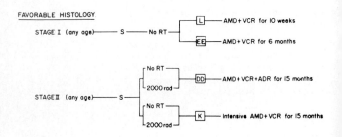

UNFAVORABLE HISTOLOGY, AND ALL STAGE IV

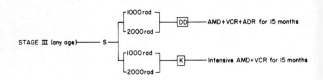

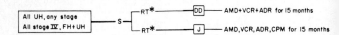

Figure 1. National Wilms' Tumor Study—3. All FH Stage IV receive 2000 rads flank RT and RT to other sites as in NWTS-2. All UH receive age-adjusted RT of 1200 to 4000 rads. Supplements of up to 1000 rads permitted to areas of bulk disease. *(From Snyder HM, D'Angio GJ, et al: Pediatric oncology. In Walsh P, Gittes RF, et al (eds): Campbell's Urology ed 5. Philadelphia: W. B. Saunders, 1986, Chap 57, pp 2244–2296.*

        d. Copious hydration with cyclophosphamide reduces incidence of fibrosing hemorrhagic cystitis.

        e. Enteral or intravenous hyperalimentation may be required.

    5. Metastases and relapses are treated with combinations adding adriamycin, or DTIC or cis-platinum, higher doses of vincristine, and/or cytoxan.

    6. Complications of therapy include bone marrow suppression, early or delayed radiation enteritis, bowel

TABLE 4. CHEMOTHERAPY

Actinomycin
   15 µg/kg/day for 5 consecutive days
   Repeat 6 weeks, 3 months, and thereafter at 12 to 13 week intervals
Vincristine:
   1.5 mg/m² weekly for 8 to 10 weeks initially; thereafter, at beginning of each
   course of actinomycin D and one week later
Adriamycin:
   20 mg/m²/day for 3 days every 12 weeks; alternate adriamycin and actinomycin D
Cyclophosphamide:
   10 mg/kg/day for 3 consecutive days; thereafter, every 6 weeks

(From Snyder HM, D'Angio GJ, et al: Pediatric oncology. In Walsh P, Gittes RF, et al (eds): Campbell's Urology ed 5. Philadelphia: W. B. Saunders, 1986, chap 57, pp 2244–2296.

obstruction, hepatic dysfunction, scoliosis, radiation nephritis, interstitial pneumonitis, cardiomyopathy with congestive failure, and sterility as well as secondary neoplasms (3 to 17% in 20–25-year survivors)

D. Prognosis (Table 5)
   1. Results of NWTS-1 and NWTS-2 are summarized in Table 6.
   2. Current efforts are directed at reducing the therapy for the favorable groups I and II, and improving survival in the UH and group IV patients.

TABLE 5. SURVIVAL IN WILMS' TUMOR

Characteristic	2-Year Survival (Percent)
Group I	95
Group II	90
Group III	84
Group IV	54
(+) nodes	54
(−) nodes	82
Unfavorable histology	54
Favorable histology	90

(From D'Angio GJ, et al: Cancer 47: 2302–2311, 1981.)

TABLE 6. RESULTS OF NATIONAL WILMS' TUMOR STUDY 1 AND 2 OUTCOME BY RANDOMIZED GROUPS AND REGIMENS

Group and Regimen[a]	No.	Percent 4-Year RFS[b]		Percent 4-Year Survival	
NTWTS-1					
I ¼ 2 yrs old					
A (RT)	38	89	$p = 0.85$	94	$p = 0.46$
B (no RT)	41	88		90	
I ½ 2 yrs old					
A (RT)	42	76	$p = 0.06$	38	$p = 0.015$
B (no RT)	42	57		81	
II/III					
A (AMD)	63	56		71	
B (VCR)	44	57	$p = 0.01$	71	$p = 0.01$
C (AMD + VCR)	63	79		84	

Percent 3-Year	No.	Percent 3-Year RFS		Survival	
NWTS-2					
I E (short)	106	96	$p = 0.21$	97	$p = 0.15$
F (long)	109	90		91	
II/III/IV C	159	65	$p = 0.0006$	74	$p = 0.06$
D (C+ADR)	155	79		84	

[a]Regimen   IA = Postoperative actinomycin D (AMD) for 15 months plus irradiation (RT).

                IB = Postoperative AMD for 15 months without RT.

                IE = postoperative AMD + Vincristine (VCR) for 6 months without RT.

                IF = postoperative AMD + VCR for 15 months without RT.

II/III/(IV)   A = postoperative RT + AMD for 15 months.

              B = postoperative RT + VCR for 15 months.

              C = postoperative RT + AMD + VCR for 15 months.

              D = postoperative RT + AMD + VCR + adriamycin for 15 months.

[b]Relapse-free survival.

(From D'Angio GJ, et al: Frontiers of Radiation Therapy and Oncology. Basel: Karger, 1982, vol. 16.)

II. NEUROBLASTOMA

A. Incidence

Six to eight percent of all childhood malignancies. Neuroblastoma is most common malignant tumor of infancy and, after brain tumors, the most common malignant solid tumor of childhood. Fifty percent of cases occur in children under age 2.

B. Etiology

Arises from embryonal cells of neural crest (''neurocristopathy'') that form the sympathetic ganglia and adrenal medulla.

C. Pathology

Gross tends to be infiltrative, micro one of small round cell tumors of childhood. May form rosettes and exhibit neurofibrils if differentiation is good. Ultrastructure shows characteristic peripheral dendritic processes. Graduated degree of malignancy from neuroblastoma (most malignant) to ganglioneuroblastoma (intermediate) to ganglioneuroma (benign).

D. Location and Presentation

Can arise anywhere along sympathetic chain from head to pelvis. Over half arise in abdomen, and two-thirds of these are adrenal. Presents as irregular, firm, nontender fixed mass often extending beyond midline. Abdominal paravertebral sympathetic ganglion origin has increased incidence of dumbell intraspinal extension, which may produce signs of cord compression. Presacral tumors may result in urinary frequency, retention, or constipation. Cervical sympathetic tumors can cause Horner's syndrome. Thoracic tumors may be asymptomatic or produce cough, dyspnea, or infection from airway compression. Up to 70% of patients have metastasis (liver most common in young, bone in older child) at presentation. Unexplained fever, malaise, anorexia, weight loss, and irritability are common.

E. Diagnosis

Anemic if disease disseminated. Bone marrow aspirate indicated in all suspected cases—50 to 70% positive. Ninety-five percent of patients have elevation of urinary catecholamines produced by tumor (vanillylmandelic acid—VMA—or homovanillic acid—HVA—or both). Can be checked on spot urine sample. Appropriate radiographic imaging will depend on site. For abdominal tumors, IVU, ultrasound, and occasionally computerized axial tomography contribute to staging tumor and determining resectability. Chest x-rays, skeletal survey, and often bone scan are routine.

F. Staging and Prognosis

1. *Stage 0*. Neuroblastoma in situ. In autopsies of children under 3 months of age, clumps of neuroblastoma cells are found 40 times more frequently in adrenals that will be later tumor incidence. Tumor apparently undergoes spontaneous maturation to benign state.

2. *Stage I*. Confined to organ or structure of origin. Surgically treatable with 80% survival.

3. *Stage II*. Extending in continuity beyond organ of origin but not crossing midline. Ipsilateral lymph nodes may be positive. Prognosis as Stage I.

4. *Stage III*. Tumor extends beyond midline ± positive lymph nodes. Tumor often involves cava and aorta and is inoperable. ''Second look'' procedures after chemotherapy and radiotherapy may be possible. Survival approximately 37%.

5. *Stage IV*. Distant metastases. Survival only 5 to 7%. Little improvement over the past 20 years.

6. *Stage IV-S*. Patients who would otherwise be in Stage I or II, but who have also metastases confined to one or more of the liver, skin, or bone marrow (with negative skeletal survey). Most common in infancy. Generally, tumor regresses spontaneously without treatment—80% survival.

G. Treatment

1. *Localized disease—Stages I–III*. Surgery offers best chance of cure. Also important for staging. ''Second look'' operation after chemotherapy and radiotherapy may result in removal of tumor. Although tumor is usually radiosensitive, prognosis is not improved in Stage I and II patients in whom tumor is completely removed. May improve prognosis if unresectable tumor becomes resectable post-XRT. Chemotherapy for Stage I and II not beneficial and as yet unproven for Stage III.

2. *Disseminated disease—Stage IV.* Little improvement in prognosis over past 20 years. No primary role for surgery. Radiation therapy has primary role in palliation of painful metastases. Combination chemotherapy can produce response in 70% of patients, but does little to change long-term prognosis. Allogeneic bone marrow transplantation following Adriamycin, VM-26, high-dose Melphalan, and total body irradiation is being studied at several centers and offers more hope for the future.

III. GENITOURINARY RHABDOMYOSARCOMA

A. General
1. Genitourinary rhabdomyosarcoma comprises about 20% of all rhabdosarcomas.
2. The incidence of connective tissue tumors is 1.2 per 100,000 children per year, of which about 50% of malignant sarcomas are rhabdomyosarcoma.
3. There is a 1.4 to 1 male predominance.
4. There are two age peaks, the first between 2 and 6 years, and the second between 15 and 19 years.

B. Paratesticular Rhabdosarcoma
1. This presents with scrotal or inguinal mass that requires exploration to establish tissue diagnosis; radical inguinal orchidectomy is performed.
   a. Histology is usually embryonic sarcoma, rarely alveolar or pleomorphic type
2. Evaluation for metastatic disease should include chest and abdominal computed tomography (CT) scan or four-view chest x-ray and abdominal CT or ultrasound.
   a. Retroperitoneal lymph node dissection is usually performed, as the incidence of nodal metastasis is 40%.
3. Staging (see Table 7).
4. Combination therapy is discussed below, as it is the same for pelvic sarcomas.
5. Prognosis: most favorable of all rhabdomyosarcomas
   a. Group I—96%
   b. Group II—90%

**TABLE 7. INTERGROUP RHABDOMYOSARCOMA
STUDY GROUPING SYSTEM**

I.	Localized disease—completely resected
	A. Confined to organ or origin
	B. Localized infiltration without nodal involvement; microscopic confirmation of complete resection
II.	Regional disease—grossly resected
	A. Microscopic residual demonstrated by involvement of margin of specimen; negative nodes
	B. Involved regional nodes or adjacent organ extension
	C. Positive regional nodes *and* microscopic residual
III.	Regional disease—incomplete resection or biopsy with gross residual disease
IV.	Distant metastases—present at onset (lung, liver, bone, bone marrow, brain, distant soft tissue, lymph nodes)

(From Snyder HM, D'Angio GJ, et al : Pediatric oncology. In Walsh P, Gittes RF, et al (eds): Campbell's Urology ed 5. Philadelphia: W. B. Saunders, 1986, chap 57, pp 2244–2296.

    c. Group III—50%
    d. Group IV—57%

C. Pelvic Rhabdosarcoma
Pelvic rhabdosarcomas include those arising in the prostate and bladder most commonly, as well as those arising in the pelvic soft tissues and vagina.
1. Tumors arising in bladder and prostate usually present with hematuria, urgency, frequency, slow stream, or frank retention, although abdominal/rectal mass is often present. Embryonal tumors of the bladder or vagina (sarcoma botryoides) grow to resemble a "bunch of grapes" and may prolapse out the urethra or vagina.
2. Tumors arising in soft tissues of pelvis or vagina usually present with a mass.
3. Many tumors can be biopsied endoscopically or percutaneously (transperineal); some require laparotomy for tissue diagnosis.
    a. Most tumors are too large or invasive for initial resection without exenteration, so that biopsy alone is done at the initial procedure.

b. Lymph node assessment and biopsy is included when laparotomy is performed.

c. Occasionally diversion of gastrointestinal (GI) or urinary tract due to obstruction is warranted as a temporary measure.

4. Pathology
   a. Embryonal type is most common in GU tract.
      (1) Botryoid subtype is submucosal tumor with papillary component
   b. Alveolar type is more common in older children and carries poorer prognosis.
   c. Pleomorphic type is rare in GU tract and is the least well differentiated.
   d. Diagnosis can be difficult and a generous biopsy should be submitted.
   e. After treatment, identifying malignant cells (rhabdomyoblasts) within fibrous stroma with certainty can be exceedingly hard even for experienced pathologists, but is crucial to management.

5. Staging is same as for paratesticular tumors (IRS) (see Table 6).

6. Treatment
   a. Over half of patients with GU rhabdomyosarcoma fall into groups III and IV (disseminated disease).
   b. Combination therapy with vincristine, actinomycin D, and cyclophosphamide usually produces detectable response within 6 weeks; therapy continues for 2 years.
   c. Radiation is added when progress with chemotherapy stops or fails to occur; or it may be used initially to improve control of bulky disease, doses in excess of 4500 rads being required.
   d. Surgery is used primarily for reevaluation (biopsies) and salvage of treatment failures by tumor excision, usually by partial or total exenteration.

7. Prognosis—Results of IRS II
   a. Overall survival approaches 80%, with two-thirds of patients retaining their bladder.
   b. Only 10% of patients have achieved relapse-free survival with chemotherapy alone.

        c. Relapse associated with ominous prognosis—only about 15% survive.

        d. Non-GU pelvic rhabdomyosarcomas have worst prognosis probably because they develop symptoms (mass most common) late when disease is advanced.

        e. Continuing trials through IRS will determine optimum regimen in future.

    8. Complications

        a. Hematologic complications similar to those seen with the same drugs in Wilms' tumor therapy occur.

        b. The high radiation dose required to control this tumor often produces severe proctitis and fibrosing cystitis, which may necessitate bladder augmentation and ureteral reimplantation.

IV. TESTIS TUMORS

A. General

1. Testis tumors are uncommon in children, accounting for about 1 to 2% of all pediatric solid tumors, and representing about 2% of all testis tumors.
2. Peak age incidence is 2 years of age.
3. There are more benign tumors and fewer germinal testis tumors than in adults.

B. Classification

1. Classification has been debated.
2. Germinal tumors constitute only about 60%—vs. 95% of testis tumors in adults.

    a. Yolk sac carcinoma (embryonal carcinoma, endodermal sinus tumor, orchioblastoma) comprises approximately 40 to 50% of all testis tumors in children. Rarely (4%) spreads to retroperitoneal nodes; more frequently (20%) spreads to lungs, especially if child is over 1 year of age.

    b. Teratoma occurs in about 10 to 12%—uniformly benign tumor in children under 2 years, even when histology appears malignant.

    c. Seminoma is extremely rare before puberty and, in essence, should be considered a postpubertal tumor.

  3. Nongerminal tumors (stromal tumors); peak age of presentation, 4 to 5 years

    a. Interstitial cell (Leydig cell) tumors comprise approximately 18% of all testis tumors, usually virilizing or virilizing with gynecomastia (rarely malignant). They must be differentiated from hyperplastic nodules that develop in testis of boys with poorly controlled congenital adrenal hyperplasia.

    b. Gonadal stromal (Sertoli cell) tumors comprise approximately 10% of testis tumors. They usually present as painless mass and are rarely malignant.

    c. Paratesticular rhabdomyosarcoma comprise about 4% of testis tumors in children (see section II).

    d. Reticuloendothelial malignancy, primarily lymphomas and leukemias, may present with testicular secondary tumor, in 2 to 3%. Patients with leukemias rarely present with a testicular mass and no evidence of systemic disease.

C. Examination

Although all boys with a testis mass will come to surgical exploration through the groin, a careful preoperative evaluation should be carried out. If it is suggested that a tumor is benign, the tumor may be removed with preservation of the gonad.

  1. Scrotal ultrasound should be done in most cases. It helps establish testis is abnormal in cases with a hydrocele. If calcium and cysts are seen, benign teratoma is suggested.

  2. Four-view chest radiographs should be done as a screen with tomography or computed tomography to follow up suspicious areas.

  3. Computerized axial tomography (CAT) is mainstay of retroperitoneal evaluation, although ultrasound can also be useful.

  4. All children should have α-fetoprotein (AFP) deter-

mination because it is a marker for yolk sac cancer, the most frequent testis tumor in children.

5. Endocrine Evaluation
   a. In cases of Leydig cell tumor, urinary 17-ketosteroids are elevated, chorionic gonadotropins and follicle-stimulating hormone (FSH) and luteinizing hormone (LH) are normal or low, and height, weight, bone age, and pubertal changes are advanced.
   b. Sertoli cell tumors evidence normal or elevated estrogens and androgens in urine and serum; 17-ketosteroids are normal, as are gonadotropins.

D. Management
1. Staging is similar to that of adult testis tumors (see Table 8).
2. Yolk Sac Tumor
   a. If child is under 1 year of age, AFP rapidly falls to normal and, unless evidence of metastatic spread exists, he receives no further treatment but is watched closely with AFP and chest x-rays for 2 years.
   b. If AFP remains elevated after orchiectomy or retroperitoneum is suspicious, laparotomy and retroperitoneal node sampling is done. Retroperitoneal exploration is not routinely carried out.
   c. If the child is older than 1 year of age, chemotherapy is usually advised even in child with apparent

TABLE 8. STAGING OF TESTIS TUMORS

I.	A. Tumor confined to testis
	B. Tumor cells in spermatic cord
II.	A. Microscopically positive abdominal lymph nodes
	B. Grossly positive/resectable nodes
	C. Massive positive/unresectable nodes
III.	Supradiaphragmatic disease (nodal, mediastinal, pulmonary)

(From Snyder HM, D'Angio GJ, et al: Pediatric oncology. In Walsh P, Gittes RF, et al (eds): Campbell's Urology ed 5. Philadelphia: W. B. Saunders, 1986, chap 57, pp 2244–2296.)

Stage I disease because of the risk of developing pulmonary metastases.

    d. If metastatic disease is present, chemotherapy is given. Vincristine, actinomycin D, and cytoxan (VAC) with or without adriamycin has been effective. Vinblastine, bleomycin, and cis-platinum are also active and have been used to salvage cases of recurrent yolk sac tumor.

    e. Radiation therapy is used when a good response to chemotherapy is not achieved, especially if bulky retroperitoneal disease is present.

3. Teratoma is treated with orchiectomy alone, or if the diagnosis is suspected, the cord can be cross clamped and the tumor shelled out for frozen section examination with testicular presentation.

4. Gonadal stromal tumors (Sertoli) are thought to be benign in almost all cases and are treated with orchiectomy alone; regression of virilizing signs is unpredictable.

5. Reticuloendothelial tumors are managed by biopsy and systemic therapy.

E. Prognosis

1. More pediatric testis tumors are benign than in adults.

2. Yolk sac tumors in children under 2 years of age have about a 90% survival. The prognosis is worse in older children.

3. Tumor registry for pediatric testis tumor has been developed by the Urologic Section of the American Academy of Pediatrics. Therapy continues to evolve.

BIBLIOGRAPHY

Batata MS, Whitmore WF Jr, et al: Cryptorchidism and testicular cancer. J Urol 124:382, 1980.

Brosman SA: Testicular tumors in prepubertal children. Urology 18:581, 1979.

Evans AE: Neuroblastoma: Diagnosis and management. Current Concepts in Oncology 4:10, 1982.

Evans AE: Staging and treatment of neuroblastoma. Cancer 65:1799, 1980.

Evans AE, D'Angio GJ, Koop CE: The role of multimodal therapy in patients with local and regional neuroblastoma. J Pediatr Surg 19:77, 1984.

Hays DM, Raney RB Jr, et al: Bladder and prostatic tumors in the Intergroup Rhabdomyosarcoma Study (IRS-I): Results of therapy. Cancer 50:1472, 1982.

Hays DM, Raney RB Jr, et al: Primary chemotherapy in the treatment of children with bladder-prostate tumors in the Intergroup Rhabdomyosarcoma Study (IRS-II). J Pediatr Surg 17:812, 1982.

Kaplan GW: Testicular tumors in children. AUA Update Series, Lesson 12, vol 2, 1983.

Snyder HM, D'Angio GJ, et al: Pediatric Oncology. In Walsh P, Gittes RF, et al (eds): Campbell's Urology, ed 5. Philadelphia: W. B. Saunders, 1986, chap 57, pp 2244–2296.

25

Enuresis and Voiding Dysfunction

William F. Tarry
Howard M. Snyder
John W. Duckett

I. NORMAL MICTURITION

Development of normal micturition is a staged process occurring between birth and 6 years of age in most children

A. Infant
In the infant, voiding to completion occurs by reflex.
1. Bladder filling stretches detrusor leading to detrusor contraction.
2. Pudendal and pelvic nerve reflex arcs coordinate bladder neck and external sphincter relaxation

B. Transitional Phase
Transitional phase voiding develops in children between 1 and 3 years of age.
1. Awareness of filling and social pressure instigate attempts at volitional control.
2. Control is achieved by voluntary external sphincter contraction upon urge to void.
3. This results in transient elevated intravesical pressure and incomplete emptying in the *normal* child.

C. Adult
Adult control of voiding develops in children between 3 and 5 years of age.
1. Detrusor contraction is voluntarily inhibited by a subconscious mechanism.

    2. Voiding is initiated by voluntary relaxation of external sphincter.

    3. Detrusor and bladder outlet activity and complete bladder emptying are coordinated reflexively by maintaining bladder outlet and external sphincter relaxation during detrusor contraction.

II. ENURESIS

Enuresis is the most common voiding dysfunction in children.

A. History
1. Nighttime bedwetting only
2. Uneventful toilet training
3. Usually dry days but may exhibit urgency reflecting imperfect cortical control of detrusor
4. No infection, normal urinalysis
5. Incidence in males greater than in females
6. Incidence: 15 to 20% at age 5 years, 5% at age 10 years

B. Physical Findings
Physical findings are normal

C. Radiographs
1. Nearly always normal
2. Not indicated except in presence of infection or when wetting is diurnal or enuresis persists beyond age 12 years

D. Pathophysiology
Immature reflex pattern of bladder emptying persists.

E. Management
1. Reassurance should be offered that spontaneous resolution is highly likely.
2. Treatment is indicated only when enuresis is embarrassing to the child or is interfering with normal social development of the child.
3. Parents should restrict fluids after dinner, have the child empty bladder before bed, and wake him or her

up to void before they retire. Goal: keep bladder empty, as it is easier to inhibit.

4. Tricyclic antidepressants: Imipramine (Tofranil) in dose to maximum of 2.5 mg/kg given 1 hour before bed helps in nearly one-half cases.

5. Wetness alarm systems are 80% successful with 3 months of persistent use.
   a. Principle: psychologic conditioning
   b. Problem: frequent heavy sleep pattern in enuretic often requires a family member to get child up and take him or her to bathroom each time alarm sounds. Thus wetness alarms are not feasible in many cases.

III. DIURNAL INCONTINENCE

Diurnial incontinence may occur separately or in combination with enuresis.

A. History
1. Onset usually after uneventful toilet training
2. Often normal nightly control
3. Usually uninfected
4. Occasional constipation
5. May have frequency, urgency-to-incontinence, "squatting" posture, "figiting"
6. Dry intervals present

B. Physical Findings
Usually absent—rule out subtle neurologic deficit in lower extremity or decreased perineal sensation or sphincter tone.

C. Urine analysis and culture
Usually negative

D. Radiographs
1. Normal
2. Indicated only in presence of
   a. Infection
   b. Absence of dry intervals
   c. Failure to respond to usual management

E. **Pathophysiology**
   Most often patients exhibit uninhibited bladder contractions.

F. **Management**
   1. Bladder training to achieve mature cortical control over bladder: timed voiding every 2 to 3 hours, relaxed voiding without straining, and voiding with steady uninterrupted stream to completion
   2. Uninhibited contractions may be assisted with anticholinergic agents (Oxybutynine, Probanthine)
   3. Improvement in bowel habits helps bladder control
      a. High fiber diet
      b. Attention to adequate evacuation
   4. Suppressive antibiotics if infections frequent: detrusor irritability from cystitis interferes with gaining cortical control of detrusor
   5. Reassurance remains important as the situation will resolve with time

G. **Follow-up**
   1. Voiding cystourethrography (VCUG) and renal ultrasound or intravenous urogram (IVU) if urinary tract infection (UTI).
   2. If wetting persists, evaluate for possible dysfunctional voiding (see below).

IV. DYSFUNCTIONAL VOIDING OR HINMAN SYNDROME

This may also be described as nonneurogenic neurogenic bladder because it has all the clinical attributes of a neuropathic situation but there is no underlying neurologic disorder.

A. **History**
   1. Usually older child or teenager
   2. Voids with intermittent stream, often with straining
   3. Both day and night wetting usually with urgency
   4. Often infected
   5. Ninety percent have constipation, often with encopresis

6. Many have had prior failed urologic surgery, particularly failed ureteral reimplantation for reflux

B. Pathophysiology
1. Felt to be persistence of a transitional phase children pass through in gaining cortical control of the detrusor. Contraction of external striated sphincter during a detrusor contraction occurs as child works to gain cortical control of detrusor. *Persistence* of contraction of external sphincter during a detrusor contraction creates syndrome of dysfunctional voiding.
2. Detrusor contractions against closed sphincter lead to hypertrophy of bladder muscle, high intravesical pressures (with possible secondary vesicoureteral reflux), and incomplete bladder emptying with high postvoid residuals. Recurrent infections common and combined with high intravesical pressure can lead to rapid renal damage.

C. Physical Findings
1. Neurologically normal
2. Tight anal sphincter and full rectum
3. Palpable or percussible bladder; high postvoid residual urine
4. Decreased or intermittent urinary flow rate

D. Laboratory Findings
Urine analysis and culture may document recurrent or persistent infection.

E. Radiographs
1. Renal/bladder ultrasound will show dilated upper tracts, often scarring from infection and thick-walled bladder.
   a. Efficient screening test when syndrome is suspected
2. IVU may show delayed visualization, dilated upper tracts, and trabeculated bladder.
3. Voiding cystourethrogram (VCU) will show "Christmas tree" bladder, large capacity, often vesicoureteric reflux, absence of valves or stricture.
   a. Failure of external sphincter to relax may be docu-

mented at fluoroscopy and may be misinterpreted
as a stricture
   b. Can be most diagnostic study if fluoroscopy carefully done and observed by urologist

F. Urodynamics

These are not essential and can be deceiving. Combined
pressure/flow study with EMG monitoring of external
sphincter may document lack of coordination between external sphincter and detrusor. Syndrome can be intermittent with synergistic voiding in the urodynamic suite and
not at home, and vice versa. Elevated postvoid residual
urine is most consistent finding.

G. Management (Table 1)

1. Infection is treated with antibiotics, and continuous
   prophylaxis is maintained.
2. In child with abnormal upper tracts, effective bladder
   emptying is best achieved by clean intermittent self-
   catheterization (CIC).
   a. As children may learn effective voluntary relaxa-
      tion of the external sphincter to facilitate comfort-
      able CIC, this procedure may assist in the learning
      of coordinated voiding.
3. Early or mild variants with normal upper tracts may be
   managed by timed voiding, double voiding, and
   efforts at relaxation during voiding, with special focus
   on maintaining an uninterrupted stream.

TABLE 1. REGIMEN FOR CHILD WITH NORMAL UPPER TRACTS

Prophylactic antibiotics if recurrent infection persists

Anticholinergic drugs

Timed voiding every 2 to 3 hours

Focus on relaxation and voiding with a sustained stream

Treatment of chronic constipation

Careful follow-up

*(From Tarry WF, Snyder HM: Urology and the primary care doctor. In Schwartz
W, Curry T, et al (eds): Principles and Practices of Clinical Pediatrics. Chicago:
Year Book Medical Publishers, 1986, in press.)*

    4. Constipation should be treated by
      a. High fiber diet
      b. Regular evacuation assisted by a gentle laxative
    5. An anticholinergic (Oxybutynine, Probanthine) may be useful to suppress uninhibited contractions.
    6. With effective emptying, continence is usually achieved and recurring infections reduced.
    7. Urinary diversion (vesicostomy) should be employed only as a temporary measure in the noncompliant patient for renal salvage.

H. Follow-up
    1. As patient learns coordinated synnergistic voiding, the postvoid residual checked by CIC will be noted to become smaller. This is the most effective indication adequate emptying is taking place.
    2. Periodic monitoring of the urinary tract radiographically or by ultrasound is carried out.
    3. Long-term follow up and periodic checks of PVR by CIC are essential as patients can regress into dysfunctional voiding patterns as long as several years after appearing to master coordinated voiding. Usually recurrence of incontinence or infection signals a problem with bladder emptying.

V. HYPOTONIC BLADDER

Hypotonic or lazy bladder is a relatively rare disorder that does not fit the spectrum of patients with tight sphincters or uninhibited detrusor contractions.

A. History
    1. Usually female
    2. Infrequent voiders
    3. Normal bowel habits
    4. Often infected
    5. Day or night wetting with dry intervals
    6. Successfully trained and previously dry

B. Physical Findings
Physical findings may be absent or bladder may be palpably distended

C. **Laboratory Findings**
   Urinalysis and culture usually positive for bacteriuria

D. **Radiographs**
   1. Cystogram shows large, smooth bladder without reflux
   2. IVU or renal ultrasound usually normal

E. **Pathophysiology**
   1. The sphincter relaxes normally but detrusor contractions are absent or ineffectual.
   2. The cause is presumed to be learned infrequent voiding habit with detrusor decompensation.
   3. Upper tract deterioration rarely occurs because the system is a low pressure one (in contrast to the Hinman syndrome)

F. **Management**
   1. Timed voiding and double voiding (achieved by valsalva) are sometimes helpful
   2. CIC may be required until the decompensated detrusor recovers
   3. Antibiotic prophylaxis may be needed

G. **Follow-up**
   Periodic urine cultures and checks of postvoid residuals

BIBLIOGRAPHY

Allen TD: Commentary on dysfunctional abnormalities of the urinary tract. Urol Clin North Am 7:357–359, 1980.

Bauer SB, Retik AB, et al: The unstable bladder of childhood. Urol Clin North Am 7:321–336, 1980.

Hinman F Jr: Syndromes of vesical incoordination. Urol Clin North Am 7:311–319, 1980.

Mandell J, Bauer SB, et al: Occult spinal dysraphism: A rare but detectable cause of voiding dysfunction. Urol Clin North Am 7:349–356, 1980.

Smey P, King LR, Firlit CF: Dysfunctional voiding in children secondary to internal sphincter dyssynergia: Treatment with phenoxybenzamine. Urol Clin North Am 7:337–347, 1980.

26

Congenital Anomalies

William F. Tarry
Howard M. Snyder
John W. Duckett

I. UPPER URINARY TRACT

A. Abnormalities of the Kidney Position and Number

1. Simple Ectopia
   a. Incidence is approximately 1 per 900 (autopsy) (pelvic 1 per 3000, solitary 1 per 22,000, bilateral 10%).
   b. Associated findings include small size with persistent fetal lobulations, anterior or horizontal pelvis, anomalous vasculature, contralateral agenesis, Müllerian anomalies in 20 to 60% females; undescended testes, hypospadias, urethral duplication in 10 to 20% males; skeletal and cardiac anomalies in 20%.
   c. No specific management is required.
2. Thoracic Ectopia
   a. Comprises less than 5% of ectopic kidneys.
   b. Origin is delayed closure of diaphragmatic anlage.
   c. Adrenal may or may not be thoracic.
3. Crossed Ectopia and Fusion
   a. Incidence 1 per 1000 to 1 per 2000, 90% crossed with fusion, 2:1 male, 3:1 left crossed, 24 cases solitary, 5 cases bilateral reported.
   b. Origin is presumed abnormal migration of ureteral bud or rotation of caudal end of fetus at time of bud formation.[1]
   c. Associated findings include multiple or anomalous vessels arising from ipsilateral side of aorta and

vesicoureteral reflux; with solitary crossed kidney only; genital, skeletal, and hindgut anomalies in 20 to 50%.

4. Horseshoe Kidney
   a. Incidence 1 per 400, or 0.25%, 2:1 males.
   b. Origin is fusion of lower poles before or during rotation ($4\frac{1}{2}$ to 6 weeks' gestation).
   c. Associated findings: anomalous vessels, isthmus between or behind great vessels; skeletal, cardiovascular and central nervous system (CNS) anomalies in 33%; hypospadias and cryptorchidism 4%, bicornuate uterus 7%, urinary tract infection (UTI) 13%, duplex ureters 10%, stones 17%; 20% of trisomy 18 and 60% of Turner's patients have horseshoe kidney.
   d. Excluding other anomalies, survival is not affected.
   e. Stones, infection may result from stasis; rarely is true obstruction present (see UPJ).

5. Bilateral Renal Agenesis
   a. Incidence is 1 per 4800 births or 1 per 400 newborn autopsies (75% are male).
   b. Origin is thought to be either ureteral bud failure or absence of the nephrogenic ridge.
   c. Associated findings include absent renal arteries, complete ureteral atresia in 50%, bladder atresia 50%, Potter's syndrome.[2]

6. Unilateral Renal Agenesis
   a. Incidence is 1 per 1100 in autopsy series, 1 per 1500 in radiographic series, 2:1 male, left kidney more often involved than right kidney.
   b. Origin is probably ureteral bud failure; there is a familial trend.
   c. Associated findings include absent ureter with hemitrigone (50%); adrenal agenesis 10%; genital anomalies in 20 to 40% in both sexes.
      (1) Müllerian anomalies in females include ureterovaginal atresia (Rokitansky's syndrome), uterus didelphys, and vaginal agenesis.
      (2) In males, the vas and seminal vesicle are absent or atretic.

      d. If the single kidney is normal, no special precautions need be taken and survival is not affected; management of the genital abnormalities is covered in section IV-B.

  7. Supernumary Kidney

     a. Incidence is unknown (approximately 61 cases described since 1656).

     b. Origin is presumed to be combined defect of ureteral bud and metanephros.

     c. Associated are hydronephrosis 50%, common ureter 40%, duplex ureter 40%, and ectopic ureter or ureter ending in pelvis of ipsilateral kidney.

B. Cystic Abnormalities of the Kidney (Tables 1 and 2)

  1. Adult Polycystic Disease (Potter's Type III)—Autosomal Dominant

     a. Adult type is most common cystic disease in hu-

TABLE 1. CLASSIFICATION OF CYSTS OF THE KIDNEY

Renal dysplasia
  Congenital unilateral multicystic kidney
  Segmental and focal renal dysplasia
  Renal dysplasia associated with congenital lower tract obstruction

Congenital polycystic kidney disease
  Infantile type
  Adult type

Cystic disorders of renal medulla
  Sponge kidney
  Medullary cystic disease
  Renal cystic disease with congenital hepatic fibrosis

Caliceal cyst

Simple cyst

Peripelvic cyst

Perinephric cyst

Cysts associated with neoplasm
  Cystic degeneration of parenchymal tumors
  Malignant change occurring in wall of simple cyst
  Cystadenoma and multilocular cysts

Cysts secondary to nonmalignant renal disease

Miscellaneous

(From Spence HM, Singleton R: Cysts and cystic disorders of the kidney: Type, diagnosis and treatment. Urol Surv 22: 131, 1972.)

TABLE 2. BENIGN RENAL CYSTIC DISEASE

Cystic dysplasia (bilateral, segmental or generalized)
    Potter Type I (infantile polycystic)   early
    Potter Type II ("classic" dysplasia)   embryonic insult
    Potter Type III (adult polycystic)
    Potter Type IV (obstructive dysplasia)   late
Unilateral multicystic kidney
Medullary cystic disease (juvenile nephronophthesis)
Medullary sponge kidney
Simple or acquired cysts (single, multiple)

---

       mans, with incidence of 1 per 1250 live births; it accounts for 10% of all end stage renal disease.

  b. Usually presents after 5th decade with pain, hematuria, progressive renal insufficiency, but can occur in children

  c. Intravenous urogram (IVU) reveals irregular renal enlargement with calyceal distortion; ultrasound shows multiple variable-sized cysts.

  d. Associated findings are liver cysts without functional impairment in one-third of patients and Berry aneurysms in 10%.

  e. Complications include uremia, hypertension, myocardial infarction, and intracranial hemorrhage.

  f. Management involves control of blood pressure and urinary infection, relief of cardiac failure, and eventually dialysis or transplantation.

  g. Pathology. Rounded or irregular cysts located in all parts of the nephron.

2. Infantile Polycystic Disease (Potter's Type I)—Autosomal Recessive

  a. Infantile type rare—1 per 10,000 live births; usually presents with bilateral flank masses in infancy, but can present in childhood with renal or hepatic insufficiency.

  b. IVU shows huge (12 to 16 times normal) kidneys with very delayed nephrogram and characteristic streaked appearance—"sunburst" pattern.

  c. May be distinguished from hydronephrosis, renal tumor, and renal vein thrombosis by IVU and ultrasound.

  d. Associated finding is congenital hepatic (periportal) fibrosis and dilatation of bile ducts with degree of hepatic insufficiency varying inversely with severity of renal disease and directly with age of presentation; cysts elsewhere are uncommon.

  e. Complications are renal and hepatic failure, hypertension, and respiratory compromise in the newborn; patients usually die within first 2 months of life.

  f. Although respiratory support, blood pressure (BP) control, and dialysis can improve survival, the longer the survival, the greater is the chance the patient will suffer from the complications of cirrhosis.

  g. Pathology is fusiform dilatation of collecting ducts and tubules.

3. Medullary sponge kidney (tubular ectasia) is an adult disease pathologically characterized by enlarged tortuous collecting ducts and occasional tiny cysts in the pyramids (75% bilateral, incidence 1 per 20,000).

  a. Diagnosis. IVU shows collections of contrast adjacent to the calyces (''bunch of flowers''), often with calcifications in the medulla.

  b. Complications. Infection, stones, distal renal tubular acidosis, and hematuria.

  c. Medical management of calculi and infections is often required.

4. Medullary cystic disease (juvenile nephrophthisis) refers to a group of disorders with various genetic patterns characterized pathologically by bilateral small kidneys, attenuated cortex, atrophic and dilated tubules, medullary cysts, and some interstitial fibrosis

  a. Patients progress to end stage renal disease by about age 20; juvenile form is said to be responsible for 20% of childhood renal failure deaths.

  b. Medical management of renal failure can delay need for transplant.

5. Unilateral multicystic dysplastic kidney is the most common cystic disease of newborn and the second most common abdominal mass in infants after hydronephrosis.

   a. The left kidney is more commonly involved, but there is no sex predilection or familial tendency.

   b. Origin is thought to be ischemic, from failure of the normal shift of vasculature as the kidney migrates, producing also the associated atretic ureter.[1]

   c. Contralateral renal abnormalities are most common when the multicystic kidney is small and/or the ureteral atresia is low. Vesicoureteral reflux may be present.

   d. Ultrasound is most diagnostic study (multiple sonolucent areas of various sizes without connections or dominant medial cyst and without identifiable parenchyma); as IVU or renal scan will usually fail to visualize, IVU and voiding cystourethrography (VCUG) are done to evaluate the remainder of the urinary tract.

   e. Pathology includes atretic artery, cysts, some solid central stroma, and some primitive nephrogenic structures.

   f. Although the cystic kidney usually does not enlarge as the child grows and thus becomes relatively less conspicuous, a few adults have had problems related to multicystic kidneys (tumor, infection, pain) and it is not unreasonable to recommend removal of the multicystic kidney—usually after 6 months of age for anesthetic reasons.

   g. Many are now detected on antenatal ultrasound but the management and the course of the pregnancy are not altered. If the kidney is so large as to interfere with delivery, antenatal cyst aspiration immediately before delivery may avoid cesarean section.

   h. This lesion is considered by many a classic example of dysplasia, but does not fit any of the four classes described by Potter; in light of Stephen's postulated etiology, it might more properly be termed dysgenesis.

6. Cystic dysplasia, Potter type II, may be unilateral or bilateral, segmental or uniform; although not exactly synonymous with the term hypodysplasia as used by Stephens,[1] it is similar in its clinical and pathologic characteristics.
   a. Pathology. Defined by the presence of small tubules lined by primitive epithelium and surrounded by sworls of acellular connective tissue—decreased numbers of glomeruli, subcapsular and sometimes parenchymal cysts, primitive glomeruli, and foci of cartilage may be seen. Hypoplasia is proportional to the degree of dysplasia and refers to reduction of the size and number of nephrons.
   b. Diagnosis. This lesion may only be diagnosed histologically or by implication from x-rays and the clinical setting; strictly, dysmorphism is the generic term for kidneys that look bizarre on x-ray.
   c. Associated findings. Reflux, ureteral duplication and ectopia, and urethral valves; this type of dysplasia is rarely associated with upper tract obstruction alone and may be seen in the otherwise normal urinary tract.
   d. Origin. It may be an abnormal location or timing of ureteral bud formation[1] or some unknown teratogenic factor;[2] dysplasia is rarely familial, except when associated with familial form of vesicoureteric reflux.
   e. It must be distinguished from cortical atrophy or oligonephronia, and hydronephrotic changes in nephron.
7. Cystic dysplasia, Potter type IV, consists primarily of subcapsular cysts and few primitive tubules that may represent the late onset of an inducing factor affecting only the last few generations of nephrons.
   a. Cystic dysplasia, Potter type IV, is present to some degree in most obstructed systems and is rarely seen alone.
   b. It is usually bilateral, classically described in patients with urethral valves regardless of presence of reflux.

C. **Collecting System Abnormalities**
1. Calyceal diverticulum occurs in 4.5 per 1000 urograms.
    a. Origin is failure of degeneration of third and fourth order branches of ureteral bud, leaving a pocket lined by transitional epithelium connected to the collecting system near the calyceal fornix.
    b. In about one-third of patients, stones will form; some will become sites of persistent infection due to stasis; the rest are asymptomatic.
    c. Treatment involves removal of stones, drainage of pus and marsupialization to the renal surface with closure of the collecting system and cauterization of the epithelium.
2. Hydrocalycosis is a rare lesion involving vascular compression, cicatrization or achalasia of the infundibulum; it rarely requires any intervention.
3. Megacalycosis is a rare lesion involving all of one or both kidneys, defined as dilated unobstructed calyces usually numbering more than 25 per kidney (normal 8 to 10). It may be confused radiographically with obstructive uropathy.
    a. Megacalycosis results from combination of faulty ureteral bud division, hypoplasia of juxtamedullary glomeruli, and maldevelopment of calyceal musculature.
    b. It may be associated with stones or infection but in itself causes no deterioration of renal function.
4. Infundibulopelvic stenosis may involve part or all of one or both kidneys.
    a. The calyces become quite large but usually no progressive functional deterioration occurs.
    b. May be associated with dysplasia and lower tract anomalies (e.g., urethral valves).
5. Ureteropelvic junction obstruction is the usual cause of the most common abdominal mass in children (hydronephrosis).
    a. Male predominance in children is 2:1, with left-sided predominance in all ages.
    b. Several etiologies have been postulated, including segmental muscular attenuation, or malorientation,

true stenosis, angulation, and extrinsic compression. Crossing vessels are implicated in about 20 to 30% of cases, but an intrinsic lesion of some sort (either noncompliant or nonconducting) is most often found.

c. Associated findings include reflux (5 to 10%), contralateral agenesis (5%), and contralateral UPJ (10%), with dysplasia, multicystic kidney, or other urologic anomaly occasionally seen.

d. Symptoms and signs include episodic flank pain, flank mass, hematuria, infection, nausea and vomiting, and sometimes uremia. In infants, the flank mass may be the only sign, whereas the older child will exhibit any of the others; very often GI distress or poorly localized upper abdominal pain are the only symptoms.

e. Radiologic findings are delayed excretion on the affected side, with variable dilatation of pelvis and calyces or even nonvisualization on the intravenous urogram (IVU); on ultrasound, multiple interconnected lucencies with dominant medial lucency and identifiable cortical rim; there is usually some measurable function on renal scan. When function is fairly good, the drainage will be delayed even in the face of lasix administration beyond 20 minutes.

f. Prompt surgical repair by excision of the narrow segment and spatulated reanastomosis of ureter to tailored renal pelvis is indicated in all but equivocal cases; these may be watched some months for a change in the scan findings.

g. Follow-up consists of an IVU at 3 months and 1 year postoperatively in most cases.

D. Ureteral Anomalies

1. Duplication of ureter occurs in 1 per 125 autopsies; 1.6:1 female, 85% unilateral.

   a. This seems to arise from two ureteral buds meeting the metanephros in most cases, but it may also be caused by a bud that bifurcates immediately after arising, before meeting the metanephros.

     b. Associated with reflux, renal scarring and dilatation (29%), ectopic insertion (3%), large kidneys with excess calyces, dysplasia/hypoplasia, infection, and ureteroceles.

     c. Duplication per se is of no clinical significance but the associated anomalies may require intervention (see ureterocele, ectopia, etc.).

2. Atresia is usually associated with multicystic–dysplastic kidney; distal segment atresia is often associated with contralateral hydronephrosis or dysplasia (50%).

3. Megaureter carries a 3:1 male and 3:1 left-sided predominance; the term has been used rather loosely to describe any dilated ureter, but there are three distinct types that should be distinguished.

     a. Refluxing type may originate because of the reflux, although some cases have an abnormal distal segment and some element of obstruction.

     b. A widened ureteral bud gives rise to a ureter dilated down to the orifice which is in the normal position, and there is no obstruction (nonreflux, nonobstructed type).

     c. The primary obstructed type is most common and results from a stenotic or aperistaltic distal short segment; the orifice is in the normal position.

     d. The refluxing type with its laterally ectopic orifice may be associated with a kidney that is dysplastic, scarred by infection, or both; the other types drain normal or hydronephrotic kidneys.

     e. The IVU will show moderate-to-severe hydronephrosis and proportionately greater ureteral dilatation; the VCUG diagnoses the reflux type; a diuretic renogram may be needed to distinguish obstructed from nonobstructed types.

     f. There are mild primary obstructed megaureters with only a spindle-shaped dilatation of the distal ureter and normal (sharp) calyces; these require no treatment.

     g. Operative correction is needed for most obstructed and refluxing megaureters. Refluxing ones more commonly require tailoring than obstructed ones which tend to decrease in caliber after excision of the aperistaltic distal segment. Tailoring by imbrication or folding may be preferable to resectional tailoring.

h. Follow-up includes IVU and VCUG at 3 months and an IVU 1 year postoperatively with further studies as indicated by findings. The reflux megaureter carries about a 40% risk of persistent reflux and 10 to 20% risk of obstruction, requiring repeat surgery.

4. Vesicoureteric reflux occurs at a rate of approximately 1 per 1000 in the general population, but is 8 to 40 times more frequent in affected families; it will be found in 50% of infants and 30% of children with a urinary tract infection.

a. It may occur because the ureteral bud arises ectopically, leading to a laterally placed orifice and short submucosal tunnel, or because the development of the intrinsic smooth muscle of the distal ureteral segment is delayed or incomplete. High intravesical pressures may cause a marginally competent ureterovesical junction to reflux and evidence is growing that voiding dysfunction may cause reflux.

b. Duplicated ureters and renal hypodysplasia may be associated with refluxing ureters with laterally ectopic orifices; infection and renal scarring are prominent findings with all types of refluxing ureters, regardless of grade; voiding dysfunction and urethral obstruction by valves are associated with an acquired form of reflux.

c. Reflux is graded I to V by the International Reflux Study system (Fig. 1).

d. All children with reflux should be placed on prophylactic antibiotics at one-quarter to one-half the therapeutic dose given once a day. Trimethoprimsulfamethoxazole and nitrofurantoin are the most commonly used drugs. They should have urine cultures every 3 to 4 months or when symptomatic.

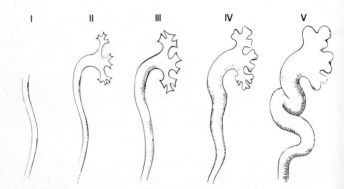

Figure 1. International classification of vesicoureteral reflux. Grade I—Ureter only. Grade II—Ureter, pelvis and calyces; no dilatation, normal calyceal fornices. Grade III—Mild or moderate dilatation and/or tortuosity of the ureter, and mild or moderate dilatation of renal pelvis *but no or slight blunting of the fornices.* Grade IV—Moderate dilatation and/or tortuosity of ureter and moderate dilatation of renal pelvis and calyces; *complete obliteration of sharp angle of fornices BUT maintenance of papillary impressions in majority of calyces.* Grade V—Gross dilatation and tortuosity of ureter; gross dilatation of renal pelvis and calyces; papillary impressions are no longer visible in majority of calyces. *(From Duckett JW, Levitt S: Medical vs surgical treatment of vesicoureteral reflux: an international collaborative prospective study. J Urol 125: 277, 1981.)*

They require periodic upper tract radiographic assessment and reevaluation of their reflux by VCUG or nuclear voiding cystourethrogram. We prefer annual follow-up and employ ultrasound or IVU and nuclear cystogram, but some centers choose a longer interval and use DMSA renal scan to visualize renal scarring.

e. Grades I to III (minimally dilated) are usually initially treated medically; the management of Grade IV remains debatable until the completion of the International Reflux Study; Grade V is usually treated surgically.

f. Reimplantation of the refluxing unit by the Cohen technique is the standard surgical management, with greater than 90% success; duplicated ureters are reimplanted in their common distal muscular sheath; other associated anomalies are covered elsewhere in text.

   g. Breakthrough infections, failure to comply with the regimen, persistent reflux into puberty in females, increasing grade, progressive scarring, and worsening renal function are all considerations in favor of surgical intervention, but there are no absolute indications for surgery for reflux.

5. The incidence of ureteral ectopia is about 1 per 1900; ectopic ureters are duplex in 80% of females, more often single in males; there is a 3:1 female predominance, and about 10% are bilateral.

   a. The etiology lies in a higher than normal origin of the ureteral bud on the mesonephric duct, resulting in a distal position for the ureteral orifice.

   b. Locations are shown in Table 3.

   c. Associated findings

      (1) Renal dysplasia correlates with degree of ectopy.

      (2) Single ectopic ureter is accompanied by contralateral duplication in 80%.

      (3) Incontinence and ureteral obstruction are variable findings; incontinence may be due to the orifice being located below the sphincter in female.

TABLE 3. LOCATIONS OF ECTOPIC URETERAL ORIFICE

Males	
Urethra	47%
Utricle	10%
Seminal vesicle	33%
Ejaculatory duct	5%
Vas deferens	5%
Females	
Urethra	35%
Vestibule	34%
Vagina	25%
Cervix or uterus	5%
Gartner's duct or urethral diverticulum	1%

        (4) Bilateral single ectopic ureters lead to poorly developed bladder and incontinence due to bladder neck incompetence.

    d. Management is most often removal of renal segment and the ectopic ureter; rarely, segment may be salvageable by ureteroureterostomy or reimplantation.

  6. Ureterocele occurs with a frequency between 1 per 500 and 1 per 4000 autopsies, accounting for about 1% of pediatric urologic admissions, and is bilateral in 10 to 15% of cases.

    a. The embryologic origin is thought to be a combination of an abnormal ureteral bud with either a stenotic orifice or involvement of the distal ureter in the expansion of the vesicourethral canal. The ureter is usually duplicated in children with the ureterocele affecting the upper pole ureter; single system ureterocele subtending a single ureter is less common in children.

    b. Associated anomalies include contralateral ureteral duplication in 50%, renal segmental dysplasia, renal fusion, ectopia, reflux (50%), and, rarely, incontinence.

    c. Classification has recently been simplified (Table 4).

    d. Caecoureterocele, a subclassification of ectopic ureterocele, differs in that a "caecum" extends beyond the orifice down the urethra; these may be associated with poor bladder neck and urethral muscularization and incontinence.

TABLE 4. URETEROCELE CLASSIFICATION

Single—adult type with single ureter.

Intravesical—entire ureterocele, including the usually stenotic orifice contained within bladder.

Ectopic—part of ureterocele, including orifice, with extension into urethra.

(From Glassberg KI, Braren V, et al: Suggested terminology for duplex systems, ectopic ureters and ureteroceles. J Urol 132:1153–1154, 1984.)

    e. Management is controversial.

       (1) Removal of associated upper pole of involved kidney with decompression but not excision of the ureterocele is generally accepted and may be sufficient in 50 to 75% of cases.

       (2) The remainder require subsequent lower pole reimplant, usually for persistent reflux, and resection of ureterocele.

       (3) Some prefer total correction [(1) + (2)] at first stage.

       (4) In rare cases, the upper pole functions sufficiently to warrant salvage, usually by ureteroureterostomy and lower pole ureteral reimplant with ureterocele resection or resection plus reimplant of both ureters. Function of upper pole on initial IVU merits consideration of upper pole salvage.

II. LOWER URINARY TRACT

A. Exstrophy/Epispadias—Spectrum of Anomalies

    1. Origin is failure of cloacal membrane to migrate toward perineum at 4 weeks' gestation, preventing ingrowth of lateral mesoderm and coalescence of genital tubercles.

      a. Most consistent finding is some degree of separation of symphysis pubis.

      b. Epispadias (30%) may be penopubic with incontinence in males (55%), penile (20%) with or without incontinence, balanitic (5%), or it may occur in females with incontinence (20%). It consists of a dorsal meatus with a distal mucosal groove, flattened glans, or bifid clitoris; in males, there is variable dorsal chordee with shortening of the corporal bodies in severe forms (penopubic).

      c. The penile and balanitic types are managed by creating a distal neourethra by Duplay tube or reversed island flap techniques analogous to hypospadias repair; the penopubic type is managed like

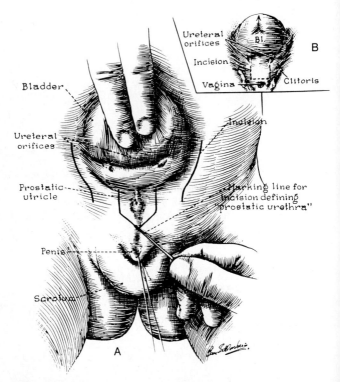

Figure 2. Diagrams of primary exstrophy reconstruction. **A.** Outline of incisions distal to the verumontanum and paraexstrophy skin areas. **B.** Similar division of urethral plate in the female. (**A,B,C,D,G** From Jeffs RD: Exstrophy. In Harrison JH, Gittes RF, et al. (eds): Campbell's Urology, ed 4. Philadelphia: W. B. Saunders, 1978; **I,J** From King LR: Exstrophy of the bladder and related disorders. In Resnick MI (ed): Current Trends in Urology. Baltimore: Williams & Wilkins, 1982; **E,F,H** From Duckett JW, Caldamone AA: Anomalies of the Urinary Tract: Bladder and Urachus. In King L, Kelalis P, Belman B (eds): Clinical Pediatric Urology, ed 2. Philadelphia: W. B. Saunders, 1984, vol II, pp 731–733.)

exstrophy in that continence and penile lengthening must be achieved, as well as cosmetic repair.

d. Classic exstrophy (60%) occurs in 1 of 30,000 births, with 3:1 male predominance; bladder and

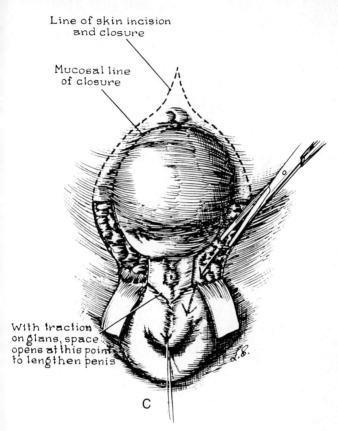

Figure 2. C. Development of paraexstrophy skin flaps and incisional lines showing excision of umbilicus.

urethra are open dorsally, and the penis is short or the clitoris is bifid.

e. Clocacal exstrophy (10%) results from the addition of failure of the urorectal septum to descend and occurs approximately in 1 of 200,000 births, about equally in males and females.

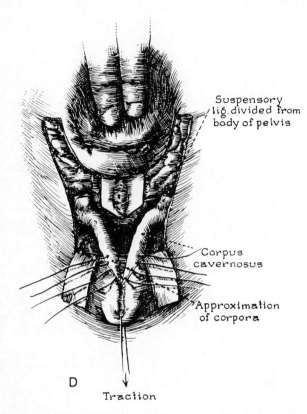

Figure 2. D. Mobilization of proximal urethral and prostate. The urogenital diaphragm is divided from the attached but separated pubic symphysis and the bladder, prostate and prostatic urethra drop down into the pelvis. Penile lengthening is done at this stage, separating the attachments to the pubic rami on either side and lengthening the penis.

2. Associated Findings
    a. In classic exstrophy, undescended testis and inguinal hernias are common; often the infraumbilical rectus fails to develop; vaginal stenosis and/or bifid uterus may be present; the upper urinary tract is normal.

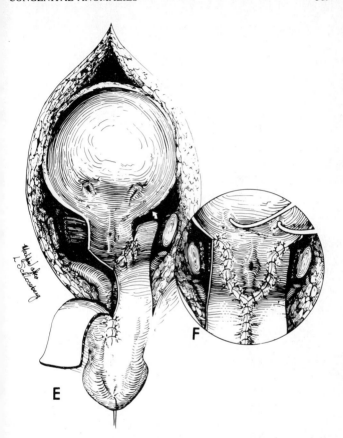

Figure 2. E. Approximation of paraexstrophy flaps in the midline and encircling the prostatic urethra and bladder neck as depicted in F.

      b. In cloacal exstrophy, there is a vesicointestinal fissure opening into the center of the exstrophied bladder, short blind distal colon, absent or duplicated appendix, and often omphalocele; two-thirds of females have absent or duplex and stenotic vagina; 50% have myelomeningocele; penis or clitoris is bifid or may be absent.

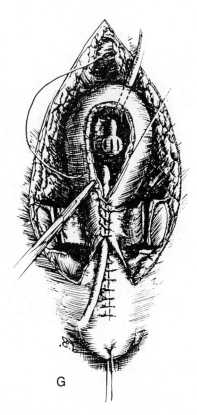

Figure 2. G. Closure of the bladder and bladder neck area. No attempt is made to tighten the epithelial tube between bladder and urethra.

3. Exstrophy is managed in stages, beginning with bladder closure in the newborn period (Fig. 2).
   a. Penile lengthening by freeing corpora from pubic bone attachments and dividing the urethral plate is accomplished at the same sitting.
   b. In cloacal exstrophy, the omphalocele and vesicoenteric fissure must be dealt with by lateral

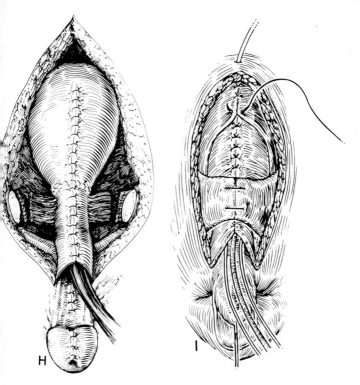

Figure 2. H. Tubularization at the abdominal wall lengthening the urethra. **I.** Closure of the symphysis pubis; in the newborn this can be done without osteotomies.

closure of the bowel and end colostomy and omphalocele repair.

4. The second stage is now epispadias repair, in most cases at about age 1 to 2 years.
   a. Some children whose bladders are too small to be functional may undergo ureterosigmoidostomy (USO) at this stage.
5. The third stage in those with functioning bladders suf-

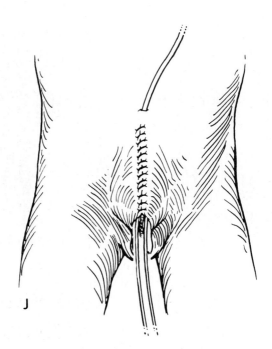

Figure 2. J. Ureteral stents French size 5F up each ureter and a small suprapubic tube. Abdominal wall closure is in a midline fashion.

ficiently large is achievement of continence by bladder neck tubularization (60% success).

a. Those who fail this are candidates for an artificial sphincter.

b. Those who do not tolerate USO can be converted to sigmoid bladder augmentation with bladder neck tubularization (Arap procedure).

c. Most cloacal exstrophy patients have undergone early ileal loop diversion but a few may be reconstructed along the same principles; virtually all males, however, should be gender converted to female because the phallus is usually unreconstructable.

6. All patients require careful follow-up throughout life with survey of the upper tracts by IVU or ultrasound, monitoring of acid–base balance with USO, renal function tests, and supportive counseling; each case must be largely individualized within this general outline.

B. Urachus

Patent urachus and persistence of portions of the urachus as cysts result from failure of fibrosis of the cranial embryonic bladder segment; they are treated by excision when symptomatic; in a few cases, they may undergo malignant transformation (adenocarcinoma).

C. Posterior Urethral Valves, Type I

1. *Incidence*. In boys, 1 per 5000 to 1 per 8000, with more than 50% diagnosed in 1st year of life, generally where the obstruction is more severe.

2. Etiology proposed is failure of regression of the terminal segment of the mesonephric duct, which is normally represented by the plicae colliculi; Type II valves are nonobstructing normal folds in the prostatic urethra; Type III valves represent either more marked anterior fusion of the valve leaflets or congenital urethral membrane (a separate embryologic entity).

3. Associated Findings

    a. Vesicoureteric reflux (40%, about one-half bilateral): resolves in about one-third generally within 2 years; persistent unilateral reflux may be associated with nonfunctioning kidney, most commonly left one.

    b. Potter type IV dysplasia is common in those with severe obstruction.

    c. Potter type II dysplasia associated with laterally ectopic, refluxing ureters, and poor renal function.

    d. Trabeculated thick-walled bladder, often with diverticula; secondary bladder neck hypertrophy, which does not require incision.

    e. Severe hydroureteronephrosis

        f. Acute renal failure and acidosis in the newborn is obstructive phenomenon; chronic renal insufficiency may be related to dysplasia or may occur when obstruction is not recognized early.

  4. Diagnosis

        a. UTI or poor stream in infant or older child; incontinence is occasionally seen in older children.

        b. Newborn with palpable bladder and kidneys; urinary ascites

        c. Voiding cystourethrography is *the* diagnostic study; excretory urography, ultrasonography, and renal scan are employed to assess the extent of upper tract damage and postoperative recovery.

  5. Management

        a. In the sick infant, bladder drainage by percutaneous suprapubic tube (angiocath) or by small feeding tube per urethra is maintained while acidosis and sepsis are treated; the VCUG may be done with this catheter in place.

        b. The healthy infant or older child may undergo transurethral fulguration of valves initially; the sick infant should wait until creatinine stabilizes and sepsis resolves.

        c. Cutaneous vesicostomy can be employed as a temporizing measure in very small infant.

        d. Lack of improvement in renal function (creatinine remains 2.0 after bladder drainage) may warrant renal biopsy and cutaneous pyelostomy or ureterostomy; ureterovesical junction obstruction, which is rare, can be documented by diuretic renography or persistent severe hydronephrosis on ultrasound or antegrade study.

        e. Nonfunctioning kidneys with refluxing ureters can be removed later in life to prevent infections and complications.

        f. Ureteral tailoring and reimplantation is sometimes necessary.

        g. Antibiotic prophylaxis is maintained as long as reflux persists or upper tract emptying is slow.

6. Results
   a. Children whose creatinine stabilizes below 1.0 mg/dl after relief of obstruction generally do well, while those with creatinines above 2.0 often "outgrow" their renal function by puberty and require transplantation.
   b. Continence is eventually achieved in virtually all cases, as long as bladder neck surgery has been avoided.
   c. About 10% of patients may develop urethral strictures from instrumentation, although recent experience with finer scopes suggests that this number will be decreasing.

D. Megalourethra
   1. This rare lesion is seen most often in association with prune belly syndrome
   2. It occurs in two types.
      a. Scaphoid type is a deficiency of corpus spongiosum allowing ballooning of the urethra during voiding; it can be repaired with hypospadias techniques.
      b. Fusiform type involves deficiency of corpora cavernosa as well as spongiosum, resulting in elongated flaccid penis with redundant skin; fortunately, this form is seen usually in stillborn infants with other cloacal anomalies, as no functional repair is feasible.

E. Miscellaneous
   1. Anterior urethral valve or diverticulum is a rare obstructing lesion with a large saccular outpouching and an obstructing distal lip of mucosa; the diverticulum is excised with careful attention to the obstructing flap distally.
   2. Enlarged utriculus masculinus is a dilated Müllerian remnant, usually asymptomatic, associated with hypospadias or intersex state; it can be excised retrovesically or transvesically if stasis leads to UTI or the full utricle interferes with bladder emptying.

3. Aphallia and diphallia are exceedingly rare failure of fusion of the genital tubercles or failure of differentiation of the phallic mesenchyme.
4. Micropenis is often associated with CNS lesions or an intersex state; gender conversion may be considered in severe cases.

III. EXTERNAL GENITAL MALFORMATIONS

A. Hypospadias

Hypospadias occurs in 1 of 300 live male births; there is a 14% incidence in siblings and an 8% incidence in offspring.

1. *Origin.* Failure of mesodermal urethral folds to converge in midline; chordee results from failure of urethral plate disintegration or fibrosis of inner genital folds (which form spongiosum and dartos fascia).
2. Associated Findings
   a. There are variable endocrine findings, such as blunted human chorionic gonadotropin (hCG) response, low androgen receptor levels in a few.
   b. Undescended testis is found in 9.3% (30% with penoscrotal or more proximal meatus); up to one-third of patients with hypospadias and UDT have intersex state, usually genetic mosaicism.
   c. Inguinal hernia is found in 9%.
   d. Upper tract anomalies—when associated with imperforate anus (46%), when meningomyelocele is present (33%), when one other system anomaly is present (12 to 50%), and with isolated hypospadias (5%) (screening IVU not needed for simple hypospadias).
3. Classification (Simplified)
   a. Hypospadias without chordee (straight erections, meatus between midshaft and corona)
   b. Hypospadias with chordee
      (1) Meatus penile or penoscrotal after release of chordee
      (2) Meatus scrotal or perineal

c. Chordee without hypospadias
   (1) With normal urethra
   (2) With short or hypoplastic urethra
4. Management
   a. One-stage correction between 6 months and 18 months of age is preferred.
   b. Type *a* may be corrected by meatal advancement and glanuloplasty (MAGPI) (Fig. 3), flip–flap (Mathieu) (Fig. 4), or onlay island flap (Fig. 5) procedure, depending upon meatal position.

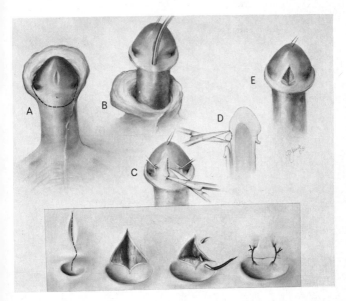

Figure 3. MAGPI procedure. **A.** Subcoronal meatus. **B.** Circumferential subcoronal incision 8 mm proximal to meatus and corona. **C–E.** Incision of bridge of tissue between meatus and glanular groove. Note the extent and depth of the incision (inset). *Inset:* Transverse Heineke-Mikulicz closure of dorsal meatal edge to distal glanular groove. *[From Duckett JW: MAGPI (Meatal advancement and glanuloplasty). Urol Clin North Am 8: 513–519, 1981.]*

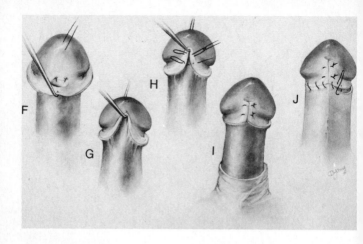

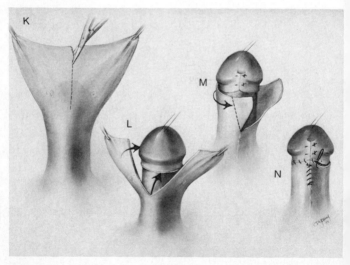

Figure 3. F, G. Traction toward the glans conforms the lateral glans edges into a V. **H, I.** Vertical mattress approximation brings the glans beneath the meatus. **J.** Sleeve reapproximation of the penile skin, with excision of excess foreskin, completes the repair. **K–N.** A Byars' flap closure is used if a ventral skin defect exists. *[From Duckett JW: MAGPI (Meatal advancement and glanuloplasty). Urol Clin North Am 8: 513–519, 1981.]*

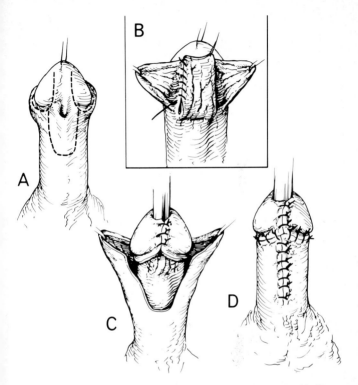

Figure 4. Mathieu procedure (flip–flap). **A.** the dotted lines outline the skin flaps. **B.** The proximal flap is rotated and the lateral glans flaps are developed. **C.** The glans flaps cover the neourethra and preputial skin is moved if necessary. **D.** Completed repair. *(From Duckett JW: Hypospadias. In Walsh P, Gittes RF, et al (eds): Campbell's Urology, ed 5. Philadelphia: W. B. Saunders, 1986, chap 47, pp 1969–1999.)*

   c. Type *b(1)* may be managed by inner preputial
      transverse island flap (Fig. 6).
   d. Type *b(2)* may require combined island flap and
      Duplay tube; it also may need secondary
      scrotoplasty for engulfment.

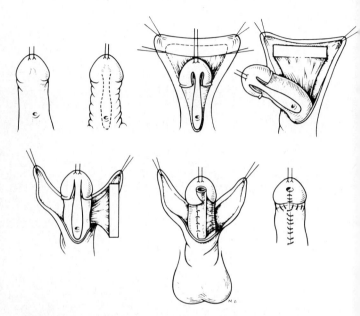

Figure 5. Onlay island flap. For cases without chordee with a meatus too proximal for a flip-flap; urethral plate left intact; onlay of inner preputial island flap with two parallel suture lines; meatus is extended to the apex of the glans; skin cover by Byars' flaps. *(From Department of Medical Illustration, Institute of Urology, London WC2, Reference No. 105211, with permission.)*

Figure 6. Double-faced preputial island flap. **A.** Outline of transverse island flap of inner preputial skin. **B.** Tubularization of inner preputial flap without mobilization. **C.** Outer preputial skin left attached to tubularized inner surface island flap as a double-faced pedicle. **D.** Mobilization of double-faced island flap to ventrum. Hatched area will be discarded so that the distal tube may be channeled through the glans. **E.** Outer preputial island flaps serve as ventral skin cover while penile skin covers the dorsum. *(From Duckett JW: Hypospadias. In Walsh P, Gittes RF, et al (eds): Campbell's Urology, ed 5. Philadelphia: W. B. Saunders, 1986, chap 47, pp 1969–1999.)*

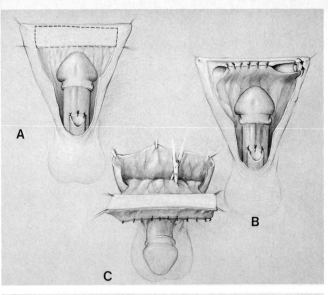

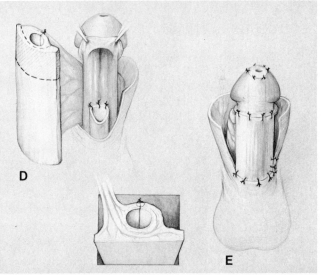

e. Type *c(1)* may be treated by degloving the penis and mobilizing the urethra.

f. Type *c(2)* requires island flap urethroplasty after chordee release due to bowstring effect of short urethra

g. Urinary diversion is employed for 10 to 14 days in all but MAGPI repairs, usually via silastic urethral stent or suprapubic tube.

h. Compressive dressing for 5 days is helpful.

5. Results and Complications (Table 5)

a. Small urethrocutaneous fistula is most common complication; it can be closed in layers without diversion with 90% success.

b. Postoperative bleeding can usually be stopped by compression.

c. UTI occurs in less than 10% and can be treated with the usual oral agents.

d. Strictures are rare, usually occur at the meatus or at the proximal end of the island flap, and are treated by Y-V meatoplasty; direct vision urethrotomy is often successful for usual short proximal stricture.

e. When carefully undertaken, the procedures outlined provide functional and cosmetically nearly normal penis and meatus in even the most severe hypospadias cases

TABLE 5. HYPOSPADIAS RESULTS (1982–1983)

Complications	
MAGPI (70 cases) 1 bleeding 1 retention (dressing) 0 fistula 0 stenosis 0 breakdown Island flap (34 cases) 5 fistula 3 stenosis 1 UTI	Mathieu flip–flap (12 cases) 1 partial breakdown 0 fistula 0 stenosis Onlay island flap (5 cases) 1 fistula

B. Cryptorchidism
1. Incidence. One per 120 live male births.
2. Origin. Aberrant testicular descent, possible failure of pituitary—gonadal axis in late gestation, i.e., absent luteinizing hormone (LH) surge or blunted testicular response.
3. Associated Findings
    a. Patent processus vaginalis occurs in 90%, with symptomatic hernia found rarely.
    b. Infertility approaching 30% in untreated unilateral UDT; surgery before age 2 and treatment with an analogue of luteinizing hormone releasing hormone (LHRH) may improve fertility.
       (1) Ectopic testis is normal histologically and not usually associated with infertility.
    c. Testicular malignancy is 20 to 35 times more common than in general population (1% for inguinal, 5% for abdominal testes).
    d. UDT is part of many syndromes, e.g., prune belly, exstrophy, genetic disorders, and intersex states (when associated with even mild hypospadias).
4. Diagnosis
    a. Retractile must be discriminated from truly undescended testis by careful examination.
       (1) A testis that can be manipulated into the scrotum with stretch of the cremaster by gentle traction and does not immediately pop up into the canal is retractile and needs no surgery.
5. Management (Fig. 7)
    a. Inguinal exploration as soon after age 1 as possible (spontaneous descent rare after 1 year).
    b. Most UDTs are palpable—85% are canalicular even if impalpable and can be brought down with conventional orchiopexy.
    c. If the canal is empty, the peritoneum is opened; either a testis or blind ending vas deferens and gonadal vessels are found overlying the psoas above the internal inguinal ring; only identification of the vessels constitutes sufficient exploration, as

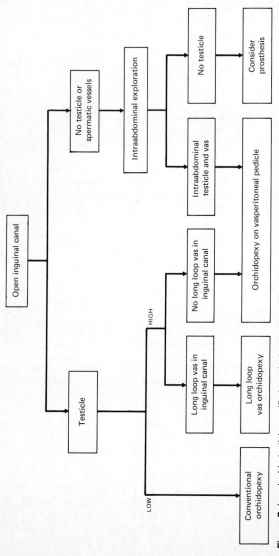

Figure 7. Impalpable testicle—unified surgical approach. *(From Snyder HM, Duckett JW: Techniques of orchiopexy. Dial Pediatr Urol 6:8, 1983.)*

the vas may embryologically be separate from the testis.

   d. Intraabdominal testis may be brought down by Fowler–Stephens orchiopexy dividing the spermatic vessels and relying on collateral flow to the testis via the artery to the vas.
   e. A testis that cannot be brought into the scrotum should be removed if the contralateral one is normally descended.

6. Results
   a. Using the Fowler–Stephens procedure, we have been 70% successful judged by palpation of a normal feeling testis in the scrotum.
   b. Results of conventional orchidopexy are better in terms of viability.
   c. Fertility seems to be improved by earlier orchidopexy but is not guaranteed. Incidence of tumor may be reduced by early orchidopexy.

C. Hernia/Communicating Hydrocele

1. Incidence is 1 to 4% of mature infants, 13% of premature infants.
2. Origin is failed closure of processus vaginalis after testicular descent; it may also be associated with incomplete testicular descent.
3. Only associated findings may be frank hernia (sac containing bowel or other organ) or undescended testis.
4. Principal differential diagnosis is with a stable hydrocele associated with a closed processus vaginalis. Stable hydroceles are often seen in infants and will usually be reabsorbed by 12 to 15 months of age. No surgery is required. A communicating hydrocele is suggested by a waxing and waning in the amount of fluid around the testicle. It is important not to confuse contraction of the dartos muscle of the scrotal wall with a change in size of the hydrocele.
5. Unlike a true hernia, which must be repaired promptly in infants due to frequency of incarceration, a communicating hydrocele may be fixed electively.

D. Appendages

1. Testicular and epididymal appendages are present usually at the upper pole of the testis or epididymis, represent Müllerian or Wolffian duct remnants, and are only significant when torsion of the appendage occurs.

2. Torsion of the appendix can sometimes be differentiated from testicular torsion by point tenderness and swelling at the upper pole, or the "blue dot" sign in which the infarcted tissue is apparent beneath the scrotal skin as a dark spot.

3. When doubt exists, exploration is essential; when the diagnosis is certain, treatment is symptomatic; pain will usually resolve in 3 to 5 days. If pain persists, excision transcrotally is needed.

IV. CLOACAL DYSGENESIS

A. General

Cloaca anomaly represents failure of the urorectal septum to descend, resulting in a single perineal opening or sinus into which rectum, vagina, and urethra enter.

1. Upper urinary tract is usually normal but should be visualized.

2. Sinogram, VCUG if possible, and cystovaginoscopy are necessary to assess the anatomy; a diverting colostomy is usually done early, as in imperforate anus, and this assessment can be performed under the same anesthetic.

3. Reconstruction via a midline posterior approach (Pena–DeVries) is carried out at age 1 to 3 years and consists of:

   a. Rectal tapering and pull-through.

   b. Urethroplasty using part or all of the urogenital sinus depending on its size.

   c. Vaginoplasty using part of the posterior sinus or by means of rotation flap from vagina or separation of vagina from bladder with vaginal "pull-through."

4. Urologic complications include urethrovaginal fistula and vaginal stenosis. Spinal anomalies and neurogenic bladders are common.

B. **Vaginal Atresia and** *Mayer–Rokitansky–Kuster–Hauser* **Syndrome**

1. Primary vaginal atresia can be distinguished from short vagina seen with testicular feminization by normal LH and follicle-stimulating hormone (FSH) levels and low testosterone levels with primary vaginal atresia.

   a. Failure of Müllerian duct to penetrate urogenital sinus or vascular acident

   b. Isolated anomaly

   c. Often presents at puberty with amenorrhea

   d. Usually atretic or agenetic uterus

   e. May treat with Frank technique (dilatation of introitus into a vagina), creation of vagina from bowel segment, or McIndoe procedure (creation of vagina from full-thickness skin graft)

2. Rokitansky Syndrome

   a. This is a combination of Müllerian duct abnormality, often duplication with vaginal atresia with ipsilateral renal agenesis.

   b. Abnormality of the Müllerian ducts may be associated with mesonephric duct absence as both structures are closely associated in early embryonic differentiation.

   c. It may present in newborn period with hydroculpos but commonly presents with amenorrhea or hematocolpos at puberty; some are discovered during investigation of a solitary kidney.

   d. Those with complete uterovaginal agenesis are managed as primary vaginal atresia; some have normal or septate uteri above obstruction requiring vaginoplasty.

   e. A special case is the patient with complete uterovaginal duplication and unilateral vaginal atresia.

      (1) Patient presents with normal menstrual periods, cyclic abdominal pain, and pelvic mass.

      (2) Management is by transvaginal marsupialization of obstructed vagina into normal one.

   f. Ultrasound is the study of choice for the evaluation of these genital anomalies; VCUG is done to rule

out reflux and cystovaginoscopy helps delineate
the introital anatomy.

REFERENCES
1. Stephens FD: Congenital malformations of the urinary tract. New York:
   Praeger, 1983, p 195.
2. Potter EL: Normal and abnormal development of the kidney. Chicago:
   Year Book, 1972.

BIBLIOGRAPHY
Duckett JW: Hypospadias. In Walsh P, Gittes, RF, et al (eds): Campbell's
  Urology, ed 5. Philadelphia: W. B. Saunders, 1986, chap 47, pp 1969–
  1999.
Duckett JW, Caldamone AA: Anomalies of the urinary tract: Bladder and
  urachus. In King L, Kelalis P, Belman B (eds): Clinical Pediatric Urology,
  ed 2. Philadelphia: W. B. Saunders, 1984, vol. II, pp 726–751.
Duckett JW, Snow BW: Disorders of the urethra and penis. In Walsh P, Gittes
  RF, et al (eds): Campbell's Urology, ed 5, Philadelphia: W. B. Saunders,
  1986, pp 2000–2030.
Fonkalsrud EW, Mengel W: The Undescended Testis. Chicago: Year Book,
  1981.
Gonzales ET, Woodward JR (eds): Symposium on Pediatric Urology. Urol
  Clin North Am 7:2, 1980. (Sections on Hypospadias, Exstrophy, Female
  Genital Reconstruction.)
Rajfer J (ed): Cryptorchidism. Urol Clin North Am 9:3, 1982.
Snyder HM: Ureteral duplication, ureterocele and ectopic ureters. In Whitfield
  H, Hendry WH (eds): Textbook of Genitourinary Surgery. London: Church-
  ill Livingston, 1985, pp 150–177.

27

Interventional Uroradiology

Marc P. Banner
Howard M. Pollack

I. RENAL CYST ASPIRATION AND ABLATION

A. Principles

1. To discriminate between simple and complex renal cystic lesions (such as cystic neoplasms) when differentiation is not possible using noninvasive imaging studies (cf. Chapter 3).

2. To obliterate a symptomatic benign simple renal cyst.

B. Indications

1. Diagnostic aspiration coupled with cytologic evaluation of cyst fluid and radiographic evaluation of the interior of the cyst is performed when a definitive diagnosis of a benign simple cyst cannot be established with ultrasonography (US) or computed tomography (CT).

2. Percutaneous ablation of a renal cyst may be indicated if the lesion, by virtue of its location in the kidney, is producing pain, obstructive hydronephrosis, renin-dependent hypertension, or pressure atrophy of the renal parenchyma.

C. Contraindications

1. An uncorrectable bleeding diathesis.

2. Very small cysts, especially if located close to the renal hilum, that cannot be well imaged with US, CT, or fluoroscopy are usually best left undisturbed for fear of inadvertent injury to adjacent major renal vessels.

Follow-up imaging studies should be obtained to ensure that the lesion remains stable and benign in appearance.

D. Technique

1. Renal cyst aspiration may be performed under ultrasonic, fluoroscopic, or CT guidance. Ultrasonic guidance is most often employed, using an aspiration biopsy transducer.
2. With the patient prone, the skin over the lesion is anesthetized and a 20-gauge needle inserted into the cyst.
3. Approximately half the volume of the cyst is withdrawn and sent for cytologic analysis. Equal volumes of water-soluble contrast material and air are injected into the cyst, with care taken to avoid overdistention.
4. The needle is withdrawn and multiple radiographs exposed with the patient in various positions so as to clearly outline the interior of the cyst with both positive and negative (air) contrast material—a double-contrast cystogram.
5. If cyst ablation is to be carried out, a small catheter or sheath is initially placed in the lesion, the diagnostic study performed (if not previously done), the majority of the cyst fluid aspirated, a sclerosing agent instilled into the cyst under fluoroscopic observation, and the catheter removed (Fig. 1). The patient is kept in the prone position for 30 to 60 minutes.
6. A variety of sclerosing agents have been employed to permanently obliterate a symptomatic cyst. The most commonly employed agents include Pantopaque (Alcon Laboratories), quinacrine, and ethanol.

E. Results

1. Diagnostic Renal Cyst Aspiration
   a. A typically benign renal cyst will contain clear, amber to yellow fluid with no abnormal cells, and exhibit a smooth cyst cavity.
   b. Hemorrhagic or infected cysts may yield dark, cloudy, or bloody fluid, but, again, should display

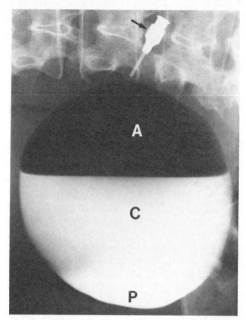

Figure 1. Renal cyst aspiration and ablation. Middle-aged female with large right lower pole renal cyst which was producing flank discomfort. Right lateral decubitus radiograph following diagnostic renal cyst aspiration and instillation of water-soluble contrast material, air and Pantopaque shows smooth interior margin of cyst as outlined by air (A), water-soluble contrast (C), and Pantopaque (P). The latter, having the highest specific gravity of the three, gravitates to the most dependent portion of the cyst. Note the metal connector (*arrow*) on the radiolucent tubing that has been inserted into the cyst. Following diagnostic examination of the cyst, the majority of its contents was aspirated, leaving the Pantopaque to sclerose the cyst lining and prevent reaccumulation of cyst fluid. Symptomatic relief was obtained following the procedure.

    a smooth lining and negative aspirate cytology to qualify as a benign lesion.

  c. Positive cytology, an irregular cyst cavity, or a fixed filling defect within the cavity suggest a cystic neoplasm and usually dictate surgical exploration.

   d. Most renal cysts reaccumulate after diagnostic as-
      piration, even if the cyst is drained completely.
2. Therapeutic Renal Cyst Ablation
   a. The majority of renal cysts can be permanently
      obliterated with the agents mentioned above, there-
      by relieving the symptoms that prompted inter-
      vention.
   b. Quinacrine and ethanol appear to be more
      effective than Pantopaque.

F. Complications
1. Complications are infrequent for diagnostic cyst
   aspiration.
2. Improper needle placement may produce pneumothorax (when an upper pole renal mass is being
   aspirated) or hematoma if a major renal vessel is inad-
   vertently punctured. Air embolism has not been
   reported.
3. Extravasation of water-soluble contrast into the perinephric tissues is innocuous; sclerosing agents, on the
   other hand, if extravasated can cause fat necrosis, soft
   tissue fibrosis, or a febrile reaction.

II. PERCUTANEOUS NEPHROSTOMY

A. Principles
1. Percutaneous nephrostomy (PCN) stands as the foundation upon which the field of interventional uroradiology has arisen.
2. PCN is widely accepted both as a safe and efficacious
   alternative to surgical nephrostomy and as a rapid
   method of gaining access to the upper urinary tract for
   a host of intrarenal and ureteral manipulations.

B. Indications
The majority of cases that benefit from PCN fall into one
of five categories.
1. Urgent renal drainage for relief of obstructive
   azotemia or anuria, especially when obstruction is ac-

companied by urosepsis. Here PCN is a temporizing measure that allows various therapies (e.g., chemotherapy, radiation therapy, surgery, or simply time) to relieve the obstructive uropathy while preserving or even improving renal function.

2. Urinary diversion when drainage from below (i.e., cystoscopic placement of a ureteral catheter) is not feasible or as clinically efficacious as percutaneous renal drainage (e.g., renal drainage required for more than a few days).

3. Urinary diversion when retrograde ureteral stenting is not possible (e.g., in patients with obstructed ureteroenterostomies or nonnegotiable ureters, or in infants and very small children, especially males, where cystoscopy is not without hazard).

4. A miscellaneous category where PCN is employed to accomplish something else in the urinary tract (e.g., manage renal and ureteral calculi, dilate ureteral strictures, place ureteral stents, or endoscope the kidney and ureter).

5. Temporary renal drainage to allow assessment of recoverable renal function of a chronically obstructed renal unit.

C. Contraindications

1. A severe and uncontrollable bleeding disorder.
2. The presence of an underlying urothelial neoplasm, if known, is a strong relative contraindication.

D. Technique

1. The renal collecting system is precisely localized, either with renal excretion of contrast medium, retrograde pyelography, or ultrasonography.
2. With the patient sedated and in the prone position, the flank is cleansed, and the skin entry site under the 12th rib in the posterior axillary line is anesthetized.
3. A needle is placed into the collecting system from the flank, urine aspirated, contrast material injected, and a guidewire passed through the needle into the kidney. The procedure is monitored fluoroscopically.

4. The needle is removed and the nephrocutaneous track enlarged by passing sequentially larger polyethylene fascial dilators over the guidewire.

5. A drainage or nephrostomy catheter, usually size 8Fr, is then passed over the guidewire and positioned in the renal pelvis. The guidewire is removed and the catheter is secured to the skin and attached to a closed gravity drainage bag (Fig. 2).

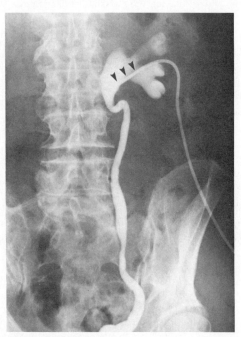

Figure 2. Percutaneous nephrostomy. Elderly male with azotemia secondary to bilateral distal ureteral obstruction from metastatic carcinoma of the prostate. Neither ureter could be catheterized cystoscopically because of prostatic enlargement and ureteral distortion by tumor. A percutaneous nephrostomy (PCN) catheter (*arrowheads*) was placed into the better functioning (left) kidney to relieve the azotemia until hormonal therapy could relieve the ureteral obstruction. Note the complete blockage of the distal ureter, in this case secondary to local spread of prostate carcinoma.

E. Results
1. Establishment of percutaneous renal drainage can be expected in approximately 99% of cases. Nondilated collecting systems and those totally filled with calculi are often technical challenges and potential sources of failure of catheter placement.
2. PCN is well tolerated by the great majority of patients and those caring for them.

F. Complications
1. Serious complications related to PCN can be expected in approximately 3 to 4% of cases and minor complications in another 10%. These include bleeding of varying severity (usually minor and transient), introduction of a new infection, exacerbation of existing sepsis, urine leak, penetration of adjacent viscera (e.g., pleura, bowel, gallbladder), and failure to establish drainage.
2. The complication rate of PCN is significantly less than that for surgically placed nephrostomies.
3. Catheter dislodgement and/or obstruction subsequent to PCN can be minimized by adequate fixation of the catheter to the skin at the time of PCN and by routinely exchanging PCN catheters every few months.

III. URETERAL STENTING

A. Principles
1. Percutaneous ureteral stenting provides urinary diversion without the need for an external collection device when cystoscopic placement of a ureteral stent is not feasible or possible.
2. Most patients find a ureteral stent catheter more convenient and cosmetically acceptable than a nephrostomy catheter.

B. Indications
1. Long-term stenting (months to years) is most frequently performed to bypass a ureteral obstruction. It is usually reserved for those cases in which retrograde ureteral stenting cannot be accomplished.

2. Short-term stenting (weeks to months) will allow post-operative pyeloureteral leaks or ureteral fistulae to close by diverting the urinary stream.

3. Temporary stenting is used in conjunction with catheter dilatation of ureteral strictures.

4. A catheter percutaneously placed in the ureter can serve as a surgical adjunct to aid in the intraoperative identification of the ureters during difficult surgical dissections (e.g., revision of an obstructed ureteroile-ostomy). The ability of a surgeon to palpate the ureter in a previously operated abdomen can reduce operating time considerably.

C. **Contraindications**

1. The presence of active renal infection.

2. Markedly diseased bladders (e.g., radiation cystitis, bladder invasion by adjacent neoplasm, or patients who are incontinent).

D. **Technique**

1. A PCN is performed and a guidewire and catheter advanced down the ureter, manipulated across the abnormal (often stenotic) ureter, and advanced into the urinary bladder or a bowel conduit if the ureter has been so diverted.

2. The catheter that has been manipulated distal to the abnormal ureter is removed over the guidewire and replaced with a ureteral stent catheter. Multiple side holes are created in the stent where that catheter will eventually be positioned in the renal pelvis. This is an *external* ureteral stent catheter. Urine from the kidney enters the catheter at the renal pelvis level, travels through the stent, and exists from its distal pigtail segment in the urinary bladder. The proximal end of the catheter protrudes from the skin a few centimeters where it is obturated externally (Figs. 3 and 4).

3. An *external* ureteral stent can be periodically irrigated, if necessary, by uncapping its proximal end, and it can be exchanged from the flank over a guidewire passed through it into the bladder.

4. Patients who require ureteral stenting for long periods

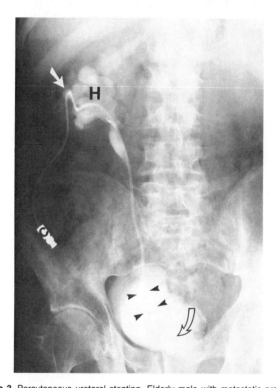

Figure 3. Percutaneous ureteral stenting. Elderly male with metastatic prostate carcinoma, azotemia, and bilateral distal ureteral obstruction. Following right PCN, a catheter could be advanced through the obstructed ureter and into the bladder. A ureteral stent catheter was then placed. Note the hydronephrotic right renal collecting system (H), contrast in the dilated, obstructed distal right ureter around the catheter (*arrowheads*), and osteoblastic bone metastases. The stent catheter enters the skin at the white arrow and traverses the kidney and ureter to terminate in the bladder (*black arrow*). Multiple side holes in the intrarenal portion of the catheter allow kidney urine to drain through the catheter directly to the bladder and permit the metal connector on the proximal end of the catheter (c) to be capped, thereby obviating the need for an external catheter drainage bag.

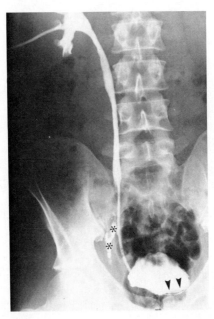

Figure 4. Percutaneous ureteral stenting. A ureteral fistula developed in this young man following open ureterolithotomy. Though the ureter could not be catheterized in retrograde fashion because of postoperative ureteral edema and distortion, a catheter could be percutaneously manipulated in antegrade fashion past the site of ureteral leak and into the bladder. By diverting the urine away from the fistula for several weeks, the ureter healed and the catheter was removed. *Asterisks* mark extravasated contrast material at the site of the fistula; *arrowheads* indicate the distal end of the stent catheter in the bladder. The catheter enters the urinary tract at the kidney level, below the 12th rib.

of time can have their urinary drainage totally internalized by exchanging the single pigtail external ureteral stent for one with a pigtail configuration at both ends, an *internal* ureteral stent. The proximal pigtail is positioned in the renal pelvis and the distal pigtail, again, placed in the bladder. Internal or double pigtail ureteral stents cannot be irrigated (as they have

been totally internalized) and must be periodically changed cystoscopically.
5. Patients who require ureteral stenting following ureteral diversion to a bowel conduit can be managed with an *external* ureteral stent that, following step 1 above, is placed in retrograde fashion. Over a guidewire that enters the kidney from the flank, passes down the ureter across the area of obstruction, and through the bowel conduit and stoma, a single pigtail catheter is advanced over the stoma end of the wire into the renal pelvis. The distal end of this catheter protrudes through the stoma to drain into the urostomy collection bag.
6. Catheters used to help identify the ureters intra-operatively are passed down the ureter to the point of ureteral obstruction following a PCN. A PCN catheter is also usually required to drain the kidney temporarily until surgical correction of the obstructed ureter has been accomplished.

E. **Results**
1. Both internal and external ureteral stents allow patients to lead as active a life as their underlying condition will permit.
2. Ureteral obstructions can often be bypassed in ante-grade (percutaneous) fashion even when retrograde ureteral catheterization is not possible (e.g., bladder tumor overlying an obstructed ureteral orifice, angula-tion of the distal ureters secondary to malignant pros-tatic enlargement or spread of prostatic malignancy, and malignant or benign distal ureteral stenoses).
3. Approximately 80% of ureteral obstructions and fistulae can be stented percutaneously. Very tightly obstructed ureters and ureters that are markedly angu-lated or encased by tumor or fibrosis just proximal to the urinary bladder or a bowel conduit are the usual causes of failure of antegrade stenting.

F. **Complications**
1. Excluding those complications related to PCN, com-plications related specifically to antegrade ureteral

stenting are infrequent and are usually related to improper positioning of the stent or placement of side holes in the catheter at the level of the renal pelvis.

2. These complications can usually be remedied by catheter repositioning (percutaneous, cystoscopic, or ureteroscopic).

IV. DILATATION OF URETERAL STENOSES

A. Principles

1. Ureteral stenting for a long period of time may be appropriate for ureters obstructed by malignant disease but is not optimal therapy for most patients who develop benign ureteral strictures postoperatively.

2. Some benign ureteral strictures are amenable to catheter dilatation.

3. If successful, this procedure can spare patients chronic indwelling stents or additional surgery.

B. Indications

An attempt at catheter dilatation of all benign ureteral strictures should be made before relegating patients to additional surgery or to chronic indwelling ureteral stents that would have to be periodically changed cystoscopically.

C. Contraindications

Ureteral strictures caused by malignant disease, either primary or recurrent.

D. Technique

1. The strictured ureter is cannulated as described above.

2. Biopsies or other imaging studies are obtained to document a benign etiology of the stricture, if doubt exists.

3. A catheter with an inflatable balloon mounted on its distal end is advanced across the stricture. The balloon is inflated under fluoroscopic control. A waist or narrowing in the balloon is usually evident at the stricture site upon initial balloon inflation. With continued inflation for a minute or two, or with multiple inflations, the waist will generally disappear (and not reappear

upon balloon deflation) if successful stricture dilatation has been accomplished.

4. The balloon catheter is removed and the ureter stented with the largest catheter that will comfortably fit in the ureter. This catheter is left in place for 1 week and serves as a ureteral stent. The stent is then removed and the efficacy of the dilatation subsequently determined prior to removal of the PCN catheter (Fig. 5).

5. Occasionally, distal ureteral strictures in females can be dilated with a balloon catheter and then stented in retrograde fashion per urethra.

6. Some ureteral stenoses can be dilated by passing progressively larger ureteral stent catheters through a stricture until a 10Fr catheter can be placed. This catheter is then left in situ for 4 to 8 weeks.

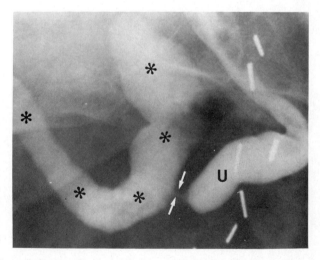

Figure 5. Catheter dilatation of benign ureteral stricture. A middle-aged female underwent cystectomy for transitional cell carcinoma of the bladder and ureteral diversion to an ileal conduit. **A.** Five years later she developed a benign stricture (*arrows*) of the distal right ureter (U) at the site of the ureterioleostomy. *Asterisks* mark the ileal conduit.

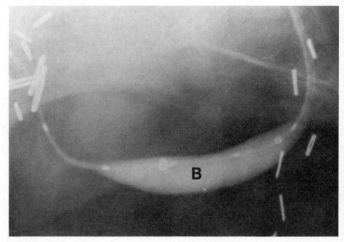

B

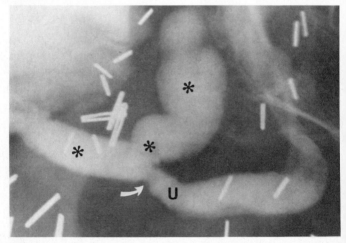

C

Figure 5. B. Following right PCN, a balloon catheter was passed through the stenotic ureteral segment and into the conduit. The balloon (B) was centered over the stricture and inflated with contrast material. **C.** Follow-up study shows a widely patent ureteral lumen at the site of the former stenosis (*arrow*). U, distal right ureter; *, ileal conduit.

642

E. **Results**
   1. Approximately 50 to 60% of all benign ureteral strictures can be successfully dilated with balloon catheters or ureteral stent catheters. Balloon catheter dilatation usually carries a greater likelihood of success than does dilatation with stent catheters alone.
   2. The etiology and duration of the stricture seem to be major determinants of the outcome of dilatation therapy. In general, fresh postoperative strictures may be dilated whereas long-standing, densely fibrotic ones usually cannot. Nonetheless, some long-standing strictures have successfully responded to balloon catheter dilatation therapy.

F. **Complications**
   No known permanent sequelae have resulted from unsuccessful dilatation therapy. Laceration of ureteral mucosa or wall may occur with balloon overdistension. These perforations heal uneventfully if the ureter is stented for a week or two and probably do not affect the outcome of dilatation therapy.

V. PERCUTANEOUS MANAGEMENT OF UPPER URINARY TRACT CALCULI

A. **Principles**
   1. Over 95% of all renal and ureteral calculi can presently be treated by means of percutaneous manipulations, obviating the need for open renal or ureteral surgery. Approximately 80% of these stones can be extracted under either fluoroscopic or nephroscopic or ureteroscopic control, and the remainder disintegrated under nephroscopic control with ultrasonic or electrohydraulic energies.
   2. Calculi of select composition (or fragments thereof) may be dissolved by direct lavage with chemical solutions instilled through one or more PCN catheters.

B. **Indications**
   1. Virtually any renal or ureteral calculus that is producing symptoms, obstruction, or medically unmanageable infection can be treated percutaneously.

2. Chemical dissolution of uric acid, cystine, and struvite (infection) calculi can be carried out as a primary therapy or, more frequently, as an adjunctive therapy for stone fragments that remain after percutaneous extraction or disintegration.

C. Contraindications

1. Absolute contraindications include patients
   a. With uncontrollable hypertension
   b. With active renal infection
   c. With an uncorrectable bleeding diathesis
   d. Who will not accept possible surgical intervention should an emergency arise
2. Relative contraindications include:
   a. A calculus that is partially embedded in the wall of the ureter
   b. Patients with an underlying congenital ureteropelvic junction (UPJ) obstruction where pyeloplasty with concomitant pyelolithotomy may be more appropriate long-term therapy

D. Technique

1. A PCN is performed through a posterior calyx (usually a lower pole or interpolar calyx) and a guidewire is passed through the collecting system and down the ureter.
2. The nephrostomy track is rapidly dilated to size 30F, either with fascial dilators of progressively larger size or with a special balloon catheter 10 to 13 cm in length.
3. A 30F-diameter, 15-cm-long Teflon sheath through which manipulations can be carried out is passed from the skin into the renal pelvis.
4. Calculi less than 1 cm in diameter are extracted from the kidney or ureter in toto with a variety of grasping forceps or helical stone baskets. This can be accomplished under fluoroscopic guidance in the radiology department or in the operating room under direct vision through a nephroscope (Fig. 6).
5. Calculi greater than 1 cm in diameter are disintegrated in the operating room by means of ultrasonic or, less

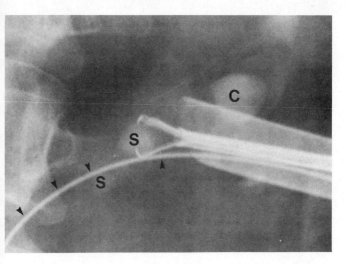

Figure 6. Percutaneous extraction of renal calculus. One of two renal pelvic stones (S) is being grasped with three-pronged forceps which have been inserted through a 30F Teflon sheath placed in a dilated PCN track. The second smaller stone was subsequently extracted in similar fashion. A guidewire (*arrowheads*) traverses the track and enters the proximal ureter. Contrast material remains in several calyces (C) from the PCN.

commonly, electrohydraulic energy applied directly to the stone or stones. Stone fragments that result are either suctioned out of the kidney through the nephroscope or extracted with forceps (Fig. 7).

6. Ureteral calculi can be extracted in antegrade fashion (percutaneously) or, in retrograde fashion, extracted or disintegrated via a rigid ureteroscope inserted cystoscopically.

7. These procedures are usually performed in two stages—performance of the nephrostomy in the radiology suite on day 1 with the patient sedated but awake, and track dilatation with subsequent stone manipulation in the operating room on day 2 with the patient under general anesthesia. Calculi amenable to

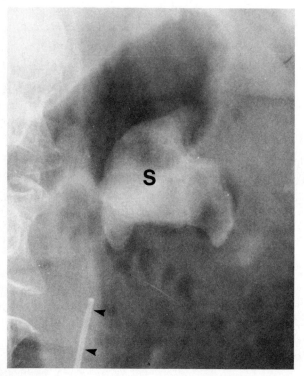

Figure 7. Percutaneous ultrasonic lithotripsy. **A.** Abdominal radiograph prior to PCN showing a large staghorn calculus (S) in the left kidney and a retrograde ureteral catheter (*arrowheads*) terminating in the proximal ureter.

percutaneous extraction can be managed totally in the radiology department on day 1, combining the skills of the radiologist (nephrostomy, track dilatation) and urologist (stone removal).

8. Following stone manipulation, a 24F nephrostomy catheter is placed in the kidney until hematuria and urothelial edema subside. The catheter is usually left in place for 1 week.

9. Fragments of uric acid, cystine, or struvite (triple

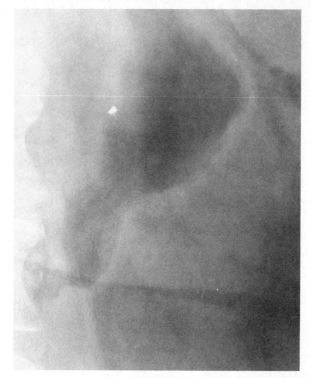

Figure 7. B. Follow-up abdominal radiograph following PCN and ultrasonic disintegration of the staghorn calculus shows that the entire calculus has been removed. White fleck overlying the left kidney is an artefact.

phosphate) calculi remaining following stone extraction or disintegration can be dissolved by infusing sodium bicarbonate, acetylcysteine or THAM-E, or Renacidin (Guardian Chemical), respectively, through the nephrostomy catheter prior to its removal.

E. Results

1. Successful percutaneous management of renal calculi can be expected in over 95% of cases. Ureteral calculi

can be successfully removed or disintegrated approximately 85% of the time, failures usually related to fixation of these stones to the ureteral wall and inability to dislodge them safely.

2. The retained renal stone fragment rate is generally less than that for open or surgical lithotomy.

F. Complications

1. Percutaneous stone manipulation carries a lower risk of kidney loss than does open surgery, particularly for patients with recurrent stones and previous stone surgery.

2. Complications occur in approximately 15 to 20% of cases, are usually transient, and, in the majority of cases, can be managed conservatively.

3. Complications include
   a. Perforation of the collecting system or ureter. These usually heal if nephrostomy drainage is adequate and, in cases of ureteral perforation, a ureteral stent is placed. Small calculi or fragments that may gain entry into the perinephric space as a result of perforation may be left undisturbed if not part of an infection-related stone.
   b. Bleeding. Hematuria accompanies all cases of track dilatation and stone manipulation. The urine generally clears in 24 to 48 hours with bed rest. Persistent bleeding may require transfusion. Major retroperitoneal or arterial bleeding is very infrequent and can usually be managed with percutaneous drainage, tamponade, or angiographic embolization.
   c. Obstruction. Transient obstruction secondary to UPJ edema or blood clots usually resolves in a few days.
   d. Infection. Routine prophylactic use of antibiotics has reduced postmanipulation clinical infection to a very low level.
   e. Retained calculi. These can be irrigated and dissolved, as discussed above, or extracted either under fluoroscopic or nephroscopic control prior to removal of the nephrostomy catheter.

4. Complications related to dissolution therapy include pain, fever, bacilluria, urothelial edema, and hypermagnesemia (when using Renacidin). Dissolution is temporarily halted until these problems are corrected.

VI. EXTRACORPOREAL SHOCK WAVE LITHOTRIPSY

A. Principles

1. Extracorporeal shock wave lithotripsy (ESWL) is the latest of the new modalities for the therapy of renal stone disease. Shock waves are produced outside the body, focused at a renal or ureteral calculus, and transmitted through a water bath in which the patient is immersed.
2. Shock waves can selectively disintegrate urinary calculi because of their brittle composition and their high acoustical impedance compared to surrounding tissues.

B. Indications

1. Although initial experience with ESWL in Germany and later in the United States was limited to relatively small opaque calculi, stones of any size and composition are presently being treated by this modality.
2. Ureteral calculi located proximal to the iliac crest that have remained in situ for less than 4 to 6 weeks are also amenable to ESWL.

C. Contraindications

1. Calcification in the aorta or renal artery that would lie near the point of maximum shock wave energy.
2. The presence of obstruction distal to the stone (not caused by the stone itself). This relative contraindication may be overcome by performing PCN in conjunction with ESWL. (See Results.)

D. Technique

1. The components of the system include a 7-×-4-foot tub, water degasser, hydraulic stretcher, shock wave generator and electrode, biplane image intensified flu-

oroscopy with image display, and control panel for activating the focused shock wave beam.

2. Following general or epidural anesthesia, the patient is placed in a semireclining position in a modified chair that is moved hydraulically to immerse the patient in a tub containing warmed degassed water.

3. Biplane fluoroscopy is utilized to localize the opaque stone and properly position the patient so that the shock waves are focused on the stone.

4. The shock wave electrode is housed in the floor of the tub. A series of shock waves are activated and focused onto the stone. The position of the stone is rechecked periodically with fluoroscopy. The shock waves pass through the water and soft biologic tissues with little loss of energy. High pressure is exerted on the stone by the shock wave. After repeated shock waves (up to 1200) the stone crumbles into tiny particles that are then passed down the ureter under conditions of forced diuresis.

E. Results

1. Ninety-nine percent of the first 1000 treated patients had satisfactory clinical results; 90% of them were stone-free.

2. Renal function in the stone-bearing kidney usually improves following ESWL.

3. Auxiliary procedures may be needed to facilitate passage of the stone debris. These include transurethral manipulation to help remove fragments from the intramural ureter or PCN to facilitate drainage or evacuate fragments in an obstructed kidney.

F. Complications

1. Risks or complications appear to be small. Evidence to date indicates little tissue effect although there may be a practical limit to total shock wave dose per volume of tissue.

2. Radiation exposure during ESWL therapy approximates that of routine urography.

3. Small subcapsular hematomas (usually not requiring therapy) have been noted on occasion.

VII. PERCUTANEOUS DRAINAGE OF RENAL AND PERINEPHRIC FLUID COLLECTIONS

A. Principles

1. Percutaneous drainage of renal and perinephric fluid collections, such as abscesses, urinomas, and lymphoceles, usually provides satisfactory clinical results with a minimum of complications, thereby obviating the need for surgical drainage.

2. Percutaneous drainage of abscesses duplicates basic surgical management principles by providing decompression, evacuation, and continuous drainage without dissemination of infection. Standard retroperitoneal approaches for operative drainage of renal and perinephric abscesses are closely duplicated percutaneously by employing cross-sectional imaging for guidance.

B. Indications

The presence of a well-defined renal, perinephric, or retroperitoneal fluid collection (abscess, urinoma, lymphocele, hematoma) that requires drainage.

C. Contraindications

1. Absence of a safe percutaneous drainage route.

2. A fluid collection containing multiple septations may be more easily and rapidly drained surgically, although a few internal septations do not represent a contraindication to percutaneous drainage.

D. Technique

1. The fluid collection and its anatomic relationship to its surrounding structures is assessed by cross-sectional imaging (CT or US). A safe percutaneous route for diagnostic needle aspiration and catheter placement is planned. The route is carefully chosen so as to avoid puncture of viscera, pleura, and major vessels.

2. Diagnostic aspiration with a 22-gauge thin-walled needle along the planned route is performed to confirm the diagnosis and the route.

3. If diagnostic aspiration yields drainable pus, a catheter is introduced under fluoroscopic control, the abscess

evacuated, and the catheter securely sutured in place to provide continuous drainage.

4. Catheters may be inserted over a guidewire passed through an 18-gauge needle placed in the abscess (PCN technique) or through a larger trocar-cannula, which obviates the need for a guidewire. The former technique is used for small, deep retroperitoneal ab-

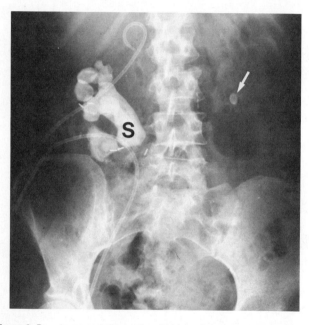

Figure 8. Percutaneous drainage of perinephric abscess. Middle-aged female with bilateral renal calculi (S, right staghorn; *arrow* on left lower pole stone) and huge right perinephric abscess secondary to xanthogranulomatous pyelonephritis. Two pigtail catheters have been percutaneously inserted into the perinephric abscess, one in its superior aspect, the other inferiorly. As the abscess was drained, the catheters were gradually withdrawn. Following percutaneous abscess drainage, her clinical condition improved considerably, thereby allowing right nephrectomy to be performed electively. Prior to the availability of percutaneous abscess drainage, the abscess would have been drained surgically and, at a later date, a second surgical procedure (nephrectomy) carried out to definitively treat the inflammatory process.

scesses and for all renal parenchymal abscesses; the latter can be employed for large or more superficial retroperitoneal abscesses where the drainage route is removed from vital strictures and has a wide margin of safety (Fig. 8).
5. Catheters usually do not require periodic irrigation.
6. Indications for catheter removal include:
   a. A satisfactory clinical response
   b. Absence of fever
   c. Return of white blood cell count to normal
   d. Cessation of drainage
   e. Follow-up imaging studies (CT or US scans, fluoroscopically controlled injections of the cavity being drained or sinograms) that indicate complete resolution
7. Drainage catheters often need to remain in place for 1 to 2 weeks to eradicate the fluid collection. The track will close following catheter removal if all infected material has been evacuated.

E. Results
1. A cure rate of 80 to 85% can be expected for percutaneous drainage of abscesses or other fluid collections with no mortality. These figures represent a tremendous improvement over cure and mortality rates from surgical drainage and reflect the abilities of cross-sectional imaging to diagnose abscesses earlier in their development and thin needle aspiration to confirm the nature of a fluid collection, as well as the efficacy of percutaneous drainage techniques.
2. Advantages of percutaneous drainage of abscesses include:
   a. Avoidance of surgery, general anesthesia and associated perioperative complications
   b. Reduction in time and expense of treatment
   c. Wide acceptance by patients
   d. Less nursing care than surgery

F. Complications
1. Urosepsis may be temporarily exacerbated immediately following placement of a percutaneous drainage catheter.

2. A less than complete clinical response may result from only partial drainage of septated collections or premature catheter removal.

VIII. BIOPSY TECHNIQUES

A. Principles

Soft tissue and visceral lesions related to the urinary tract can be percutaneously sampled for cytologic analysis when knowledge of the nature of the abnormality in question (benign or malignant) affects patient management. Biopsies can be obtained through a needle percutaneously placed into the lesion or via a catheter inserted into the urinary tract percutaneously or endoscopically (transcatheter).

B. Indications

1. Primary diagnosis of upper urinary tract malignancy in those sites where a percutaneous or transcatheter biopsy will not compromise future therapy.
2. Accurate staging of neoplastic disease by direct biopsy of radiologically visualized abnormal lymph nodes or soft tissue and visceral masses.
3. Diagnosis of the etiology of ureteral obstruction in patients with a known current or past malignancy.

C. Contraindications

1. Contraindications to needle aspiration biopsy include:
   a. A hemorrhagic diathesis
   b. A suspicion of an arteriovenous malformation in the area to be biopsied
2. Local dissemination or needle tract implantation of tumor is a theoretical possibility but is extremely rare with the small bore needles used for urinary tract biopsies.

D. Technique

1. Needle biopsy
   a. The proposed biopsy site is localized by one of several imaging modalities, including fluoroscopy, excretory urography, retrograde pyelography, ileal loopography, ultrasonography, computed tomo-

graphy, cystography, lymphangiography, and even manual palpation.

b. A 22- or 23-gauge thin-walled (Chiba or "skinny") needle is positioned through surgically scrubbed and locally anesthetized skin and advanced to the lesion being biopsied. Depth of insertion is ascertained by imaging the needle tip on CT or US (with an aspiration biopsy transducer) or, if fluoroscopy is being employed, by comparing the position of the needle tip with the biopsy site in various oblique fluoroscopic views.

c. The needle is placed directly into soft tissue or visceral abnormalities or immediately adjacent to

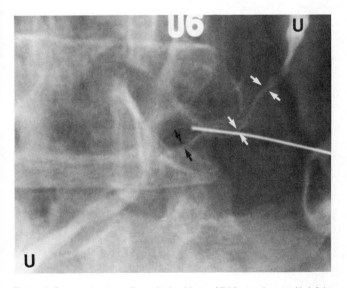

Figure 9. Percutaneous needle aspiration biopsy. Middle-aged man with left hydronephrosis following cystectomy for bladder cancer and ureteroileostomy. Loopogram demonstrated reflux into the left ureter (U) and outlined a long segment of irregular ureteral narrowing (*small arrows*). Thin-needle aspiration biopsy of the periureteral tissues at the site of obstruction yielded recurrent transitional cell carcinoma in the retroperitoneum. Note the tip of the 22-gauge thin-walled needle adjacent to the narrowed ureter.

an obstructed ureter at the point of narrowing or
blockage. Most needle biopsies are obtained trans-
peritoneally (Fig. 9).

    d. Aspiration is done with a 20-ml syringe and short
up-and-down movements of the needle. The aspirate is sent for cytologic study. If particulate tissue
is obtained, it is fixed and a cell block preparation
is made.

2. Transcatheter Biopsy

    a. This approach is most frequently employed to ob-
tain a brush biopsy of pyelocalyceal or ureteral
lesions suspicious for transitional cell carcinoma
on excretory urography.

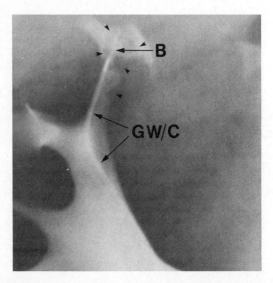

Figure 10. Transcatheter brush biopsy of transitional cell carcinoma. An irregular
filling defect in the upper pole calyx and infundibulum (arrowheads) is being
sampled ("brushed") for cytologic analysis with a nylon brush attached to a
guidewire. The brush and wire are passed through an open-ended catheter that
has been passed up the ureter cystoscopically. Under fluoroscopic control, the
brush is advanced beyond the end of the catheter and the lesion biopsied. GW/C,
guidewire inside of catheter; B, nylon brush.

    b. An open-ended catheter is passed cystoscopically into the ureter or kidney. A guidewire on which is mounted a nylon brush is then passed through the catheter and the suspicious abnormality "brushed" under fluoroscopy. The cells retrieved by the brush are then subjected to cytologic analysis (Fig. 10).

    c. Other biopsy instruments, including forceps and snares, can be employed through catheters larger than those passed cystoscopically, such as those percutaneously inserted into the kidney or ureter.

E. Results

1. A positive result (Class V cytology) generally will alter patient management by:

    a. Obviating other more invasive diagnostic techniques

    b. Eliminating the necessity for a surgical biopsy or staging procedure

    c. Upstaging the disease such that curative therapy is eliminated from consideration or changed in type or scope

2. Negative findings do not exclude the presence of disease in the area biopsied or elsewhere. Therefore, thin-needle aspiration or transcatheter brush biopsy are of value only when positive results are obtained.

3. The value of the results obtained from such biopsies depends on the abilities of the guiding diagnostic procedure to localize the area of pathology to be biopsied, the physician performing the biopsy to obtain material of diagnostic quality, and the cytopathologist to interpret the specimen correctly.

4. Biopsy of lymph nodes containing filling defects on lymphangiography has a 70% correlation with surgical lymphadenectomy results. On the other hand, positive aspirations may be obtained in up to 15% of normal appearing nodes.

5. Needle biopsy of soft tissue and visceral lesions and transcatheter brush biopsies yield true positive results in approximately 90% of cases. False-positive results are very infrequent.

F. Complications

1. Significant complications from biopsy procedures are rare. Surgical exploration following percutaneous needle biopsy with a 22- or 23-gauge needle has almost invariably failed to identify tissue damage at the biopsy site or in adjacent areas.

2. Spread of urinary tract malignancy along the biopsy needle track is exceedingly uncommon.

3. Although complications following transcatheter brush biopsy of urothelial abnormalities have not been reported, perforation of the collecting system or ureter, with subsequent spread of tumor, is a theoretical possibility.

IX. PERCUTANEOUS TRANSLUMINAL RENAL ANGIOPLASTY

A. Principles

Percutaneous transluminal renal angioplasty (PTRA) is the most commonly employed vascular interventional procedure designed to increase renal blood flow. It usually serves as a nonoperative treatment alternative to renal artery bypass grafting in patients with renovascular hypertension. Other angiographic techniques that increase renal blood flow include intraarterial thrombolysis and transcatheter thromboembolectomy.

B. Indications

1. Indications for PTRA are the same as those for surgical correction of a renal artery stenosis that has been shown (by renal vein renin determinations) to be responsible for the patient's hypertension.

2. Goals
   a. A cure of the renovascular hypertension
   b. Facilitation of the medical management of the hypertension by permitting reduction or elimination of the patient's antihypertensive medications
   c. Prevention of renal failure due to impending renal artery occlusion
   d. Reversal of renal failure in patients with recent thrombosis of a stenotic renal artery

    3. PTRA may be performed in patients with renal atherosclerotic stenosis or occlusion, renal artery fibrodysplasia, renal artery neurofibromatosis, Takayasu's arteritis, and arterial anastomotic stenosis of renal transplants.

    4. Intraarterial infusion of streptokinase can lyse a thrombus that has occluded the renal artery. Following thrombolysis, PTRA can then be performed to dilate the underlying renal artery stenosis.

    5. Transcatheter thromboembolectomy may be an effective nonsurgical technique for immediate restoration of renal blood flow with minimal risk in patients with acute thrombotic or embolic occlusion of the renal artery, especially in those having underlying medical problems that would make surgical thromboembolectomy more risky.

C. Contraindications
Contraindications are the same as those for surgical correction of a renal artery stenosis producing hypertension.

D. Technique
    1. All antihypertensive drugs are reduced or eliminated if possible to prevent hypotension after a successful angioplasty.

    2. PTRA is usually performed following diagnostic renal arteriography via the initial femoral puncture site. Occasionally an axillary approach is required when a stenotic renal artery forms an acute angle with the abdominal aorta or if the femoral arteries are markedly diseased.

    3. A catheter is selectively engaged in the renal artery and a guidewire used to cross the stenotic lesion.

    4. The catheter is removed and replaced with a double-lumen balloon catheter. The balloon is centered over the stenosis and inflated with contrast material under fluoroscopic control. Persistent narrowings in the inflated balloon often suggest the necessity for multiple balloon inflations (Fig. 11).

    5. Prior to and following angioplasty, pressure measurements across the stenosis are obtained. These are fol-

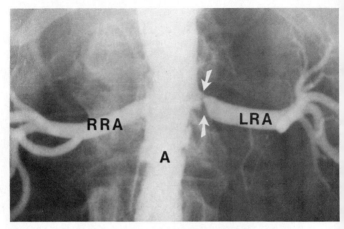

A

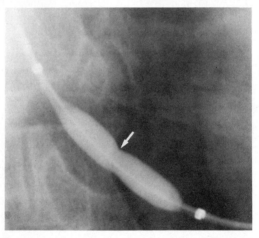

B

Figure 11. Percutaneous transluminal renal angioplasty (PTRA). Elderly male with hypertension, atherosclerosis, and renal artery stenosis. **A.** Midstream aortogram shows a tight stenosis at the origin of the left renal artery (*arrows*) and irregularity of the abdominal aorta attributable to atherosclerosis. A, aorta; RRA, right renal artery; LRA, left renal artery. **B.** PTRA was performed via the axillary artery because of concomitant femoral artery stenoses. A balloon catheter positioned across the stenosis is being inflated with contrast material. Note the indentation on the balloon catheter (*arrow*) at the site of the stenosis.

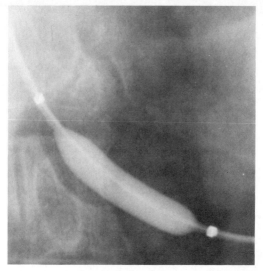

C

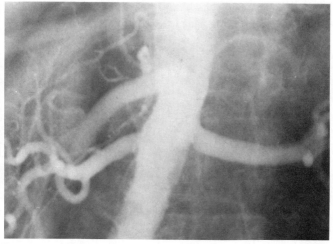

D

Figure 11. C. Continued inflation has effaced the indentation suggesting a successful dilatation. **D.** Postangioplasty aortogram shows a widely patent left renal artery. The stenosis has been successfully dilated and the patient's blood pressure reverted to normal.

661

lowed by aortography to assess the anatomic success
of the procedure.

6. Antispasmodics and vasodilators may be injected prior
to crossing a renal artery stenosis. These medications
prevent or diminish the frequency or severity of renal
artery spasm.

7. Intraarterial administration of a fibrinolytic agent,
such as streptokinase, may be used to lyse pre- or post-
PTRA thrombotic occlusions.

8. Patients are anticoagulated prior to, during, and following PTRA with one of several agents, including
aspirin, persantine, heparin, and coumadin.

E. Results

1. A technically successful PTRA (i.e., the procedure
has resulted in either a cure or an improvement in the
hypertension) occurs in 85 to 90% of cases.

2. Recurrent stenoses that occur in between 5 and 22% of
patients may be redilated percutaneously.

3. The success and long-term patency rates of PTRA are
greater in fibromuscular renal artery stenoses than in
atherosclerotic lesions.

4. Technical failures occur most commonly when lesions
are at a surgical anastomosis or at the origins of the
renal arteries. Other failures are due to the inability to
cross the lesion with a guidewire and/or catheter.

5. Advantages of PTRA over surgical treatment include:
   a. Decreased morbidity and mortality
   b. Shorter hospital stay with decreased recuperative
      period
   c. Restenoses following PTRA can be redilated per-
      cutaneously or corrected surgically.

F. Complications

1. Although complications may occur, most are easily
managed and do not result in permanent deterioration
of renal function or in nephrectomy. Rarely is there a
need for emergency surgical intervention. To date no
deaths have been associated with PTRA.

2. Nonocclusive dissection of the renal artery usually requires nonemergent surgical bypass grafting.

3. Occlusive dissection of the renal artery requires surgical bypass.

4. Puncture site hematomas or thrombosis may or may not require surgery.

5. Transient renal failure and nonfilling of segmental intrarenal branches on the post-PTRA arteriogram, probably due to transient spasm or thrombosis, may occur but do not usually produce clinical sequelae.

X. TRANSCATHETER EMBOLIZATION

A. Principles

Transcatheter techniques for vascular occlusion in a variety of sites throughout the body can be used to treat selected acute and nonacute clinical problems. Renal abnormalities account for most urinary tract embolizations. A variety of embolic materials may be introduced through angiographic catheters; these agents may be particulate, mechanical, polymerizing, or sclerosing. Most particulates provide temporary vascular occlusion (hours to weeks). All other agents produce permanent occlusion.

B. Indications

1. Decrease the vascularity of renal or other vascular retroperitoneal tumors prior to surgical extirpation.
   a. Devascularization facilitates surgical removal of the tumor.
   b. Preoperative renal embolization may enhance the patient's immune response and/or diminish possible seeding of metastasis at the time of nephrectomy.

2. Embolic obliteration of tumor vascularity may relieve symptoms in patients with nonresectable tumors and thereby control intractable bleeding, pain, and paraneoplastic syndromes. The growth of a renal cell carcinoma may be temporarily halted (months to years) by total obliteration of the renal vascular bed and tumor.

3. Control of renal hemorrhage secondary to trauma, aneurysms, and arteriovenous malformations.

4. Control of pelvic hemorrhage secondary to trauma.
5. Control of intractable vesical hemorrhage secondary to radiation cystitis when conservative urologic management is not effective or is contraindicated.
6. Occlusion of the internal spermatic vein in patients with testicular varicocele.

C. **Contraindications**
   1. Lack of a valid indication for embolotherapy.
   2. The presence of untreated renal infection.

D. **Technique**
   1. An angiographic catheter is selectively introduced into the vessel or vessels supplying the tumor, malforma-

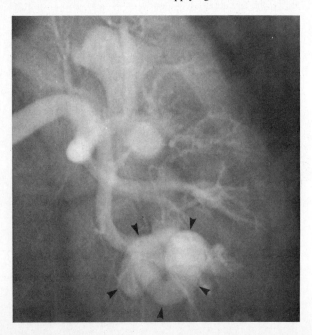

Figure 12. Renal embolization. Massive hematuria and hypertension in a young man. **A.** Selective left renal arteriogram shows a large serpiginous vascular structure in the lower pole (*arrowheads*) that drained prematurely into the renal vein, representing an arteriovenous malformation (AVM).

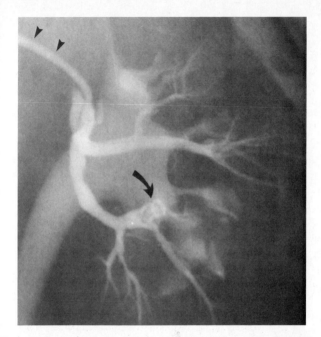

Figure 12. B. The AVM was selectively embolized with a stainless-steel coil (*arrow*) placed in the artery supplying the malformation. Contrast injected through a catheter (*arrowheads*) selectively placed into the lower pole artery shows complete cessation of flow through the AVM and preservation of blood flow to the majority of the remainder of the lower renal pole. The patient became normotensive following embolization.

tion, organ, etc., to be devascularized and one or more embolic agents introduced. These include:

a. Particulates, e.g., autologous clot, Gelfoam, polyvinyl alcohol (Ivalon)

b. Mechanical agents, e.g., stainless steel coils, detachable balloons

c. Polymerizing fluids, e.g., isobutyl-2-cyanoacrylate (Bucrylate)

d. Other agents, e.g., absolute alcohol, hot contrast material

2. An occlusion balloon catheter is often employed in the renal vessels when performing transcatheter embolization in order to prevent reflux of the embolic agents elsewhere in the renal vascular or systemic circulations.
3. A postembolization arteriogram is obtained to ascertain the effectiveness of embolotherapy (Fig. 12).
4. Therapeutic embolization should be performed at least 1 day after a diagnostic angiogram in order to decrease the contrast medium load to the remaining kidney.

E. Results
The efficacy of embolotherapy is apparent on the postembolization angiogram. Complete vascular occlusion may require the use of more than one embolic agent. For localized renal abnormalities (e.g., aneurysms, vascular malformations), segmental vessel embolization preserves the maximal amount of functioning renal tissue.

F. Complications
1. Postembolization syndrome. Most patients experience transient pain in the area of the embolized vessel. This may be accompanied by nausea, vomiting, or a febrile response lasting 24 to 48 hours. These symptoms may be related to the tissue ischemia and infarction that result from embolization.
2. Reflux of embolic material with undesired embolization of other vessels is the most serious complication of embolotherapy. Reports of spinal cord and bowel infarction during renal artery embolization as well as occlusion of the contralateral renal artery and peripheral vessels dictate the use of occlusion balloon catheters, slow injection of small quantities of the embolic material, and frequent test injections of small amounts of contrast material to determine the extent of embolization and help to prevent the complication of reflux. The rate of clinically significant reflux is generally 1% or less.

BIBLIOGRAPHY
Athanasoulis CA: Therapeutic applications of angiography. N Engl J Med 302:1117, 1179, 1980.

Banner MP, Pollack HM: Dilatation of ureteral stenosis: techniques and experience in 44 patients. Am J Roentgenol 143:789, 1984.

Banner MP, Pollack HM: Fluoroscopically guided percutaneous extraction of upper urinary tract calculi. Radiol Clin North Am 22:415, 1984.

Banner MP, Pollack HM: Percutaneous antegrade renal drainage techniques. In Carson CC, Dunnick NR (eds): Endourology. New York: Churchill Livingstone, 1986.

Barbaric ZL, MacIntosh PK: Periureteral thin-needle aspiration biopsy. Urol Radiol 2:181, 1981.

Chaussy CH, Schmiedt E: Extracorporeal shock wave lithotripsy (ESWL) for kidney stones. An alternative to surgery? Urol Radiol 6:80, 1984.

Eckstein MR, Waltman AC, Athanasoulis CA: Interventional angiography of the renal fossa. Radiol Clin North Am 22:381, 1984.

Gerzof SG: Percutaneous drainage of renal and perinephric abscess. Urol Radiol 2:171, 1981.

Gill WB, Lu C, Bibbo M: Retrograde brush biopsy of the ureter and renal pelvis. Urol Clin North Am 6:573, 1979.

Lang EK: Diagnosis and management of ureteral fistulas by percutaneous nephrostomy and antegrade percutaneous stent catheter. Radiology 138:311, 1981.

Lang EK, Price ET: Redefinition of indications for percutaneous nephrostomy. Radiology 147:419, 1983.

LeRoy AJ, May GR, et al: Percutaneous ultrasonic lithotripsy. Radiol Clin North Am 22:427, 1984.

Newhouse JH, Pfister RC: Renal cyst puncture. In Athanasoulis CA, Pfister RC, et al (eds) Interventional Radiology. Philadelphia: W. B. Saunders, 1982, p 409.

Sos TA, Pickering TG, et al: The current role of renal angioplasty in the treatment of renovascular hypertension. Urol Clin North Am 11:503, 1984.

Stables DP: Percutaneous nephrostomy: Techniques, indications and results. Urol Clin North Am 9:15, 1982.

Wein AJ, Ring EJ, et al: Applications of thin needle aspiration in urology. J Urol 121:626, 1979.

28

Specific Infections
Philip M. Hanno

I. GENITOURINARY TUBERCULOSIS

A. General Considerations

1. Forty thousand new active cases of tuberculosis occur every year in the United States, the majority arising from reactivation of previously healed loci.

2. Approximately 9 percent of patients with pulmonary tuberculosis and 26 percent of those with miliary disease have associated infection of the kidney, ureter, or genital organs.

3. Among the extrapulmonary organs, involvement of the urogenital tract is the leading secondary site.

4. Urinary tuberculosis is primarily a disease of young adults.

B. Pathogenesis

1. Tuberculosis of the kidney arises from infection of the lungs or hilar lymph nodes. The infection is blood borne equally to both kidneys.

2. Involved sites may be dormant for many years, eventually beginning to spread and develop caseation and cavitation.

3. Tubercles in the glomeruli may heal or spill into the nephrons and may be caught in the narrow loop of Henle, where they form tuberces.

4. Tubercles caseate and slough into the calyceal fornix. Bacilli are spilled down the ureters with potential stricture formation and bladder inflammation and contracture.

5. About 4% of initial tubercles result in destructive tuberculosis. When caseation is progressive, the disease

may involve the entire renal pelvis, leading to a calcified mass of caseous material called a ''putty
kidney.''

6. If early renal lesions do not heal (the response of each
kidney is independent of the other) the passage of
infected urine through the urogenital tract can lead to
involvement of the ureters, bladder, prostate, seminal
vesicles, vas deferens, epididymis, and testis. Rarely,
the primary hematogenous lesion in the urinary tract
may be the prostate.

C. Pathogenesis and Diagnosis (Table 1)

1. Renal involvement is largely silent. In the male the
earliest indication may be tuberculous epididymitis or
cystitis. Females may present with bladder pain and
dysuria. Back pain and hematuria are not uncommon.
2. The severity of symptoms does not correlate with the
degree of urinary tract involvement.
3. The diagnosis is made by finding *Mycobacterium tuberculosis* in the urine or semen.
   a. Three consecutive early morning urines are
   cultured; repeat if results are negative.
   b. Acid-fast stains on concentrated urinary sediment
   from 24-hour specimen may be positive in 50 to
   60% of cases, but culture corroboration is
   essential.

TABLE 1. SOME CLINICAL FINDINGS IN GU TUBERCULOSIS

''Sterile'' pyruria
History of present or past tuberculosis elsewhere in body
Hematuria unexplained
Chronic cystitis unresponsive to antibiotics
Chronic epididymitis with epididymal nodularity and/or beaded or thickened vas
  deferens
Prostate nodularity, shrunken ''bean-bag'' prostate
Induration of seminal vesicles
Dull flank pain/renal colic
Chronic, draining scrotal sinus

       c. A negative tuberculin skin test makes the diagnosis unlikely.

       d. Radiographs alone are not sufficient for diagnosis.

       e. Drug sensitivity testing is essential.

    4. Differential Diagnosis

       a. Chronic nonspecific cystitis or pyelonephritis.

       b. Acute or chronic nonspecific epididymitis.

       c. "Urethral syndrome," interstitital cystitis.

       d. Necrotizing papillitis of one or both kidneys.

       e. Schistosomiasis.

D. Therapy (Table 2)

    1. General Considerations

       a. The size of the bacillary population is related to the extent of the disease.

       b. Multiple drugs work synergistically against resistant organisms in early treatment.

       c. Close follow-up of upper tracts is essential during therapy, as asymptomatic ureteral strictures (especially lower third) may occur during healing phase. Tuberculous strictures lend themselves to percutaneous or transurethral dilatation techniques. Steroids may be beneficial.

       d. Surgical intervention may play an increasing role with trends toward shorter duration of chemotherapy.

    2. Standard Therapy (Subject to Sensitivity Results)

       a. INH 300 mg daily
          Ethambutol 1200 mg daily
          Rifampin 600 mg daily
          Pyridoxine 100 mg daily

       b. Duration of treatment—2 years

       c. Surgical procedure *if necessary* to drain perinephric abscess, remove nonfunctioning renal tissue, bypass ureteral strictures, and augment severely contracted bladders.

    3. Short-Course Chemotherapy

       a. Popularized by Gow in Britain.

       b. Pyrazinamide 25 mg/kg daily up to 2 g for 4 months; INH 300 mg daily for 2 months, 300 mg

TABLE 2. COMMON ANTITUBERCULOSIS CHEMOTHERAPEUTIC AGENTS

Drug	Dose	Side Effects	Remarks
Isoniazid (INH)	5–10 mg/kg/day up to 300 mg daily	Peripheral neuritis, Hepatitis	Bactericidal, pyridoxine for neuritis
Rifampin	10–20 mg/kg/day up to 600 mg daily	Hepatotoxicity; transient leukopenia, thrombocytopenia; hypersensitivity reaction	Bactericidal, urine turns orange
Ethambutol	15 mg/kg/day	Retrobulbar neuritis; color vision changes	Tuberculostatic, baseline visual acuity tests
Streptomycin	Up to 1 g daily IM for 1 month; then 25 mg/kg twice weekly	Vestibular damage, deafness, nephrotoxicity	Tuberculostatic
Pyrazinamide	15–30 mg/kg up to 2 g daily	Hepatotoxicity—may be fatal. Elevates serum uric acid	Monitor uric acid, liver function every 3 weeks
Para-aminosalycilic acid	150 mg/kg up to 12 g daily	GI distress, hypersensitivity, hepatotoxicity	Bacteriostatic
Cycloserine	10–20 mg/kg daily up to 500 mg	Psychosis	Contraindicated in epileptics

three times weekly for 2 months. Rifampin 450 mg daily for 2 months, 900 mg daily three times weekly for 2 months.

c. Surgery, when indicated, is performed 4 to 6 weeks after chemotherapy begun.

d. Nephrectomy for grossly diseased nonfunctioning kidney, or diseased kidney and secondary hypertension.

e. Partial nephrectomy for calcified polar lesion increasing in size.

f. Reconstructive surgery as necessary.

II. SCHISTOSOMIASIS

A. General Considerations

1. Caused by a blood fluke, this disease was first recognized by Egyptian physicians of the XII Dynasty (1900 B.C.).

2. About 300 million humans are infested with *Schistosoma mansoni*, *S. japonicum,* or *S. haematobium,* an estimated 500,000 living in the United States.

3. Intestinal schistosomiasis caused by either *S. mansoni* or *S. japonicum* is common in East and South Asia, South America, and in certain parts of Africa.

4. Genitourinary schistosomiasis is caused by *S. haematobium* and is endemic mainly in Africa and certain areas in the Middle East.

B. Etiology

1. Adult schistosomes are delicate cylindrical worms, 1 to 2 cm in length, that are adapted for existence in venules.

2. Humans are infected through contact with infested water in small canals, ditches, or drains. The infective larval stage—free-swimming cercariae—penetrate the skin or mucous membranes.

3. Cercariae reach the general circulation and are pumped by the heart throughout the body. Only worms that reach the portal circulation live.

4. Adult worms reaching their definitive destinations mature and mate, females laying eggs in the submucosa of the involved tissues—the bladder, lower ureters, and seminal vesicles in genitourinary (GU) schistosomiasis.
5. Ova are eliminated in human feces and urine. If they reach freshwater they hatch, and the contained larvae, ciliated miracidia, find a specific freshwater snail that they penetrate. There they form sporocysts that ultimately form the cercariae that leave the snail and pass into the freshwater to begin the cycle.

C. **Pathogenesis of GU Manifestations**
  1. Stage I—Generalization or Incubation Period
      a. Young schistosome rapidly acquires host-derived antigenic materials on its body surface and is immunologically camouflaged.
      b. Secretions and excretions of the worms may engender hypersensitivity and general manifestations of illness.
      c. Allergic skin reactions, cough, fever, malaise, body and bone aches, and gastrointestinal symptoms may be present.
  2. Stage II—Deposition of Ova by Mature Worms in Target Area
      a. Since female worms may lay eggs for years, the disease is slowly progressive.
      b. Toxic and antigenic products of a viable miracidium pass through the shell of the egg and cause a minute abscess wherever the egg lodges.
      c. Inflammatory infiltrate progresses to granulomatous pseudotubercle.
      d. Painful terminal hematuria, hemospermia, vesical irritability.
  3. Stage III—Late Complications
      a. End result of repeated, chronic infection.
      b. Infection of urinary tract—usually coliform organisms (*Escherichia coli, Klebsiella, Pseudomonas*). Definite association with *Salmonella typhi* infections.

    c. Schistosomal bladder polyps, secondary infection stones, urinary tract calcification.

    d. Fibrosis is ultimate result of infection—involves bladder, urethra, ureters leading to hydronephrotic renal atrophy, bladder contraction.

    e. Relationship to bladder malignancy—usually squamous cell carcinoma.

D. Diagnosis

1. Diagnosis of Infection

    a. Urine sediment reveals terminally spined eggs of *S. haematobium* (midday urine sample best).

    b. Rectal or bladder mucosal biopsy to look for eggs.

2. Diagnosis of Sequelae and Complications

    a. Plain x-ray of abdomen classically reveals bladder calcification. Seminal vesical, urethral, distal ureteral calcification may be seen.

    b. Intravenous urogram essential to look for obstructive uropathy.

    c. Cystoscopic appearance

E. Treatment

1. Medical Management

    a. Praziquantel, a heterocycline prazinoisoquinoline is the drug of choice for treatment of all species. Dosage for *S. haematobium* is 40 mg/kg by mouth in single oral dose.

    b. Niradozole (Ambilihar) is a nitrofuran given orally in two divided daily doses of 25 mg/kg/day for 5 to 7 days.

    c. Stillbocaptate (Astiban) is an antimony dimercaptosuccinate given intramuscularly 8 to 10 mg/kg weekly for 5 weeks.

    d. These drugs may have many side effects, and in edemic areas one must be cognizant of risk–benefit ratios, as low-level infection is well tolerated by many persons and generally will not produce symptomatic chronic disease or chronic obstructive uropathy.

2. Surgical Management
   a. Surgical procedures are reserved for complications of infection such as ureteral stenosis, bladder fibrosis, and bladder carcinoma.
   b. Procedures include ureteral dilatation, ureteral reimplantation, partial cystectomy, bladder augmentation, and cystectomy and diversion.

III. GENITAL FILARIASIS (BANCROFTIAN FILARIASIS)

A. General Considerations
1. About 300 million people are infected with filaria.
2. Although numerous filarial species cause human disease, urologic problems are most common with *Wuchereria bancrofti*. *Onchocerca volvulus*, the agent of African river blindness, can also cause scrotal elephantiasis.
3. *W. bancrofti* is a human parasite without known animal reservoirs.
4. Periodic bancroftian filariasis is found throughout tropical Africa, North Africa, tropical coastal borders of Asia and Queensland, the West Indies, and northern South America.

B. Etiology
1. Adult filarial *W. bancrofti* are 4- to 10-cm worms about 0.2 mm in diameter; they reside in the lymphatic system and live for decades.
2. The female worm is viviparous, producing microfilariae that are found in the peripheral blood at night (nocturnal periodicity) and in the lungs during the day. Microfilariae live 3 to 6 months.
3. If ingested by suitable mosquitoes, microfilariae develop in the thoracic muscles of the insect and move to the mouth parts in 2 weeks.
4. They enter the skin of humans through puncture wounds of a mosquito bite and move to lymphatics where males and females meet and mate and mature— 1 year later microfilariae appear in the blood.

C. Pathogenesis and Manifestations
1. Severity of Lesions Related to
   a. Load of adult worms.
   b. Site of infection.
   c. Host susceptibility.
2. Maturing adults in the lymphatics cause fibrotic and inflammatory changes producing lymphatic obstruction.
3. "Filarial fever" involves fever, headache, lymphadenopathy, and urticarial rash.
   a. It occurs in acute phase.
   b. Often no history of this can be obtained.
4. Chronic phase—lymphatics affected include inguinal region, upper arm, and spermatic cord.
   a. Chronic lymphadenopathy.
   b. Retrograde lymphangitis.
   c. Lymphatic obstruction and resulting edema (elephantiasis), especially in lower limbs and scrotum, hydrocele formation.
   d. Bacterial and mycotic superinfection.
   e. Chyluria from renal lymphaticourinary fistula formation.

D. Diagnosis
1. In early stages, microfilariae are usually present in smears of blood obtained at night.
2. In long-standing, chronic disease, blood smears are usually negative.
   a. Look for eosinophilia.
   b. Look for microfilariae in hydrocele fluid or chylous urine.
   c. Filarial complement fixation tests.
3. Differential diagnosis includes congenital lymphatic defects, tuberculous inguinal lymphadenitis, schistosomiasis, and lymphatic obstruction from malignancy.

E. Treatment
1. Even though chemotherapy is effective in eliminating *W. bancrofti*, structural changes may not be reversible.

2. Diethylcarbamazine (Hetrazan)
    a. Mainstay of treatment.
    b. Mechanism of action unknown.
    c. Toxicity (anorexia, nausea, vomiting, pruritis) may be due to dying microfilaria.
3. Suramin (Antrypol, Moranyl)
    a. Complex derivative of urea.
    b. Used after failure of diethylcarbamazine.
    c. Toxicity—renal damage, urticaria, shock.
4. Management of Chyluria
    a. Correction of urostasis.
    b. Intrapelvic instillations of silver nitrate 1 to 2% solutions.
    c. Rarely—surgical interruption of renal pedicle lymphatics.

IV. GU CANDIDIASIS

A. General Considerations
1. *Candida albicans* is the most prevalent and the most pathogenic of the fungi affecting the genitourinary tract.
2. Normally inhabitants of mucocutaneous body surfaces, candidas will overgrow and invade tissues when permitted by alterations in the host.
3. Virulence is related to this species' ability to transform in tissues into the mycelial phase, a form more resistant to the cellular defenses of the host than the yeast phase.

B. Pathogenesis and Manifestations
1. Predisposing factors include extended use of broad-spectrum antibiotics, diabetes mellitus, corticosteroids, indwelling catheters, immunosuppressive drugs, antineoplastic drugs, and an immunocompromised host.
2. Bladder involvement may be asymptomatic, or present with urgency, hematuria, frequency, nocturia, severe dysuria, and suprapubic pain.

3. Upper tract involvement may be signaled by signs of pyelonephritis or obstruction from fungus balls.
4. Systemic candidiasis may be sudden or insidious—fever, shaking chills, hypotension, lethargy, petechiae, and embolic phenomena.

C. **Diagnosis**
1. Blood or urine cultures must be evaluated in the context of the clinical setting, as candidemia and candiduria may occur as transient phenomena.
2. Diagnosis of fungal cystitis based on clinical presentation of irritative symptoms, history of predisposing factors, positive fungal cultures ($>10^4$ colonies/ml), negative bacterial and acid-fast cultures, cystoscopy and bladder biopsy to rule out tumor, and tissue cultures.
3. Blood cultures, ophthalmologic examination, and serum agglutinin titers may help diagnose systemic involvement.
4. Intravenous urography may show calyceal defects and ureteral obstruction (fungus masses).

D. **Treatment**
1. Asymptomatic candiduria implies a colonization of the urinary tract without tissue invasion.
   a. It will usually disappear when predisposing factors (antibiotics, indwelling catheters) are removed.
   b. Urinary alkalinization with sodium bicarbonate to a pH of 7.5 is helpful.
2. Symptomatic or intractible vesical candidiasis can be treated with intravesical amphotericin-B instillations (100 mg in 500 ml of 5% dextrose solution three times daily).
3. Renal and Systemic Involvement
   a. Flucytosine (5-FC, Ancobon)
      (1) Oral agent.
      (2) Interferes with fungal synthesis of DNA.
      (3) Toxicity—rash, diarrhea, hepatic dysfunction, bone marrow suppression.
      (4) May use alone with urinary candidiasis; use with amphotericin B in systemic disease.

b. Amphotericin B (Fungizone)
 (1) Intravenously administered macrolide antibi-
     otic—combines with sterols in fungal cell
     membranes.
 (2) Mainstay of treatment in systemic infection.
 (3) Toxicity noted in greater than 85% of pa-
     tients—fever, hypotension, dyspnea, and
     nephrotoxicity.
 (4) Synergistic with flucytosine.

BIBLIOGRAPHY

Al-Ghorab MM: Schistosomiasis of the bladder. In Kaufman JJ (ed): Current Urologic Therapy. Philadelphia: W.B. Saunders, 1986, pp 248–251.

Barrett-Connor E: Drugs for the treatment of parasitic infection. Med Clin North Am 66:245–255, 1982.

Eisenberg H: Chemotherapy of tuberculosis. In Edberg SC, Berger SA (eds): Antibiotics and Infection. New York: Churchill Livingston, 1983, pp 191–197.

Gow JG, Barbosa S: Genitourinary tuberculosis. A study of 1,117 cases over a period of 34 years. Br J Urol 56:449–455, 1984.

Hamory BH, Wenzel RP: Hospital-associated candiduria: Predisposing factors and review of the literature. J Urol 120:444–448, 1978.

Kazura J: Filarial infections. In Edberg SC, Berger SA (eds): Antibiotics and Infection. New York: Churchill Livingston, 1983, pp 105–108.

Lattimer JK, Wechsler M: Genitourinary tuberculosis. In: Harrison JH, Gittes RF, et al (eds): Campbell's Urology, ed 4. Philadelphia: W. B. Saunders, 1978, pp 557–575.

Lichtenberg FV, Lehman JS: Parasite diseases of the genitourinary system. In Harrison JH, Gittes RF et al (eds): Campbell's Urology, ed 4. Philadelphia: W. B. Saunders, 1978, pp 597–639.

Mahmond AAF: Schistosomiasis. In Edberg SC, Berger SA (eds): Antibiotics and Infection. New York: Churchill Livingston, 1983, pp 110–112.

Marsden PD: Lymphoreticular filariasis. In Hoepvich PD (ed): Infectious Diseases. Hagerstown, Md: Harper & Row, 1977, pp 1100–1103.

Michigan S: Genitourinary fungal infections. J Urol 116:390–397, 1976.

Naude JH: The natural history of Ureteric Bilharzia. Br J Urol 56:599–601, 1984.

Rohner TJ, Tuliszewski RM: Fungal cystitis: Awareness, diagnosis, and treatment. J Urol 124:142–144, 1980.

Weller TH: Schistosomiasis. In Hoepvich PD (ed): Infectious Diseases. Hagerstown, Md: Harper & Row, 1977, pp 658–665.

Wise GJ, Goldberg PE, Kozinn PJ: Do the imidazoles have a role in the management of genitourinary fungal infections? J Urol 133:61–64, 1985.

Index

Italic letters following page numbers refer to tables (*t*) and figures (*f*).